A Philosophical Basis of Medical Practice

A Philosophical Basis of Medical Practice

Toward a Philosophy and Ethic of the Healing Professions

Edmund D. Pellegrino
David C. Thomasma

New York Oxford
OXFORD UNIVERSITY PRESS
1981

Library of Congress Cataloging in Publication Data

Pellegrino, Edmund D
A philosophical basis of medical practice.

Includes bibliographical references and index.
1. Medicine–Philosophy. I. Thomasma, David C., 1939- joint author. II. Title. [DNLM: 1. Ethics, Medical. 2. Philosophy, Medical. W50 P386p]
R723.P3813 610'.1 80-36735
ISBN 0-19-502789-2

Printed in the United States of America

For our wives
Clementine and Lynne
—who share a larger part of this book in ways
only we and they can appreciate.

Preface

If there is any possible means of increasing the common wisdom and ability of mankind it must be sought in medicine.

Descartes

Health and virtue are fundamental aspirations of human beings. Enormous effort and resources in every culture are devoted to achieving some particular notion of being-well and being-good. Both aspirations presume a basic judgment: that human life is at once fragile and perfectible.

To seek health and virtue is, moreover, a creative interference in the given, a taunting of fate and nature. In our day medicine is asked increasingly to do the taunting. Doing so, it takes on some of the spirit of Aristotelian tragedy, forcing us to realize those things we forgot to take into account. With each tragic realization there is an act of discovery–unique, concrete, and individual. Each act offers the possibility of a reinterpretation of the nature of humanity and the world, of life and death.

This special form of tragic insight gives shape to the central focus of all medical theory and practice: how can general and non-personal laws of science be formed from, and applied to, the being-well and being-good of unique persons? At issue is the essential nature of the clinical enterprise: what it is, what distinguishes it from other human enterprises, and what kind of knowledge it handles with what logic and under what obligations.

Because so much of medicine is oriented to practice, to caring for human beings, we have decided to focus on the philosophical implications of medical practice. This approach necessarily neglects some important theoretical considerations, not the least of which is a thorough discussion of concepts of health and disease. However, it is our conviction that the practice of medicine is at the base of all theoretical considerations. The focus on practice, therefore, not only places the theoretical discussion in proper perspective, but also permits a natural discussion of implications in terms of ethics and norms for the conduct of modern medicine. Hence, the theory discussed in this volume stems from our understanding and description of the realities of medical practice.

Medicine is as fundamental as any human endeavor for the revelation of what it means to be human. As such, it offers a fruitful source for philosophical reflection. Medicine, in turn, needs philosophy. Critical reflection on the "style" and content of medicine will aid its own self-understanding and the patient's self-understanding as well.

A philosophy of medicine is needed: to organize medicine's rapidly increasing number of successes; to form an integrating principle for its splintering specialties; to offer a rational, scientific explanation of its methods; and to discover the relationship between Eastern and Western medical systems so that each can function in an expanding world community. Most important, perhaps, a philosophy of medicine is needed to help clarify medicine's goals in relationship to those of a technological civilization. Medicine suffers from an abundance of means and a poverty of ends. Medicine really cannot be successful until it knows exactly what it is trying to achieve, whether this achievement is possible, and whether it reflects a desirable goal of contemporary human culture.

"It is a source of strength as well as weakness," E. B. Strauss has written, "that there is no real philosophy of medicine so far as orthodox European medicine is concerned."[1] As we will show in the first chapter, philosophy and medicine have had a tenuous relationship. No vital philosophy of medicine has existed in the twentieth century. The reason for medicine's strength in this century is well-known: it has been enormously successful in curing. This success is due to knowledge and technique based on experience, not theories and philosophical speculation.[2]

But the lack of a philosophy is now being felt as a weakness. Without the reasonable restraints imposed by philosophical critique, medicine and its practitioners may unintentionally convert science and medical method into a muddled philosophy of human life. It would be inappropriate, not to say false, to consider human beings merely collections of organ systems and deposits of disease entities. Therefore medicine must begin questioning its conceptual framework. Holman has suggested that "some medical outcomes are inadequate not because appropriate technical interventions are lacking but because our conceptual thinking is inadequate."[3]

There are several reasons for the absence of a philosophy of medicine in our day. We have already mentioned that the successes of modern medicine stem from empirical method and not from philosophical theorizing. This success encourages the positivistic bias in medical literature, at least in England and the United States.

And, unlike theoretical scientists, medical practitioners are wary of philosophical speculation. Although a few medical practitioners delve into the history and philosophy of their craft, most hesitate to become embroiled in the philosophical aspects of their profession. This hesitation is understandable in light of the deleterious effects of nineteenth-century Romanticism on medicine,[4] the physician's lack of formal, logical and philosophical training, and the pragmatic concerns for patients that must govern physicians.

Ironically enough, the professional philosophers have also neglected philosophies of medicine. Like Plato, they often use medicine as a source of examples to make a wide variety of philosophical points in morals, politics, or social philosophy. But only a few, such as Descartes, have shown the same kind of interest in medicine that they exhibit in philosophies of history, law, religion, education or art.

If a philosophy of medicine is to meet the needs of both philosophy and medicine, it must somehow unite the concreteness of clinical experience with the critical method of philosophy. While physicians and philosophers might share the same concerns for clarity, each has a tendency to retreat to previous successes: the philosophers into the philosophy of science and the physician into the concreteness of clinical medicine. Yet neither can fashion a credible philosophy of medicine without moving toward the other and away from the safety of traditional positions.

Finally, experience in clinical settings, from the perspective of both medical and philosophical practice, confirms the need for "decisional space" for health care practitioners. Medicine must engage in a kind of empirical-inductive reasoning that cannot conform solely to the canons of scientific correctness established over the long years of the history of science.[5] It must make experimental judgments about human life. This may be yet another reason why physicians react negatively to concepts and ideas created by a philosophy of science primarily concerned with physics or actuarial logic.

The health care practitioner, particularly the physician, is held responsible for the scientific, medical, legal, and moral implications of his decisions. The intrusion of a critical philosophy into the process of decision-making is perceived by many as both dangerous and confining.[6] At a time when the physician's responsibility to make decisions is being narrowed rapidly by governmental intervention, any philosophical critique of decisions would initially appear as a limitation. This responsibility remains closely guarded by physicians because they rightly view the clinical decision as central to their craft.

We hold that a philosophy of medicine is as important for philosophy as it is for medicine. Our culture and our society have yet to synthesize a working philosophical anthropology that could form the basis for our ethical, economic, and political considerations. Agreement on goals and means in medicine as in other human endeavors presupposes some agreement on the nature of a human being. Medicine can offer the verifiable, empirically sound phenomena upon which contemporary philosophical anthropology might be based. These phenomena abound in contemporary medical science as well as in medicine in the clinical encounter. Though the pluralism of our society might seem to negate such an agreement, the problems that modern medicine uncovers offer an unavoidable challenge.[7]

Line of Argument

Chapter One: Medicine and Philosophy

The status of the relationship between philosophy and medicine throughout history demonstrates a current intellectual and cultural urgency for a philosophy of medicine in our day. While philosophy and medicine have had periods of mutual enrichment, at times medicine has been dominated by a particular form of philosophy. This domination has been to its detriment. The crisis of modern medicine lies in the lack of a suitable philosophy of practice whereby nonmeasurable clinical factors and values can be treated with the same attention as clinical indicators of disease. Contemporary concern, therefore, dictates the search for a philosophy of medicine developed *from* the practice of medicine itself, and not from external imposition of one or another existing philosophies.

Chapter Two: A Philosophical Method

Given the complexity of modern medicine and the requirement we imposed that the philosophy of medicine be developed from the practice of medicine, Chapter Two deals with a realistic methodology of philosophical analysis. This methodology must be eclectic, since no one philosophical stance is capable of completely exploring the substance of medicine. The method borrows from Aristotle the search for a definition that can lead to a discipline, and it is enriched by phenomenological description, an ontology of practice, and a practical aim.

Chapter Three: What Is Medicine?

In this chapter it is argued that medicine is a discipline in its own right and that a philosophy of medicine is a philosophy of an identifiable human activity, a form of unique relationship in which cure may take place. A definition of medicine is presented that includes the importance of the body in any philosophical consideration of medicine. A definition of medicine as a science of skill or craftsmanship is proposed.

Chapter Four: Critique of Medicine

The argument in this chapter yields the empirical or pragmatic a priori condition of medicine, i.e., the necessary and sufficient condition for medicine to take place. We explore the epistemological problem of medicine in its classical and modern form. Review of this problem demonstrates that the epistemological challenge for medicine throughout its history has been the explanation of how scientific theories of diagnosis, prognosis, and therapy can be derived from and applied to individual living human bodies.

Chapter Five: An Ontology of the Body

Critical reflection in this chapter produces an important ontology of the living body as the a priori condition of medicine. Philosophy itself can be enriched by this "reintroduction" of the body as a condition of practice and, therefore, of theory.

Chapter Six: The Anatomy of Clinical Judgments

In Chapter Three it is argued that medicine is essentially a relationship. For the physician, medicine is a habit of clinical judgment. The ontology of the body presented in the preceding chapter reveals that clinical judgment must include attention to the human condition and the corporeal individualities of patients. In this chapter the physician's clinical judgment is examined as the distinguishing feature of medicine; the role of patients is not highlighted.

Chapter Seven: Discretionary Space in Professional Judgment

The clinical judgment analyzed in the previous chapter does not take place in a vacuum, but rather in the context of a growing institutionalization of health care. This institutionalization shrinks the discretionary space normally afforded professionals, and it may alter radically the nature of current medical practice. If the observations about clinical judgment are correct, then the nature of professional judgment and making right and good decisions requires a degree of responsible freedom in clinical matters. This is the first chapter that applies the philosophical explorations of the earlier chapters to ethics and policy questions.

Chapter Eight: Philosophy of Medicine and Medical Ethics

We argue that the relationship between medicine and values is intrinsic. The application of a philosophy of medicine to moral agency is required by the purpose of medicine as a craft of healing. In this chapter we attempt to ground medical ethics in a philosophy of medicine so that its proper context can be recognized. Hence, we do not draw upon previously developed moral theories, but rather upon the conditions imposed by the ontology of the body in medicine itself. Further, three axioms are developed from an ontology of a living body in need of help. These axioms are: Do no harm; Respect vulnerability of patients; Treat all patients as equal members of the human race.

Chapter Nine: A Philosophical Reconstruction of Medical Morality

Based on the three ethical axioms proposed in Chapter Eight and the nature of the medical transaction, this chapter develops a philosophical basis for professional ethics in medicine, a feature largely missing in the history of medical codes. We argue that a professional code should not be based primarily upon religious or cultural values, but upon the responsibilities of physicians and patients in the medical relationship. These responsibilities follow from the aim of medicine to heal, the obligations resulting from the three axioms, and the current abilities of modern medicine.

Chapter Ten: The Social Ethics of Primary Care

Having established the framework of a professional ethics stemming from the axiom of vulnerability, the argument now turns to human need and the obligations that may arise therefrom. We argue that primary care responds to such human need and should therefore be universally accessible. This accessibility does not rest on political exigencies but is a moral requirement of medicine itself.

Chapter Eleven: Social Ethics of Institutions

The moral obligations of institutions is a topic rarely addressed in philosophical reflections on medicine, yet it is important because medicine increasingly is practiced in institutions. This topic embraces the relationship of the patient to health care institutions and the appropriate theory of team health care obligations to patients that must guide this relationship.

Chapter Twelve: Medical Morality and Medical Economics: The Conflict of Canons

In this final chapter, the growing use of economic theories of health care is explored. On the basis of medical and professional ethics developed in the previous chapters, primary emphasis is placed on the axiom of vulnerability. A call is made for the establishment of moral policy regarding health care in the United States. The touchstone of this policy is compassion toward those in need.

The book therefore develops the notion of medicine as an integral discipline in its own right.[8] The philosophy of medicine we seek is a philosophy of an identifiable human activity, not a philosophical hodgepodge of the sciences and arts that medicine employs. We hold that medicine is not reducible to biology, physics, chemistry, or psychology; nor is it only what doctors do or what patients expect; nor is it simply a rigorous science or solely an art of making good on clinical hunches. Instead we argue that medicine is a form of unique relationship.

Medicine teaches us about human existence because it deals with a fundamental aspiration of man to be healthy. And it teaches us about human existence because it deals with a corresponding tragedy of life. Often when we become sick, our lives come to a halt. We are forced to look at ourselves as fragile, mortal beings; normal independence cannot be reconciled with our new dependence on health care professionals, drugs, hospitals, and insurance companies. What was once private now becomes public. Our self-image is shattered.

As our self-image is disrupted, and our existence is questioned, we become aware of the moral basis of medicine. For the values professed by patients and physicians are derived from the meaning of human existence and the reality that as we have navels, so must we have graves.

Acknowledgments

Many of the ideas set forth in this work were subjected to the criticism of our colleagues and students. In the spirit of the best philosophical discourse they examined our propositions vigorously and rigorously. From them we have gained much and have modified and clarified our initial conceptions materially as a result.

It is impossible to single out one of our critics for special thanks without doing some injustice to the others. So we thank all our friends and colleagues who took us seriously enough to criticize our ideas with care. To these must be added our editor James J. Anderson, Helen Greenberg, and Melanie Miller at Oxford University Press, for their expert help in clarifying many inept phrases and for their suggestions to develop some inconclusive arguments.

We are also indebted to the University of Tennessee and the National Endowment for the Humanities through the Institute for Human Values in Medicine for their support of summer study and travel.

The staff of the Yale University Libraries deserve our gratitude for their gracious assistance in our bibliographic searches.

The arduous tasks of typing and preliminary editing were cheerfully and expertly carried out by Carol McVety of the Yale University Medical Center, Gloria Smith, Debra Strong, and Lois Dickson of the University of Tennessee Center for the Health Sciences, and Nancy Anzelmo of the Catholic University of America who also assembled the final version of the manuscript.

Washington, D.C. E.D.P.
Memphis, Tenn. D.C.T.
July, 1980

Contents

A Philosophical Basis of Medical Practice

Prologue: Some Notes on Method

This book is a first step toward what we hope will become a systematic philosophy of medicine. In it, we have tried to define what we believe the nature of medicine to be, and then, what the conception means for medical practice and medical morality. Our emphasis is primarily on metaphysical, ontological, and moral questions. Logical and epistemological issues are touched on only tangentially. These must be aired in future volumes if we are to move toward a comprehensive philosophy of medicine.

We hope with this work to contribute to the development of a contemporary theory of medicine. Is there a philosophy of medicine distinct from the philosophy of science or biology? To many, such a distinction will seem dubious, problematic, or nonexistent. However we may classify the effort, there is an undeniable need for a theoretical formulation upon which the practical activities of physicians can be philosophically grounded. The capabilities of modern medicine are so impressive and so pervasive that everyone is affected by the way we construe medicine and justify its ends and purposes. These matters cannot be left solely to individual physicians or even the profession as a body.

Our mode of philosophizing is eclectic. Though it leans most heavily on the moderate realism of the Aristotelian-Thomist tradition, it is supplemented by some of the analytic tools and insights of phenomenology and empiricism. This combination seems best suited to the kinds of problems encountered in our attempt to philosophize about medicine. The combination we have chosen, however, is not sufficiently distinctive to warrant its own classificatory rubric. When we do refer to this eclectic approach, we will call it a "practical ontology."

Thus, we share with empiricism a starting point in real, experienced entities sufficiently external to the observers to be shared among them. Like James, we regard the relations between things (in medicine, the relationship between the persons in a healing transaction) as "matters of direct particular experience."[1] But we do not accept his radical generalization of the categories applicable to experience to all reality. While grounding our analyses in experience, we seek meanings and essences deducible from the experienced realities.

We share with phenomenology its view of critical philosophy and its starting point in the phenomena exhibited by things in themselves—the activities, behaviors, and relations peculiar to medicine.[2] Especially helpful are the insights in Merleau-Ponty's notions of embodiment and the lived body with which the physician so directly deals. We differ from phenomenology in not making the subject's perceptions of these phenomena the first reality, and in not observing the strict demands of the phenomenological methods of epoché and reduction.

We appreciate fully the susceptibility of any eclecticism to criticism. Those who see their own methods of philosophizing as universally applicable must of necessity reject any admixture with alien systems of thought. Our primary aim, however, is to understand the nature of medical activity, not to elaborate a philosophy of philosophy. We are grateful for the insights both phenomenology and empiricism may cast upon those activities, even while retaining our own central commitments to perennial and more traditional modes of philosophizing. We trust that our eclecticism will not discourage the serious examination our major theses, conclusions, and line of argument deserve.

We have therefore taken some pains to make our line of argument as clear as possible by two devices: (1) a summary at the beginning of each chapter which links it to the preceding, and (2) a summary of our whole argument in the Preface entitled "Line of

Argument." Thus, we begin with an empirical description of the realities and phenomena which characterize medical activity. From these we derive those which make medicine a distinctive human activity. We locate that specificity in a human relationship–the relationship of healing in which one person in need of healing seeks out another who professes to heal, or to assist in healing. The acts of medicine tie these two persons together. It is the nature of this action in the presence of the healing relationship that gives medicine its special character among human activities.

All health professionals enter, in some degree, into this nexus of relationships; therefore we include all health professions in our concerns. We use medicine and the physician-patient relationship as our paradigm because of its moral, legal, and historical precedents. What we say of the healing relationship is equally significant for nurses, pharmacists, dentists, clinical psychologists, medical social workers, and allied health workers. We hope they will recognize their inclusion, although we do not make repeated specific reference to every one of the health professions. With certain modifications, however, the conclusions we draw for medicine are pertinent for the others.

This is especially true of our search for a philosophical foundation for a common ethics of healing. Such an ethics, with minor emendations, should serve in the reconstruction of all professional codes of healing, and in a common code of ethics of the healing professions. That is why we have titled this book: *A Philosophical Basis of Medical Practice: Toward a Philosophy and Ethics of the Healing Professions.*

I

Principal Features of a Philosophy of Medicine

1

Medicine and Philosophy

> *Phaedrus:* Hippocrates the Ascelepiad says that the nature even of the body can only be understood as a whole.
>
> *Socrates:* Yes, friend, and he is right–still we ought not to be content with the name of Hippocrates, but to examine and see whether his argument agrees with his conception of nature.
>
> *Phaedrus,* 270

Medicine and philosophy oscillate about each other like the strands of a complex double helix of the intellect. They are intermittently drawn together by their immersion in man's existence and driven apart by their often opposing preoccupations with that existence. Special tensions arise from their conflicting claims to universality–medicine divinizing the body and the particular, philosophy the intellect and the abstract.

In this first chapter, we will examine the relationship between philosophy and medicine in ancient and modern times, the benefits and obstacles which can accrue from that relationship, the dangers posed by historical antecedents, current objections to any notion of a philosophy of medicine, the basic modes of engagement of philosophy with medicine possible today, a list of urgent issues for a philosophy of medicine, what the philosophy of medicine ought not to be, and a conclusion. All of these topics are intended, however, to

This chapter originally appeared as "Philosophy of Medicine: Problematic and Potential," *Journal of Medicine and Philosophy,* Vol. 1, No. 1 (March 1976), 5–31. It has been altered and expanded in places from its original form.

present the thesis that the relationship between philosophy and medicine is of profound cultural significance. When medicine and philosophy converge, they can greatly advance man's search for a unified image of himself and the world; when they diverge, that image becomes fragmented, puzzling, and even absurd. Today, the intersection of medicine and philosophy is fraught with uncommon possibility and urgency. The problematic state of that intersection is one of the most significant challenges our culture faces.

While it is generally agreed that our culture is split between scientific and more traditional humanistic world views, it is not as clear to observers that a profound human experience of the world is the only common root of science and the humanistic disciplines.[1] The crisis of culture caused by the rise of science and a corresponding scientism has provoked serious study by thinkers as widely diverse as Husserl and Huxley. Responses to the crisis predictably range from suggestions for a wholesale adoption of a scientific utopianism to a wholesale rejection of science and technology. Only Van Rensselaer Potter, of the many prominent thinkers who have been concerned about the cultural split, has suggested that bioethics might be the bridge spanning the two cultures.[2]

However, our cultural urgency calls for a more fundamental linkage between science and humane studies, one which medicine could provide. Medicine, because it bridges both scientific study of man and deeply rooted human values, offers a field for a resolution of tension between abstract and concrete, science and humanities, the search for knowledge and the search for well-being. It is in this context that a philosophy of medicine is called for by our cultural crisis. But, as Claude Bernard observed long ago, there is nothing more sterile than philosophy divorced from real scientific information.[3] A philosophy of medicine divorced from the realities of theory and practice in medicine would be as useless to culture as it would be emaciating to both philosophy and medicine.

It is also important to note that medicine itself represents a tension between therapeutic aims and explanatory theory. Thus accounts of disease, the theoretical aspect of medicine, are formulated along physiological and pathological scientific lines while simultaneously aimed at the practice of healing. Therapeutic and preventive concerns are framed in scientific and abstract terms in order that medicine parallel scientific explanation. This tension between theory and practice, between abstract and concrete, makes medicine particularly susceptible to popular theories and myths about disease as well as to current philosophical claims about man. We regard the clinical exerience of medicine as the watershed of all theories about medicine. Clinical experience functions as a check on abstractions.

Ambiguities and Tensions

The ambiguities and tensions inherent in the links between medicine and philosophy have been expressed in ancient and modern terms:

Plato, with his usual prescience, exposes these ambiguities. In the *Protagoras,* the *Gorgias,* and elsewhere, he stresses the close congruity of medicine and philosophy as practical disciplines aimed at promoting the good life. For both Plato and Aristotle, medicine and philosophy share a concern with the normative–medicine prescribing the right conduct of the body and philosophy the right conduct of the soul, as well as of the social and the political life.[4] In Chapter Four we will show how *sophrosynē* (happiness) enters both medicine and philosophy in the Greek view.

In the *Symposium,* however, the emphasis is on the antithetical claims of medicine and philosophy. Eryximachus, the physician, is a symbol of technicism, promulgating the cultivation of the body as the true end of human life: "And this is what the physician has to do, and in this the art of medicine consists: for medicine may be regarded as the knowledge of the loves and desires of the body, and how to satisfy them or not. . . ."[5] While the physician exalts the body, the philosopher tends to dream of a form of perception which would transcend the body. Later in the dialogue, for example, Diotima speaks for Socrates of a higher form of Eros: "But what if man had eyes to see the true beauty–the divine beauty, I mean, pure and clear and unalloyed, not clogged with the pollutions of mortality and all the colors and vanities of human life?"[6] Or, as Socrates says to Simmias in the *Phaedo,* ". . . the body is always breaking in upon us, causing turmoil and confusion in our inquiries."[7]

This early debate highlights the importance of a theory of man and the proper aims of human life to both medicine and philosophy. For the Greeks, the answer to the question about the ends of a good human life directly fed into the aims of medicine and the role of speculation therein.[8] Thus, while Hippocrates cites the importance of theorizing in medicine if it is grounded "in incident" and "deduces its conclusions in accordance with phenomena,"[9] he also disallows speculative metaphysics from playing a central role in medicine. He argues against those philosophers who claim that medicine can be practiced only by those who know (from philosophy) what man is.[10] It is perhaps this concern that led Aristotle to observation and scientific theory.

These dichotomies are expressed in more modern terms as an opposition of method, the antithesis between contemplation and understanding, and fact and observation. Claude Bernard stated what is still a dominant medical view: ". . . philosophy does not teach anything, and is unable to teach anything itself, since philosophy makes neither experiment nor observation."[11] Scott Buchanan, calling for a philosophy of medicine, says: ". . . it [medicine] stands at the head of the natural sciences, and does not know which way to go. It has a record maximum of knowledge and a minimum of understanding. It has art, and wonders if it has science. It is suffering from an intellectual imbalance of virtues."[12]

A glance at the history of the opposition between observation and a priori theories in medicine reveals how important Hippocratic caution about abstractions are for any philosophy of medicine. Plato attempted, in later life, to base all bodily functions in geometry.[13] Descartes, who became fascinated with medicine toward the end of his life, predicted, on the basis of his a priori philosophy, that he could live 150 years.[14] This prediction's failure often obscures Descartes' methodological advances over Galenic postulates about vital spirits.

Reductionism, such as Descartes' mechanistic theory, while cleaning out unwarranted postulates, frequently leaves medicine with a dearth of hypotheses and overly simplistic explanations of complex processes. The search for a single cause of cancer is one such current example.

While the relationship between philosophy and medicine in culture continues, each discipline is also subject to its own special intellectual hubris, and these pretensions have complicated their interaction for centuries. Today, medicine's temptation to technicism is greatly enhanced by its obvious technological abilities, while philosophy's temptation to detachment is nourished by its recent analytic and linguistic bias. Paradoxically, the very triumphs of technicism have revealed how urgently medicine needs understanding and wisdom, just as the limitations of its analytic stance have revealed philosophy's urgent need for a reimmersion in the realm of practice.

Contemporary medicine and philosophy are, therefore, at the moment in their intellectual histories when each needs the other to redress an internal imbalance. It is the context, the quality, and the parameters of this new engagement of medicine and philosophy that shall now be examined.

Mutual Benefits and Attitudinal Obstacles

In every culture, medicine rests on a substructure of concepts which determine its character–that is, its method and practice as well as its ethos, ethics, and ideology. These are the ideas used to justify the expectations and the behavior of physicians, patients, and society. They are the source, too, for an idea or image of man which inevitably flows from medicine to color the whole of culture. Never have the conceptual bases of medicine had a wider impact on mankind than today, and never has it been more urgent to examine them critically, dialectically, and speculatively–i.e., philosophically.

Philosophy, then, has a special cultural and social responsibility to help redress the "imbalance" of intellectual virtues in medicine to which Buchanan alluded. It possesses the intellectual tools–its own traditional and contemporary *tekné*–to make the whole matter of medicine an examined activity. By *tekné* is meant an activity coupled with the knowledge of how that activity is to be applied and why it works. This is the sense in which Plato used the word. If philosophy can be seen as such a *tekné,* it can bring the understanding and clarification necessary to forestall the easy seductions of technicism tempting contemporary medicine.

Few issues are more fundamental to human well-being than the humane use of medical knowledge. But the validity of the ends and means of medicine and of the models of man that emerge from them is a "trans-medical" matter–one not susceptible to the methods of medicine itself. Medicine does not have the tools within its methodology to critique its goals and values. This must be the task of an external discipline, such as philosophy.

Philosophy's engagement with questions raised by medicine provides significant benefit to its own enterprise. Anglo-American philosophy, more so than European philosophy, has too assiduously eschewed a concern with the central issues of human existence and daily life. As it moves to reengage those issues, philosophy will need fuller input from what medicine has learned about man's encounters with his body, his world, and his psyche. Medicine abounds in concrete, verifiable, and measurable data about human life and offers these as ground for cogitation and inquiry. Out of this ground, philosophers can find new stimuli to their traditional concerns for apprehending human existence, thought, knowledge, and value. As Wartofsky has put it: "I believe philosophy has to get beyond philosophy to remain philosophical."[15]

For the dialogue between medicine and philosophy to be mutually beneficial, each discipline must overcome temptations to universalize its method as a standard for human existence. Life cannot be completely explained by either philosophy or medicine.

Philosophers must learn to see the immediate and grave issues in medicine as philosophically legitimate and no less respectable for their origin in such a practical domain as medicine. Neither the fastidiousness of analytic and linguistic modes nor the return to metaphysical system building will suffice. To be of service to medicine, and to itself, philosophy must learn to turn to medicine even to understand some of the issues with which it is itself concerned. A refurbished and less precious–though no less rigorous–image of philosophy needs to be fashioned.

For its part, medicine must overcome its antiphilosophical bias and its own claims to preciosity and sacerdotal privilege. These barriers to a critical examination of the conceptual structures of medicine are already breached by the searching reevaluations now underway of the social purposes of medicine. The most effective way medicine can generate a new and more realistic image of itself is through the kind of scrutiny philosophy can bring. This scrutiny does not entail an abandonment of the scientific fundamentals of medicine. In fact, a realistic appraisal of what medicine is, and must be, should reinforce the validity of that effort.

The dialogue between Eryximachus and Diotima is entering a new phase–one in which competing claims of medicine and philosophy to universality may have to be compromised in the interests of the mankind each presumably serves.

Medicine and Philosophy—The Historical Antecedents

Medicine began as a discipline under the domination of religion and myth. In the Western world it freed itself from this influence by becoming a part of pre-Socratic Ionian natural philosophy, from which it imbibed an interest in the explanation of the natural world through reason, as well as a fascination with the ideas of cause and effect and change. In this period, physicians and philosophers–as well as medicine, science, and philosophy–were largely indistinguishable.

Medicine became an independent profession in the fifth century B.C. with the appearance of the Hippocratic school. As Edelstein points out, medicine took on two distinct features: It emphasized the importance of basing its art on the observation of individual patients, and of doing so in an ethical framework.[16]

Medicine and philosophy became independent and strong disciplines. Because of this fact, Hippocratic medicine and Attic philosophy enjoyed their most fruitful relationship–one not equaled since. Each contributed conceptually to the other, and their congruence eventuated in *Paideia,* the ideal of Greek culture, as Werner Jaeger so well documents.[17] It was in the spirit of this felicitous conjunction that Hippocrates likened the physician who was a philosopher to a demigod,[18] Aristotle posited that philosophy properly ended in medicine,[19] and Galen insisted that the best physician was a philosopher.[20]

But even in that most salubrious of relationships, there were discordant notes. The treatise *On Ancient Medicine* in one sense fortifies the analogies between medicine and philosophy, as exemplified in the *Protagoras*. But in another sense, that same treatise warns explicitly against speculations undisciplined by direct observation of patients. Hippocratic medicine even developed some of the attributes of a philosophy of its own. Thus, even at the moment of their happiest conjunction, the tensions which Plato symbolizes in the *Symposium* were clearly discernible.

The more usual pattern over most of its history was for medicine to come intermittently under the influence of whatever philosophical school had currency in a given era. It took the methodological potency of modern science to fortify medicine against overspeculation and philosophical domination. This theme has been sketched in "Medicine and Philosophy," an annual oration delivered to the Society for Health and Human Values by one of the co-authors, November 8, 1973. A brief summary of the concept is presented below.

In the Hellenic and Greek worlds, whole medical systems were fashioned out of bits and pieces of the philosophies of Aristotle, Plato, Pythagoras, or Zeno–as the multiple and successive schools of Dogmatism, Methodism, or Eclecticism attest. In the Middle Ages, scholasticism and Christian theology suffused medical thought and practice. Later, the power of Descartes' mechanistic biology became–and remains today–an enormous influence, from the iatromechanists, iatrochemists, and iatrophysicists of the seventeenth and eighteenth centuries to the biological reductionists of our time.

Of more recent memory is the influence of German Idealist philosophy on the medical systematists of the eighteenth and nineteenth centuries such as Hoffman, Stahl, John Brown, and William Cullen. Risse and Galdston have documented how such notions as nervous ether, animism, or vitalism could derive from readings–or misreadings–of Hegel, Kant, Schelling, or Fichte.[21] Systems of diagnosis and treatment unrestrained by empirical or scientific observations proliferated in the Romantic era and for a time inhibited the growth of scientific medicine.

As a reaction to these transfers into medicine of poorly comprehended philosophical models, modern medicine has become distrustful of philosophical intrusions. Its historical susceptibility to the tyranny of philosophical systems derived from the lack, for so many centuries, of a scientifically verifiable base of knowledge. Thought unopposed by fact was too powerful to be gainsaid. But in the last century, the triumph of Bernard's experimentalism, and the infusion of the chemical and biological sciences into clinical medicine, have reduced this susceptibility to a very large degree. The philosophical threat to medicine today is not excessive and unrestrained system building but an excessive faith in reductionistic and positivistic modes of thought and explanation. Medicine is again strong enough and independent enough, as it was in Greece, to engage philosophy as an equal and is quite capable of resisting domination.

Philosophy has reacted for more than a century to the speculative excesses of Idealism and the Romantic philosophies. Through the media of logical positivism, the constraints of the Vienna Circle, and the analytic and linguistic emphasis of Anglo-American philosophy, speculative metaphysics in the United States has been neutralized. Philosophy, like some of the social sciences, has sought a nonproblematic base in the logic and method of science. Philosophy's own crisis now arises out of an overemphasis on analysis, the limitations of which are in turn being unfolded by the philosophers of science themselves. These limitations, as McMullin shows, are leading them toward more traditional metaphysical concerns.[22]

Contemporary medicine and philosophy are becoming aware that their zeal in overcoming the Idealists' enthusiasm for system building may have led them too far. There is renewed interest in the fundamental issues of value, purpose, ontological meaning, and the central questions of human existence. Contemporary medicine is overextended in the direction of reductionism and contemporary philosophy in the direction of analysis. Medicine manifestly cannot grasp the full reality of its object, man, or learn how to use its knowledge morally and humanely without relaxing its positivist bias–which persists even though it is losing its grip in philosophy. Philosophy, in its turn, cannot deal with the new questions about man–the specifically human issues–by an uncompromising adherence to the verification criteria of the Vienna Circle or by too narrow a focus on linguistic usages, rules of "meta-issues."

The serious normative issues in medical ethics, for example, demand more than the ministrations of "meta" ethics in the analytic sense of that term. If these issues are not treated philosophically, they will be resolved in the crisis of the clinical situation and by individual practitioners in the light of their own pragmatic leanings.

These issues are too important for society to be decided without serious critical reflection and the participation of thinkers outside, as well as inside, medicine. Philosophy will have to refocus its interest on questions of the value and purpose of human life and on the uses of professions as instruments of personal and social purpose, a point we raise in Chapter Nine. Without decrying the advances in philosophy made by the analytic and positivist schools, the issues raised by medical progress are more often closer to the concerns of traditional philosophy than they are to those of contemporary Anglo-American philosophy.

European philosophy, with its phenomenological and existential emphases, has turned to some of the nonscientific dimensions of human existence and has grappled with some of the issues medicine is examining. One thinks notably of the work of Marcel, Merleau-Ponty, Lain-Entralgo, Foucault, and E. Straus. These thinkers observe a conscious fastidiousness about ontological questions and generally eschew the ancient idea of a "first" philosophy which confronts the unanswerable but perennially relevant questions. European philosophy, however, has on the whole been responsive to the fact that questions of another kind must now be addressed, and those questions must bear once again on this human condition, its meaning, and the central questions of what man "is." The grapplings of Marcel, Camus, and Sartre with the complexities and absurdities of the human existence at least face the questions, even if, for some, their solutions are not acceptable.

Even at this late date in the English-speaking world, there is no recognition of a formal discipline under the rubric of the philosophy of medicine. We do acknowledge the philosophies of law, education, science, religion, and history. But even Edwards' comprehensive *Encyclopedia of Philosophy* has no article under this heading; nor is there an article on medical ethics. Indeed, its only reference to medicine is an article on Hippocrates.[23]

In continental Europe, the philosophy of medicine has had a more definable status. Beginning in the nineteenth century, a substantial number of studies under this category have appeared in Germany, France, Poland, Italy, and Russia—as Szumowski's valuable review attests.[24] A wide variety of topics is covered—such as the logic and epistemology of medicine, the concepts of health and disease, medical ethics, causality in medicine, the mind-body problem, mechanism, and vitalism. Several chairs of philosophy and medicine were established in Polish universities in the twenties.

The significance of the European efforts is not to be denied. They represent, however, a rather all-encompassing notion which suffers from diffuseness and includes much that would not be strictly defined as the philosophy of medicine. They are notable exceptions to the predominantly antipathetic attitude of the majority of physicians toward philosophical exercises.

No doubt, many thinkers in both fields will continue to see an impassable gulf. The stereotypes of philosophy contemplating the world of untestable ideas, and of medicine confined to practical and technical concerns, are too comfortable to be speedily abandoned, although we will try in the next two chapters. The artificiality of these extreme positions is becoming plain in light of the kinds of issues medicine now raises and the kinds of questions philosophy must itself confront. As their interests reach beyond the peripheral intersections we now observe, a true dialogue must emerge–one which will require each to break out of its immediately past traditions and biases.

The need for a genuine dialectic is increasingly obvious. The philosopher cannot really clarify the ontological status of man without reliance on the most accurate statement he can obtain on man's existence. Much of this can be found in the kind of data medicine alone can provide. The physician, on the other hand, needs an ontological conception of man which can give order and intelligibility to his objective search–and this is the business of philosophy. The ontological encounter between science and philosophy, which de Waelhens feels is so important for our understanding of each, can have its paradigm in the encounter of medicine and philosophy.[25]

The possibilities inherent in such an encounter are exemplified by the increasing number of philosophers in recent years who have examined questions highly pertinent to medicine or the medical context. We can cite only a few to make the point: the deep interest in the philosophy of the body evidenced in the work of Marcel,[26] Merleau-Ponty,[27] Dewey, and contemporaries such as Spicker and Zaner;[28] the philosophical foundations of psychiatry, psychology, and perception in the works by Straus,[29] Natanson, and Ey,[30] and Grene;[31] Engelhardt's concern with concepts of health and disease and the philosophical bases of medical ethics;[32] Buytendijck's fusion of physiology and anthropology;[33] Lain-Entralgo's analyses of the patient-physician encounter;[34] Wartofsky's inquiry into human ontology and medical practice;[35] and Zaner's series of papers underscoring the character of the human self, interpersonal bonds (as exemplified in medical contexts), and the concept of "enabling" in medical education.[36] Of note, too, are the works of Price, Taylor, Fabrega, Feinstein, and Murphy on the logic of disease taxonomy and clinical judgments. The search in these works is for a formal process of decision making underlying medical practice.

These explorations speak eloquently to the genuinely philosophical nature of many medical issues. They underscore the need for an orderly and detailed inquiry into the matter of medicine, from its prelogical assumptions to its method and modes of thought and their applications to persons and society. Serious philosophers are now examining this totality with a variety of philosophical tools. The increasing frequency and depth of these engagements raise the possibility of the philosophy of medicine as a formal discipline, distinct from other branches of philosophy. The subject is still in an inchoate state. It is toward its maturation that Engelhardt and Spicker have established their series on philosophy and medicine,[37] the *Journal of Medicine and Philosophy* has been initiated, and the American Philosophical Association has formed a Committee on Philosophy and Medicine.

The historical wariness of the two disciplines is being overcome, and the ground between them is again being actively tilled. We are entering a new era of dialogue—perhaps one as promising as that between Greek medicine and philosophy. Given the historical antecedents, the relationship will be a delicate one nonetheless.

Philosophy of Medicine—Discipline or Philosophical Mélange?

Do the medical forays of philosophers in Europe and the current interest in the United States prefigure the emergence of a definable discipline—the philosophy of medicine? Opinions range from flat denial to all-encompassing acceptance. Jerome Shaffer categorically denies the possibility, Toulmin regards it as problematic, and Szumowski accepts the notion, going so far as to define it. We will first examine these opinions and then lay out the requirements the philosophy of medicine must satisfy if it is to be a distinguishable discipline.

Shaffer's denial of the possibility is unequivocal.[38] He doubts there are any problems common to medicine and philosophy. Those alleged to be at the interface are either misclassified or not philosophical problems at all. He would reduce all philosophical efforts in the medical context to philosophy of science, philosophy of mind, or moral philosophy. Schaffer freely acknowledges the significance of the issues for philosophy but sees nothing to distinguish medicine from a mere summation of biology and psychology.

Toulmin partially agrees with Shaffer by finding no real distinction between medicine and physiology.[39] Physiology is itself a derivative of physics and chemistry. Physiology, however, deals with the "special field of life" whose laws are not independent of chemistry and physics but still not fully equated with them. Thus the somatic elements in medical science are subsumed under the philosophy of science or of biology. Toulmin, however, allows for the possibility of a philosophy of medicine based on the psychosocial dimensions of medical practice and the whole realm of values and choice which remain outside the concepts of medicine as science.

Szumowski, who traced the history of medical philosophy in Europe, is the least critical and proposes a very broad definition as follows:

> The philosophy of medicine is a science which considers medicine as a whole; it studies its position in humanity, society, the state and the medical school; it embraces at a glance the totality of the history of medicine; it sets forth the most general problems of philosophy and biology; it analyzes the methodological forms of medical thought, mentioning and explaining the logical errors committed in medicine; it borrows from psychology and metaphysics the knowledge and ideas of moment to the whole of medicine; it touches on medical praxeology; it discusses the principal values in medicine; it formulates the principles of ethics and medical deontology; finally it discusses aesthetics in medicine. (Authors' translation)[40]

None of these views is really adequate. Shaffer ignores too much; Szumowski embraces too much; and Toulmin occupies a halfway house which, on further analysis, must either move toward Shaffer or accept the philosophy of medicine as a discipline—though not necessarily in the diffuseness of Szumowski's definition. Toulmin is right in believing that the first step is to distinguish medicine from science. Then we must show what specific philosophical issues are contained within medicine which are susceptible to comprehension by no discipline other than philosophy.

In recent times, philosophy has examined many special disciplines for their meaning and essence, their modes of explanation, the metaphysical assumptions upon which they are based, and the possibility of some unifying theory of the realities they encompass. Thus the logical, epistemological, and metaphysical examinations of what historians, lawyers, or scientists do, and the meaning of what they study, comprise the philosophy of history, law, or science. One can ask the same questions about philosophy itself—the philosophy *of* philosophy. Indeed this has been a preoccupation of some major thinkers, such as Ortega, Heidegger, Husserl, and Merleau-Ponty.[41]

Special difficulties do arise when we consider adding the philosophy of medicine to this list. Medicine does, in fact, derive much of its method, logic, and theory from the physical and biological sciences, so it is to a certain extent a branch of those sciences. But medicine is also a *praxis* in the Aristotelian sense—knowledge applied for human ends and purposes. In this sense, medicine can be classed among the technologies. But medicine also sets out to modify the behavior of individuals and societies, and thus has roots in the behavioral sciences. Finally, medicine operates through a personal, and therefore an ethical, relationship intended to "help" the person to "better" health. It is a value-laden activity, with roots in ethics and the humanities.

At first glance, it would seem that Schaffer's position is correct—medicine is totally derivative. It has no distinctive subject matter, and its "philosophy" is therefore nothing but the sum total of the philosophies of biology, mind, and moral science. But is this so? Let us see if we can distinguish medicine from science first, and then from the social sciences and the humanities. Only then can we speak properly of a philosophy of medicine. What follows is only an initial discussion, designed to outline the need and the dimensions of a philosophy of medicine. We will further describe medicine and its uniqueness as a discipline in Chapter Three.

Medicine is, in part, a truly scientific endeavor. It shares with chemistry and physics the aim of understanding physical processes. Medicine as science studies man by observation, mensuration, hypothesis formulation, and experiment under controlled conditions. In studying *man as object,* it follows the canons of good science—proper experimental design, validity of observation and method, correct logic, and verifiable conclusions. This surely is the content of the basic sciences of medicine, even though they pursue these ends in the most complicated of biological systems. Granting that the "special field of life," as Toulmin suggests, imparts special features to the laws of chemistry and physics, the basic sciences of medicine could indeed be subsumed under the philosophy of biology.[42]

But the basic sciences by themselves are not sufficient to constitute medicine either as clinical science or medical practice. As clinical science, medicine must study the human entity, in which purpose, values, consciousness, reflection, and self-determination complicate the laws of chemistry and physics even more than do the special micro-environments of living things in general. Medicine, even as science, must encompass the special complexities of *man as subject* interacting with *man as object* of science. Physiology, unlike the clinical science of medicine, studies physical processes while ignoring the lived reality of the experimental subject—his or her self-perceived history, uniqueness, and individuality. Thus even when it functions as clinical science, medicine must correlate the explanatory modes of the physical sciences with those of the social and behavioral.

But neither the basic sciences nor the clinical sciences can be properly considered as medicine until they are used in a particular clinical context, in a particular individual, and for a particular purpose to effect the attainment of health. The purpose of medicine *qua* medicine, then, transcends that of medical science per se—which is primarily to know. Medical science, basic or clinical, becomes medicine only when it is used to promote health and healing–that is, only when it is an intervention in an individual human life to alter the human condition. Medicine, thus construed, has a telos which distinguishes it from its component sciences, whose telos is to understand physical processes in as general a way as possible, and certainly not to particularize that knowledge in an individual human life. For medicine *qua* medicine cannot deal with general scientific laws as such, but must locate them in a time, place, and person. This thesis is defended in Chapters Three through Five.

Medicine is, in short, a practical theory of human reality. It is a moral activity, since it operates through a personal interrelationship in which physician and patient are co-participants in defining the goal and achieving it–cure of illness or promotion of health. The patient is not a passive object to which a technique is applied, since he or she seeks advice and help and modifies his or her behavior in conformity with the physician's advice. This dimension impinges directly on the person and his or her values. It involves two persons interacting, each in his own socio-historical moment. The intersection of their values, together with those of medicine, science, and society, creates a nexus of choices and priorities. It is the unraveling of that nexus for this patient, here and now, that constitutes medicine. The resultant synthesis is more than the sum total of the component sciences–physical, social, and moral–which contribute to that unraveling.

This synthesis, moreover, is constrained by the fiduciary responsibility which imposes itself on the physician by the very nature of the contract between him and the patient. The physician is *presumed* to help and not to harm, and to advocate the "good" of the patient at all times. Our concern that this moral axiom rest on more than professionalism or the glossy patina of cultural expectations leads to the matter in Chapter Eight on the link between medical ethics and the philosophy of medicine. The patient presents himself in a state of wounded humanity. He has lost some of his freedom since he must come to the physician; he must give consent when he is in pain and discomfort, and he does so in the presence of an information gap which can never be closed fully. Medical science, therefore, becomes medicine only when it is modulated and constrained in unique ways by the humanity of physician and patient.

Its telos takes it out of the realm of *theoria* and puts it into the realm of *praxis.*

It is the totality of this unique combination which constitutes the clinical moment and the clinical encounter, without which authentic medicine does not exist. No simplistic neo-Cartesian reduction of medicine to sciences of mind, arithmetically added to science of the body and tied together with a ribbon of moral science, is adequate to explain this synthesis. Nor is this merely biology. Neither plants nor animals–granting that they become ill as well as humans–can enter into a relationship with the healer in which the patient participates as subject and object simultaneously.

Medicine might be considered in one sense a technology, since its purpose is the application of techniques to meet specific human needs. But technology cannot be the same as medicine, since the way technology is used is determined by the clinical encounter as we have outlined it above, and not by technology itself. Technology, like the sciences, becomes part of a larger synthesis when it is used within medicine. The further question, "Usefulness for what?", is beyond both medicine and technology and resides in philosophy, as Jonas points out.[43]

We have thus far said nothing of medicine as art. Here too, medicine has an autonomy very much like that of music, for example. Music depends upon physics, acoustics, and mathematics. But it operates with an autonomy which results in an entity called "music," which is not completely definable in terms of its derivatives.

The same kinds of distinctions can be made between medicine and the social sciences and humanities, upon which it also depends. Medicine differs from psychiatry because it works in and through the body to affect health, while psychiatry works through the senses only, to affect the psyche–as does religion to affect the spirit. Medicine differs from the humanities, which also deal with values and human existence. But they do not do so with the direct purpose of affecting health or curing illness through manipulation of the body. The philosophy of medicine, therefore, is not congruent with the philosophy of the humanities, any more than it is with the philosophy of the sciences.

Finally, we must add the social dimensions of medicine *qua* medicine–the applications of medical knowledge on an aggregate of humans rather than an individual. This "social encounter" is a parallel of the clinical encounter with an individual patient. Without taking the time to carry out a parallel analysis, it is clear that scientific knowledge can also be used to improve the health of the community. Here medicine is concerned with values, choices, and priorities which relate to the "good" of society. Such issues as the distribution of health services, the purposes for which medicine is used, for whom, who decides, and upon what principles, would constitute the elements of a social philosophy of medicine.

Medicine, then, is an activity whose essence appears to lie in the clinical event, which demands that scientific and other knowledge be particularized in the lived reality, of a particular human, for the purpose of attaining health or curing illness, through the direct manipulation of the body, and in a value-laden decision matrix. It is in this sense that medical theory is a theory of practical reality and not just the theory of the sciences which contribute to it. Chapter Six will support this thesis.

Up to this point, we have tried to distinguish among three levels of meaning of the term "medicine": (a) the basic sciences component, which seeks to understand physical processes in a living being, healthy or ill; (b) the clinical sciences component, which seeks to understand physical processes in a perceiving subject in whom mind and body are united; and (c) medicine per se, or medical *praxis,* in which the clinical and basic sciences are particularized in the clinical moment or encounter, with all the complexities outlined above. In medicine *qua* medicine, the sciences are not only means of understanding but also means to intervention in the lives of persons or societies. It is for this reason that we chose the title for this book, to stress the importance of medical practice.

Thus we would agree, with Shaffer, that the basic science portions of medicine are derivative, and that their philosophy is the philosophy of biology or the sciences. Clinical sciences, however, attempt to understand a larger totality which includes the entities of mind and psyche. The contemporary Cartesian would consider even clinical science completely derived from the physical sciences and psychology, and its philosophy to be some combination of the philosophies of biology and psychology. We prefer to consider clinical science as a synthesis which cannot be encompassed by biology and psychology, so that its philosophy would be a philosophy of clinical science. Finally, medicine *qua* medicine–i.e., medical practice as we have outlined it in the clinical encounter–could not be totally congruent with either basic or clinical sciences. Hence the philosophy of medicine could not be congruent with the philosophy of biology, added to the philosophy of mind, added to moral science.

Medicine clearly is a domain of activity which is distinctive and distinguishable as science, art, and *praxis*. It comprises a set of legitimate philosophical issues and questions which derive from the unique nature of the clinical encounter. It is precisely the clinical encounter that constitutes the singular ordering concept which distinguishes medicine from the sciences and which is the ground for the logic, the epistemology, and the metaphysics of medical practice. It cannot be reduced to the philosophy of science, mind, and morals, as Shaffer proposes; nor is it so all-embracing, as Szumowski's definition would have it. By failing to place emphasis on the clinical moment, Szumowski's definition would include everything about medicine–not only its philosophy but also its sociology, economics, politics, education, and aesthetics. In his definition, both "philosophy" and "medicine" are too loosely used.

Philosophy and the Modes of Engagement with Medicine

The philosophy of medicine must emphasize genuinely philosophical questions, and these must be defined with care. These are the questions not answerable by medicine itself or by any of the other scientific or humanistic disciplines which enter into it. It is important, therefore, to elaborate somewhat the sense in which the term "philosophy" is used here. The term has been particularly misused by medical writers, as Temkin's observations about even so revered a figure as William Osler make clear.[44] Osler's *Way of Life* is an example of a large number of works of opinion and belief written by eminent physicians about medicine, which are commendable but which have been too gratuitously termed "philosophy."[45]

The nonphilosopher cannot presume to enter into the question, "What is philosophy?", which has engaged almost every major modern philosopher. Nor would we exalt one mode of philosophizing above the others as most suitable to the specific issues raised in medicine. The number and variety of problems are sufficient to challenge the whole range of philosophical methods. Some problems are best approached phenomenologically, others analytically, and still others speculatively. This is not to sanction an undiscriminating collage of philosophical notions or some mysterious process of intellectual *épluchage*. However, in the nascent state of the inquiry a pluralistic methodology has certain advantages. The precise nature of the questions may be more clearly revealed by divergent modes of inquiry–particularly if they eventuate in similar formulations. Thus, in the next chapter, we will attempt a philosophical methodology which aims at realism but allows one to categorize elements of reality. For want of a better term, we call this approach an "ontology of practice."

There is little room for an autocratic notion of philosophy, sitting in judgment above the special disciplines. This tendency is too easily manifest in dealing with medicine, whose immersion in the practical may range from the sublime to the sordid. There is already something of a backlash among medical practitioners, as a consequence of misunderstanding the intent of some philosophers who have ventured into the troubled arena of bioethics.[46]

What is needed is a systematic set of ways for articulating, clarifying, defining, and addressing the philosophical issues in medicine. The philosopher can contribute by his capacity for critical discussion of the physician's thoughts and action, and by dialectical dissection of the presumptions behind them. The aim is the same as in philosophizing about any human activity–to grasp something of its reality, of the value of the things which comprise it, and of the nature of man as it is revealed in the medical act, the clinical encounter. It is the act of philosophizing on the whole domain of the clinical moment that is essential–not the particular mode of that philosophizing.

There are three distinct ways by which philosophy as philosophy can engage medicine. We have devoted most attention to one of them–the philosophy *of* medicine–because it is the problematic and also the most in need of delineation. There are two others–

philosophy *in* medicine and philosophy *and* medicine. They can be distinguished by the ways in which medicine and philosophy address each other and the types of issues with which they deal.

These distinctions are a modification of the distinction our colleague Robert Straus has made between sociology *in* and *of* medicine.[47] He did not make a third distinction, sociology *and* medicine, which we shall add in the case of philosophy.

Philosophy *and* medicine comprises the mutual considerations by medicine and philosophy of problems common to both, or problems which exist in medicine but are not limited to the special rubric of the philosophy of medicine as we have outlined it above. Here the effort is collaborative. Medicine and philosophy retain their identities. Each draws on the resources of the other, is enriched, and elaborates some new medical or philosophical concept of its own. Some of the recurrent problems of philosophy–the mind-body debate; the meanings of perception, consciousness, language; the special or nonspecial character of chemical and physical laws in living things–are susceptible to this type of collaborative attack. The findings of neuropathology, neurosurgery, and the physiology and pharmacology of the nervous system are essential, for example, to any serious deliberation on the philosophy of mind or psyche. It was just such a study which led Merleau-Ponty to philosophize upon the phantom limb syndrome as an element in his phenomenology of perception. Out of the interaction of medicine *and* philosophy may come part of a synthesis of the constellation of interpretations which now constitute the idea or image of man. A true philosophical anthropology must start with the full range of observations medicine makes of individual humans in health, in illness, and when they face their own death. It cannot end there, of course.

Philosophy *in* medicine refers to the application of the traditional tools of philosophy–critical reflection, dialectical reasoning, uncovering of value and purpose, or asking first-order questions–to some medically defined problem. The problems can range from the logic of medical thought to the epistemology of medical science as science, the problem of causality, the limitations of observation and experiment, and, of course, the whole range of vexing issues in the active field of biomedical ethics. These are problems which medicine shares with other sciences, professions, and technologies. The philosopher serves an invaluable function *in* medicine—that is, in the medical setting as educator and trained thinker exhibiting the way philosophy can illuminate and examine critically what physicians do in their everyday activity.

This is a common form of interaction in the United States, especially on those medical campuses and in hospitals which have formal programs in medical ethics. Philosophers in these medical settings are making significant contributions without necessarily addressing the question of the theory of medicine as medicine. Most of the problems of the basic clinical sciences as sciences can fall under this rubric.

When philosophy turns, as we do later in this book, to the meaning of medicine as clinical practice and examines its conceptual foundations, its ideologies, its ethos, and the philosophical bases of medical ethics, then it becomes the philosophy *of* medicine. The questions examined by philosophy *in* medicine are then carried to the unique realm of the clinical encounter with a human being experiencing health, illness, neurosis, or psychosis, in a setting which involves intervention into his existence. The questions then transcend the philosophy of science per se and grapple with the meaning of medicine—its nature, concepts, purposes, and value to society—what can be called the philosophical problem of medicine. The philosophy of medicine seeks explanations for what medicine *is* and *ought* to be, in terms of the axiomatic assumptions upon which it is based. This is the realm of the transmedical meaning of medicine, the realm which neither medicine nor any other science can explore by itself. "And yet, there is another side in every science which that science as such can never reach: the essential nature and origin of its sphere, the essence and essential origin of the manner of knowing which it cultivates. . . ."[48]

These three types of engagement are rarely separable in actual fact, and philosophers can, and do, engage in all three. We have dissected them to underscore the central importance of the philosophy of medicine—i.e., the philosophical issues embedded in the theory of medicine as a practical human activity. Ultimately, the more proximate issues dealt with by philosophy *and* medicine, and by philosophy *in* medicine, must rest on the philosophy *of* medicine.

Some Urgent Philosophical Issues Arising in Medicine

Whatever mode or level of philosophizing one chooses, there are a series of interesting and genuine philosophical problems arising in contemporary medicine. We will choose only a few to illustrate some of the points we have been making thus far.

First, there is a set of questions which medicine shares with the philosophy of science–such as the analysis and meaning of medical language and explanation, the verifiability criteria of medical theories, the notion of causality, the logic of discovery and experimental design, and the limitations of statistical and stoichastic analyses. These questions are modulated in medicine, since they must be examined in reflecting, conscious subjects in the clinical context. Some mode of explanation must be found which overcomes the pretensions of reductionism and vitalism. How, if at all, is the scientific enterprise to be modified in medicine?

There is another set of questions, not usually part of the philosophy of science, which demands philosophical inspection. These relate to the unique existence of humans as a unity of mind and body. The meanings of the phenomena of embodiment and corporeality, and their perception by the subject, have a deep impact on medical theory and practice. Both Cartesian dualism and monistic materialism are glaringly deficient in satisfactory explanations of these phenomena. Still, no alternative to these polarities is at hand. Resolution of the deficiency is fundamental to any theoretical development of medicine. Our inchoate efforts at describing health and disease without reference to a dualism of mind and body should be judged against this background.

To what extent are the methods and modes of explanation of sociology, psychology, and philosophy valid in grappling with the realities of man's existence as a thinking being? Is intelligence, for example, reducible to engineering concepts, and totally simulable as artificial intelligence by the computer? Or, as Dreyfus suggests, are the metaphysical assumptions upon which such an assertion rests in error?[49] Medicine and philosophy should be able to reinforce each other in dealing with such issues. Philosophy is still far from drawing fully on the large base of neurophysiological, neuropsychiatric, and neuroendocrinological data medicine has collected.

Medicine has yet to appreciate the insights metaphysical or phenomenological analysis can contribute to the interpretation and intelligibility of these data. This conjunction should help to reconcile the scientific with the commonsense images of man.

This reconciliation is a most important step in the persistent search for a philosophical grasp of the idea of man. Philosophical anthropology is still a diffuse exercise of quite recent origins. The "image of man" is fractured and in need of restoration, as Buber, Scheler, and Cassirer have told us.[50] There is a growing need to weave together the numerous separate strands of information about human existence. In this regard, Stent, an unusually philosophical biologist, has sketched the limitations of both the positivist and structuralist formulations of man.[51]

Difficult as the effort may be, such a scientific-philosophical synthesis is fundamental, and prior, to the choices we must make about human life, death, health, and disease. There must be some idea of man to order our definition of what is "good" for the person and society, and for the optimal relationships between them. Individual and social bioethics both derive from this context of our idea of man.

Intimately related to the philosophical conception of man are the definitions of health and disease, of cure, and of disability. The presuppositions physicians hold about these conceptions shape medical theory and practice. Since health is the end and purpose of medical knowledge, the clearer the definition we can give to that term, the more order and priority we can give to our uses of medical knowledge. The intersection of human, societal, and historical values which characterizes the medical encounter can be dealt with rationally only if both physician and patient understand each other's presuppositions about the purposes and perfection of human existence.

The idea of man underlies a whole set of humanistic issues which arise out of the technological potencies of modern medicine. Matters formerly the concern of the speculative and imaginative intelligence are now technological realities. Medicine can prolong or terminate life, control conception and fertility, elevate our moods, or blunt our pain and anxieties. To apply these measures is to challenge traditional meanings of the value and dignity of individual life, of the family, of suffering and dying, or of individual versus social good. The ancient metaphysical question, "What is 'the good?,' " has resurfaced with an unprecedented urgency. We cannot use medicine for the attainment of health or the "good life" unless we clarify these conceptions in light of our technological possibilities. We plan this explanation in Chapters Five and Six.

The philosophical foundations of contemporary biomedical and professional ethics also derive from the ideas of man the person and the balance which should obtain between the life of man as an individual and as a member of society. Samuel Gorovitz has sketched out a very complete topography of the philosophical issues at the heart of medical ethics. He underscores the urgent need for a closer examination of the assumptions about the primarily philosophical questions which underlie medical decisions and calls for their examination by philosophers. In fact, Gorovitz puts the matter squarely in terms of social responsibility: "That science exists in the final analysis, for the pleasure and for the benefit of society, is a point to which philosophers generally accede readily. What is perhaps less often noted by them is that philosophy, too, is a social enterprise supported in the final analysis by the public, to whose interest it accrues."[52]

But what value system should we use in addressing these humanistic questions? Do we follow the ideology of modern science, which has influenced so many medical men today? Bronowski and Holton have ennobled the community of science, and the pursuit of science is an ethic of unique proportions in itself. Bronowski praised the value system of science–the capacity to tolerate dissent, to foster freedom and independence of thought.[53] Holton holds that the scientist has no choice but to pursue creativity and new knowledge, even if we have not the means at hand to cope with the challenges to human values created by the scientist's activity.[54]

Hans Jonas, on the other hand, calls for an ethic of limits, prudence, and restraint to balance the ethics of endless progress.[55] The more a technique has the possibility for modifying human life, the less free is the scientist to pursue it without some restraint. This is in direct contradiction to the freedom which the ethics of science holds as a fundamental requisite: "The demand of each discipline to choose its own problems and fit them to its own concepts and techniques and instruments, suggests that science is not eager to undertake to solve the problems of society, as society would define them."[56]

The ethos, as well as the ethics, of science and medicine demands critical examination. How do we reconcile the image medicine has developed of itself and the concept society holds of its functions? The ideology of science has taken firm hold in medicine. But can medicine provide answers to the questions it creates using only the method of science? Medicine must be reintegrated with all the humanities, as one of us has argued elsewhere.[57] Isolation of technique from purpose poses an antinomy whose perpetuation can only confuse, and possibly subvert, the humane use of medicine.

The process of modernization is associated with bureaucratization and technology, which have become values in themselves. They are prime shapers of the cognitive style of our culture and of modern medicine. They are part of what Foucault calls our *epistemé*—the aggregate history of a human endeavor which enables it to occupy a specific space in a given culture.[58] Has the *epistemé* of medicine arising from its own bureaucratization already determined what society seeks from medicine, and created a self-reinforcing cycle carrying man ever further from what is distinctly human? Will this distorted view contribute further to man's philosophical infirmity?

These are some of the questions which might constitute the content of the philosophy of medicine as a formal intellectual endeavor. This topography is necessarily incomplete. What it illustrates is that there are several sets of truly philosophical questions which medicine can neither pose clearly nor discuss critically if it relies only on its own modes of inquiry. These questions are susceptible to deeper exploration by the methods of ancient and modern philosophy. The choice of any particular set of questions and the emphasis placed on them will depend upon the philosopher's own conception of his subject and of the act of philosophizing. Only some of these questions can be addressed in a book of this length. The others must be left to further explorations by the many thinkers active in the area of the philosophy of medicine.

What the Philosophy of Medicine Ought Not to Be

Several dangers occur in any effort to use the critical and speculative intellect on the matter of medicine. Risse and Galdston, as noted above, have both shown how medical theory, when not securely based on the data of experimental science, can become a vast speculative enterprise which inhibits the growth of medical science. These authors used the example of the eighteenth-century German physicians who hoped to find "ultimate" causes of life, health, and disease. The resulting conflict between those physicians who sought truth in speculative constructs and those who sought it at the bedside was a vigorous one, felt even today. The deleterious effects of thus turning medicine into philosophy have been only too evident in the history of medicine. The greatest disservice to modern medicine would be done by a resurgence of that error today. Medicine should not become bad philosophy, or philosohy bad medicine.

MacIntyre warns against the unrealistic expectation the public and physicians might have of philosophy.[59] The philosopher, and particularly the ethicist in medicine, cannot hope to provide ready answers or formulas for all the moral problems of modern medicine; nor can ethicists be society's only monitors over the actions of health professionals. Some medical people are too eager to delegate moral guidelines to philosophers or ethicists, while others would resist even the asking of ethical questions by those outside medicine.

Philosophers cannot, on the other hand, avoid their responsibility as "delegated intellects." They must not, however, compromise the integrity of their discipline or be lured by sudden prominence and attention to indulge in pontifications beyond the limits of the method they master. Philosophers are as susceptible as others to the temptation of all intellectuals to see their special mode of inquiry as the universal way to truth. One way to balance this tendency is to place philosophers in medicine in the company of other humanists. Historians, theologians, and specialists in literature are also entering the medical setting. Their interaction with philosophers may be salubrious for all.

Nor should the philosophy of medicine become *medical* musing–that is, ruminations and meditations of physicians on the state of medicine, the professions, health, or other related matters. These intuitions serve a hortatory, interpretive, and inspirational purpose, important in education and practice. They might become a matter for pondering in the philosophy of medicine, but they must not be confused with the philosophy of medicine.

The philosophy of medicine should also not become a quest or crusade for *the* philosophy–some unified theory for all of medicine which would explain all human, biological phenomena. We seek rather to emphasize the continual examination of the crucial philosophical questions which arise in the substance of medicine, not a final system of medicine which will put an end to all questioning. We can conceive of *a* philosophy of medicine–some theoretical construct put forth tentatively to be tested against experience on the one hand, and dialectical reasoning on the other. *A* philosophy of medicine, as a set of propositions *about* medicine, is valid only as a hypothesis is valid in experimental science.

The philosopher contemplating medicine must be careful to avoid the twin seductions of overly serene detachment, on the one hand, and total submersion in medicine, on the other. He should remember the unfortunate plight of some social scientists who have weakened their identity in the medical setting, losing credibility as social scientists and contributing little to the medical milieu. The philosopher will be helpful to medicine and advance his own discipline only if he remains a bona fide philosopher.

Some Educational Implications

If there is any cogency in this explication of the necessity and nature of the philosophy of medicine, then its nurture becomes a concern of educators and practitioners as well as scholars. Wartofsky's recent analysis of the impact of human ontology in shaping the concept of disease, and thus of medical practice, illustrates clearly how important the seemingly academic considerations of the philosophy of medicine can be in the practical world.[60]

The questions subsumed under the three forms of engagement of medicine with philosophy outlined here will have varying degrees of immediacy for physicians and other health workers. Practitioners need, most of all, to develop some capacity for critical examination of their own value systems and their concepts of man.

Teachers of medicine will require a deeper understanding of theological and epistemological questions in medical science and clinical practice. Those who make public policy decisions will require a better grasp of the social ethics of medicine. The medical scholar will want to probe the more ontological and metaphysical issues.

It would be palpably unwise to attempt to make every physician a philosopher, in Galen's or Plato's sense. But every physician, since he is involved with values, concepts, and ideas of medicine, must have some philosophical *sense*. It does seem reasonable to expose every student to critical discussion of the issues outlined here, particularly those relating to medical and professional ethics. Medical schools are becoming more cognizant of the centrality of issues of human values in medical practice. By 1977, approximately eighty schools had developed formal programs to integrate ethics, philosophy, and the humanities into professional education.[61] Similar efforts have been initiated to involve the practicing physician as well.

A minimal aim for all students in the health professions should be to sensitize them to the reality and meaning of their personal value presuppositions, so that they can understand more clearly the basis of their own daily decisions and recommendations. Some exposure to the rigor of philosophical inquiry may possibly balance some of the antiphilosophical bias of medical education. For those students who wish to probe more deeply, opportunities for extended study, research, or a career in the problems at the interface of medicine and philosophy may help to expand the number of physicians able to take responsibility as educated men in the consideration of how medicine shall be used to advance human purposes.

What is needed is the cultivation of the humanities and philosophy in the medical and health care setting with something like the vigor we dedicate to the basic sciences. Indeed, for the greater number of practitioners, the utility and importance of humane studies equal those of the clinical and basic sciences. Charles Fried has shown how philosophical, legal, and economic values and principles overlap in practical decision making–not only in human experimentation but also in personal health care and in the social ethics of medicine.[62] Few physicians who wish to be more than technicians can ignore the philosophical bases of these practical, daily choices so integral to their authenticity as professionals.

Summary

The congruence between medicine and philosophy which we find in the *Protagoras* and the *Treatise on Ancient Medicine,* as well as the tensions symbolized in the dialectic between Eryximachus and Diotima, will always be with us. The congruence and the divergence of these ancient disciplines are both important to human well-being. By opposing one another, medicine and philosophy can each balance the other's pretension to universality. By converging, they illuminate some of the most important questions of human existence.

This chapter has examined ways in which medicine and philosophy can converge in our time as philosophy *and* medicine, philosophy *in* medicine, and philosophy *of* medicine. The present moment in our intellectual history is particularly propitious for the nurture of the engagement of medicine and philosophy. The most fruitful form of that interaction may be in the philosophy *of* medicine, which is a definable discipline with a set of issues specific to it. If the obvious intellectual dangers can be avoided, those who practice medicine, those who think about it, and those who are served by it can gain deeper insight into the nature and the purpose of medicine, as well as the nature of the profession and of man himself.

In the next two chapters, we will examine philosophy and medicine in more detail, paying special attention to a suitable methodology with which to examine medicine philosophically and the nature of medicine as a unitary discipline, distinct from the numerous arts and sciences from which it borrows. These chapters are preparatory to Chapters Four, Five, and Six, the former two offering an ontology of medicine and the latter the development of clinical judgment. We intend these chapters to serve as an example of a philosophy of medicine, not *the* exclusive philosophy of medicine, in the sense discussed above. However, we find it difficult not to perceive medicine, positioned as it is at the intersection of the sciences, the humanities, and technology, and a clinically based discipline, as "a medium and the focus in which the problems of wisdom and science meet."[63]

2

A Philosophical Method

Introduction

In order to make sense of the plurality of opinions about philosophy, we propose that for this book, the fundamental understanding of philosophy be a structured dialogue for the purpose of critical understanding. Put another way, philosophy is a disciplined, critical reflection following logical rules. Defense and discussion of this point of view occupy a significant portion of this chapter.

First, we must show that the most general category for the philosophical enterprise is dialectic. That is, at root, philosophy deals with a problem or set of problems in a disciplined manner. The problem or set of problems can range from concrete objects to criteria for thinking, from the history of philosophy to the nature of disciplines present in culture today, from man to logical rules. The disciplined manner of philosophy sets it squarely among the humanities and distinguishes it from mere fanciful thinking. Because the problem or set of problems varies so widely, the language, function, and goal of a particular philosophy will also vary widely. Because any particular philosophy is a dialectic with a problem or set of problems, the latter operate as limiting factors on the philosophical inquiry. The broader the set of problems, the greater the chance for generally true statements to emerge from philosophical inquiry. In any case, the inquiry itself is colored by the limits the problem or set of problems imposes on the dialectic.

Because we are interested in deriving a suitable methodology for inquiring into the philosophy of medicine, our interests in this chapter do not include even a minimal resolution of the question: "What is philosophy?" However, a brief discussion of the present situation in philosophy and the tensions inherent in the philosophical enterprise will prepare the way for our choice of a starting point, a methodology, and a realistic philosophy of experience. Recalling what we said already, our choices in philosophical methodology are largely circumscribed by the nature of the medical enterprise which poses the problems. In no case would we wish to claim that the philosophical approach herein taken be applied without modification to other disciplines or even to other problems.

A second consideration in the argument that philosophy be viewed as a dialectic is to develop the notion that the purpose of philosophical activity is disciplined, critical reflection on problems. We therefore argue that an authentic philosophical approach to a problem or set of problems occurs when commitment to thinking about problems is coupled with a choice of a starting point. Observing that a starting point must be congruent with a practice and theory of any set of problems, we then argue that a philosophy of medicine must be open to medicine as a discipline of experience. Noting that both philosophy and medicine begin as an inter-human event, we argue that a proper starting point for a philosophy of medicine must be based upon a choice of what is important from a field or world of matters of fact. We consider "cure" to be what is important about medicine.

Our final consideration indicates how a philosophy of experience must deal in practical problem solving that results from paying attention to the world of practice. Congruent with the experimental aims of medicine, this philosophy has four functions: (a) description, producing modes of medicine; (b) radical reflection, reproducing forms and the form of medicine; (c) critical reflection, producing the structures of medicine; and (d) practical reflection on ethics and policy considerations. It is from the third function that we mold an ontology of the body. In this third part of our argument, we indicate how a philosophy of experience is guided by the realm of practice, starting from this realm and returning to it. The validity of our reflections will depend less on canons of scientific rigor and more on how these reflections truly describe what takes place in the clinical relationship. Ideas prove hollow if not rooted in what William James called "the thickness of reality."

Philosophy of Philosophy

Philosophers today are in sharp disagreement about the nature of the philosophical task. Very few, for example, would dare suggest, as did St. Augustine, that philosophy is an attempt to understand the world. Fewer still would describe it as a "love of wisdom," however etymologically justified that description might be.

Philosophy today suffers from an identity crisis comparable to that found in all of the humanities. Steven Marcus, in "The Demoralized Humanists," explains why:

> Although it would be false to say that the humanities today are in a state of crisis—they are too diverse and diffuse for that—they are undeniably experiencing a loss of self-confidence. Increasingly the parameters of social change are being set by technological and scientific innovations, while explanations for human action are being provided through statistical findings and the behavioral assumptions of the social scientists.[1]

The humanities have always emphasized reasoned criticism of culture. But to use them to create a "new order" is a suspect activity. Thus, while being in touch with the real human problems encountered in, or even caused by, medicine, a philosophy of medicine should remain cautious about marketing new values, or as Marcus puts it, engaging in "mental management of society."[2]

To satisfy these conditions in a philosophy of medicine, it is necessary first to describe which philosophical approach will be taken in this book. Despite the garbled chorus of opinions about the nature of philosophy, some methodology must be chosen which would aid the understanding of medicine. In the process of choosing, we are forced to opt for one mode of philosophizing over others. The task of choosing is aided, however, by the following points:

We have shown that philosophy does and can enter into a dialogue with medicine and that a contemporary philosophy of medicine is desirable, if not mandated, by the increasing complexity of medicine today. Furthermore, we intend to show that major philosophical importance should be attached to the epistemological problem facing medicine: How can one extract from, and apply to, specific individuals the more universal knowledge of biological science and pathogenesis practiced by modern medicine?

What philosophical approach should be chosen then? What current or traditional method would be helpful? To answer this question, one must turn to the current state of philosophy as described in *The Owl of Minerva: Philosophers on Philosophy,* edited by Bontempo and Odell. Philosophers are shown to disagree not only on what conclusions they should reach but also on what they should be talking about. The editors suggest that philosophy is an art, not a science, since no discoveries are made and no real discipline is formed.

In the body of the book, Ayer argues that philosophy deals with what can be put into words, while Watts counters that philosophy occupies itself with the transcendent, that which cannot be put into words. An even more disturbing disagreement is that between Smart and Marcuse. Smart posits that philosophy is conceptual analysis, avoiding all attempts to change concepts, while Marcuse argues that philosophy precisely does change concepts. The more influential philosophers tend to be those who reject speculative metaphysics for an imitation of the rigors of science. Philosophy is thereby driven into professionalism and specialization, disqualifying itself as a critic of such specialization.[3]

Whenever such professional disagreement occurs within a discipline, there is always an irenic voice or two proclaiming tolerance of divergent points of view. Paul Schaff takes this stance when he says that there is no way to "prove" the correctness of one approach over another, since all philosophical generalizations are hypothetical. He is able to argue persuasively because he holds a philosophy (Marxism) open to change without sacrifice of absolutism!

Philosophy will probably survive these inconsistencies, as it always has—and, indeed, has thrived on them. But its effectiveness is certainly diminished by the lack of a common language, by the trivia of some of its subject matter, and by the crossword puzzles it plays while critical problems face contemporary human beings and the societies they form.

Can any sense be made out of the current state of philosophy? Can divergent philosophical enterprises be embraced simultaneously —for example, enterprises which range from the study of transcendence to concept formation, from thought divorced from action to thought in the service of action, from synthesis of insights to analysis of differences? We propose that the fact that so few philosophers agree about what they do is itself a clue to the nature of the philosophical task. Attempts to understand a set of problems must be relative perspectives on that set of problems. These perspectives are conditioned, at the very least, by the questions asked, the matters of interest upon which the discipline is focused. These concerns can be judged to be intrinsically important, simply interesting to the philosopher, or highlighted in a culture. We consider problems raised by modern medicine to be in this last category.

The reason philosophers disagree about philosophy is that each is determined by perspective, which in turn is created by the problems with which the philosophy entered the dialogue. Our explanation of this conviction turns on the dialectical nature of philosophizing.

The connotations of "philosophy" carry several dialectical tensions in its use as a word, in its origins, and as a method. We will examine each of these in turn.

As is commonly known, the term "philosophy" comes from the Greek word meaning "love of wisdom." Our English word "love" is at once vaguer and more complicated than the Greek "Philo." The latter meant an all-consuming, passionate commitment. By contrast, the search for wisdom, the other pole of the philosophical enterprise, was considered a higher form of knowledge in which one came to understand the basic meaning of things, activities, life, and nature. In its original meaning, then, philosophy dangerously coupled a commitment with a special quest for understanding, a passion for life with the task of intellectually organizing it. Philosophy is, therefore, an infrequently achieved balance between these opposing tensions. It is dialectical.

In its origins as well, philosophy involved a dialectical tension. Seeking to understand the world, the Greeks had at their disposal religious myth and slowly burgeoning skills in science. Therefore, philosophers simultaneously sought understanding of systems of meaning regarding human affairs (myth and, later, other philosophical systems) and of systems of meaning regarding the laws of nature (the early sciences, especially metallurgy, cosmology, and medicine).

The inherent tension between the decision to "love wisdom" and the dialectical sources of meaning (systems of meaning either about human affairs or about nature) generates conflicts over the starting point of philosophy and the proper limits of its concerns. This disagreement is as sharp today as it was for the Greeks.

Does philosophy begin with the obviously changing structure of nature (Democritus and Aristotle)? Should philosophy be continually concerned to protect change as an ultimate reality (Democritus) or to search for the principles of change (Aristotle)? Should philosophy, instead, begin with the permanent laws which allow one to predict–indeed, to trust–that tomorrow will be much like today (Parmenides)? Are these laws mathematical principles (the Pythagoreans), or are they ideas (Plato)? Should one start, instead, with doubt (Descartes), with the mistrust of reason itself (Hume), with a priori scientific statements (Kant), with the tricks of language (linguistic analysts), or with that which cannot be objectified (some existentialists)?

Should one neglect nature and turn, instead, to human affairs as a starting point for philosophy (Socrates, the Stoics)? Should one examine logic and language, politics, economic systems? Or should one begin with the opinions of others, balancing them again in dialectical fashion?

If it is true that one becomes a philosopher through choosing a passionate search to understand, then everyone who seeks understanding for no other purpose than that is a philosopher. But there is surely a stricter sense of being a philosopher which we encounter in trying to select a starting point and focus of concern. When one decides on a proper starting point, one is not only a self-conscious philosopher, one is doing philosophy. Philosophy begins with a reasonable, inductive hunch about what most possibly is the case. In this sense, philosophy is analogous to a laboratory experiment in chemistry or an initial diagnosis of a patient. The choice of a starting point is a critical measure in philosophy, for it will determine the language of that philosophy, its concerns, and its impact.

Space and our purpose preclude a more complete treatment of this point. However, we have suggested that philosophers disagree about philosophy because each has chosen a different starting point, a different problematic, which in turn organizes the discipline and provides it with a language different from other special philosophies. Determined in this way, philosophy is circumscribed not only by the matter chosen for discussion and exploration, not only by the dialectical tension between commitment to the topic and its critique, but also by a focus of concern. This last point leads to a discussion of the functions of philosophy and some considerations of methodology.

Philosophy is dialectical in its methodology as well as in its meaning as a word and its origins as a discipline. The tools of philosophy are both analysis and synthesis. Each philosopher differs in the extent to which he uses one or the other of these tools, as his starting point and interests dictate. Thus, Parmenides, interested in accounting for permanence, analyzed the Greek *esti,* which could mean "there it is, it is real," "the truth of what is," or "being." His analysis led him to synthesize a philosophy of Being over a philosophy of Becoming. Wittgenstein analyzed the use of the word "time" in our language, but did not choose to synthesize his puzzles about time into a logically coherent system. Aristotle analyzed change and specific difference to inaugurate initial sciences of physics and biology, which later led to a metaphysics of act and potency. Democritus before him analyzed change and apparently accounted for it by positing atoms of change.

One may also analyze other systems of meaning, including other philosophical systems, reverentially, as did the early Scholastics of the Middle Ages, or scornfully, as did Bertrand Russell. One's purpose in this analysis might simply be to rest with the discoveries or to construct another system of meaning. At any rate, the choice of tool and the extent of its use depend upon self-satisfaction wrought by the philosopher's makeup and the questions and interests he might have. To repeat, now from the methodological standpoint, philosophy is perspectival.

Because philosophy is a dialogue for the purpose of critical understanding, it produces dialectical tension. This tension arises within, and between, philosophers in a desire to achieve a balance between understanding a set of problems and being committed to that set of problems as a portion of life itself. That is, the philosopher seeks to avoid understanding remote from the reality studied. His articulations must remain true to the reality of the set of problems he is studying.

Thus the philosopher can err in three ways: (a) by immersion in the set of problems, in which case he ends up saying nothing at all; (b) by remaining too abstracted from the set of problems, in which case he says too much; or (c) by not being committed enough to the set as an aspect of life, in which case he does violence to reality. In our view, an example of the first error is the intuitive approach to ethical problems without establishing criteria. An example of the second error is the overintellectualization of problems into neat categories without a sense of their complexity. An example of the third error is idealism in any of its forms. The first approach produces ethical inertia–no new criteria are established. The second approach produces principles and precepts so remote as to be inapplicable to concrete situations. The "ethical backlash" described by Callahan among physicians derives from a failure to avoid this second mistake.[4] The third approach actually neglects the self-critical function of philosophy–which, as a last step in its analysis, should review the ideas presented against the backdrop of real, everyday life.

To conclude this section, therefore, is to note that philosophy is a discipline. It takes discipline to do philosophy, not to fall into the traps cited above. Its takes discipline not to extrapolate beyond the matter cited and the problems with which a particular philosophy deals. It takes discipline to offer concrete suggestions for problem solving when flights of fancy would entertain one's mind better. In a more rigorous sense of discipline, philosophy requires logical rules, rules of coherence, predictability of theory, and other forms of proper reasoning which lead to the production of knowledge. Despite the opinion of Odell and Bontempo that philosophy is merely an art of thinking which does not produce knowledge, if one curtails the temptation to flee beyond the borders of the established set of problems, knowledge of the problem, its underlying structure, and practical applications can be discerned through philosophy. This knowledge, of course, varies in its certitude, depending upon the nature of the set of problems, the polish of reasoning and soundness of the assumptions, including the starting point and focus of concern. It is for these reasons that philosophy is called by us a disciplined, critical reflection following logical rules.

From the reflections so far, a philosophy of medicine would start with an explanation of a starting point about a field of problems called "medicine." Following the explanation of the starting point, a gradual delineation according to rules of thought would take place regarding what is considered important or interesting. In order to establish a dialectic with a set of problems called "medicine," it would be necessary to argue that medicine is a unified discipline, or at least a recognizable human activity distinct from other activities. We attempt this in the next chapter.

A Suitable Philosophical Method

The proper philosophical method in approaching a set of problems should be congruent with the status of that set in any given age. Since medicine is a science in the making, the philosophy chosen must be open-ended and capable of adapting to an ever-expanding complex. Additionally, medicine is above all a discipline of experience. Any philosophical method chosen must pay attention to *praxis* as well as *theoria*.

What should this philosophy be? Where to start? These questions are, perhaps, the most difficult we ask in this book. Medicine is capable of a variety of interpretations. The lack of agreement among philosophers about what is philosophy would seem to make a philosophy of medicine hopeless. If we are to make some headway, then our starting point must be congruent with medical practice and theory. The dialogue must follow rules of thought that are consistent with both the reality of medicine and standard logical patterns.

A Starting Point

Both medicine and philosophy as dialogue begin with an inter-human event. This inter-human event is, as Merleau-Ponty observes, the locus of meaning. Thus philosophy is not just the history of ideas, nor is it a dialectic of ideas (Hegel) or of matter (Marxism).

Both philosophy and medicine share a common function as a dialectic of human beings. Man's creative efforts produce a set of symbols, a language, a dialectic of men. In this way, meaning, including historical meaning, is immanent in the inter-human event. This is the locus of philosophy.[5] Similarly medicine begins with a dialectic of human beings, a dialogue about sickness and health. From this inter-human event both disciplines develop.

This inter-human locus of meaning and language gives rise to interpretations about the world. Philosophy, by focusing upon this locus, is actually an interpretation of interpretations of the world. It is already a second-order reality. Its roots lie in the verbal dialectic about a set. But philosophy criticizes this dialectic and thus offers interpretations about the interpretations of sets. At this point, medicine and philosophy diverge. Philosophy seeks understanding; medicine seeks cure.

Basically, then, philosophy is a search for the origins of meaning in interpretative signs, be they mathematical symbols or theories of disease. Merleau-Ponty calls this unearthing task an "architectural" function of philosophy.[6] If, indeed, philosophy focuses upon the inter-human event located in a particular history, then its search uncovers certain meanings expressed now in a new language removed from that historical event. This new language, or set of interpretative signs, is like an algebra of history–symbolic abstractions from everyday life in which philosophy is rooted.[7]

Our task would be greatly simplified if there were a standard anthropology upon which to base philosophical and medical "interpretive signs." But such an anthropology is nonexistent. In fact, it is one of the eventualities one might hope for in devising a philosophy of medicine. Cassirer quotes Scheler on this point:

> In no other period of human knowledge has man ever become more problematic to himself than in our own days. We have a scientific, a philosophical, and a theological anthropology that know nothing of each other. Therefore we no longer possess any clear and consistent idea of man. The evergrowing multiplicity of the particular sciences that are engaged in the study of man has much more confused and obscured than elucidated our concept of man.[8]

The starting point of a philosophy of medicine is the interhuman event. But there is no common anthropology upon which to base such a philosophy. A philosophy of medicine must, perforce, be based on choice. Yet this cannot, and need not be a blind choice. The philosophy of medicine must be based on a choice that is guided by an initial hunch about what is important in medicine.

The choice which grounds philosophical thought in certain assumptions or hypotheses is, as Whitehead put it, a choice to consider what is important about matters of fact. The distinction is grounded in the binary nature of experience.[9] Simultaneously with an experience of something, there is a corresponding experience of reflexive meaning for the subject of that experience.

Explaining the concept of importance versus matters of fact, Whitehead observes that "importance" is an ultimate experimental notion, a kind of presystematic assemblage carved out of the priorities of matters of fact.[10] Although there is a freedom of selection from matters of fact implied in the concept, that same freedom is guided by the priorities of one's own experience, and the past experience and theories of others, as well as by the pressing needs of one's culture. Thus, the choice of what is important is not blind. Neither is it a full-scale theory or concept.

Matters of fact, then, are the immediate, rich, vast experiences which inundate each moment of existence. The choice to select what is important (or even merely interesting) is largely dictated by cultural concerns, present and past, and by personal concerns of the philosopher.

Applying this concept to medicine, the starting point is an interhuman event, the relationship between physician and patient. Successive steps in the examination of this set of problems will consist of judgments about what is important in this relationship versus those aspects which must remain just matters of fact. More will be said on this point when we articulate the steps to follow at the end of this chapter. However, it is sufficient to note here that we consider what is important about the physician-patient relationship to be healing, or more specifically, cure. An example of matters of fact which are left untouched in this book would be current cancer chemotherapy.

Method and Practice

Once the matters of fact rooted in human experience have been identified as a starting point for a philosophy of medicine, how can such a philosophy remain open to the new experiences developed by modern medicine? How is the philosophical method to be tied to medicine?

After choosing what is important about medicine as a starting point, successive descriptions are necessary about this reality, the doctor-patient relationship. In particular, the descriptions focus on the formal conditions necessary for its effectiveness. However, the effectiveness of medicine, either cure or healing, is a *praxis*. Therefore, the method of philosophy must begin in practice and return thereto for a test of its meaning. In other words, a philosophy of medicine must be an ontology of practice, a search for meaning in the practice of medicine, and specific applications of the results of this search.

It is the practice of medicine today which raises many of the difficult moral and metaphysical questions of our time. As Stuart Spicker remarks about Hans Jonas, "Medical ethical issues cannot, as Professor Jonas points out, be understood apart from an analysis of fundamental issues in ethics and ontology."[11] After all, it is medicine in practice which raises questions about the beginning of human life (abortion) and its end (determination of death), the relationship of man's mind to his body (in psychosurgery, for example, or pharmacy), the nature of practical judgment and its connection with moral ends (in clinical judgment), and so on. In every case, there is embodied a wealth of values and social commitments by both the patient and the physician, all of which immerse one in the realms of philosophical reflection on action.

On this point, we depart from many of our contemporaries who find it fruitful to apply a particular philosophy to medicine, especially those who find the presuppositions and methods of a philosophy of science helpful. We will take up these opinions in Chapters Four and Six. In our view, however enlightening this latter approach, it carries with it a serious flaw. That flaw is that it presupposes medicine to be a science and consequently neglects the richer reality of medical practice. This is not to deny that insights gained about the scientific aspects of modern medicine are helpful. But these insights do not comprise the kind of general base needed. Modern medicine is criticized because it neglects the nonmeasurable factors brought to the clinical relationship by the patient, physician, and the institutional and cultural environment. The requirements of a philosophy of medicine must embrace these factors and their impact on both the theory and the practice of medicine.

We would liken the movement of our philosophical methodology toward practice to the important strain of empiricism manifested in American pragmatism and some forms of continental phenomenology. William James called for a reaction against Idealism by returning to what he called "the world of the street." In phenomenology, Husserl introduced the *Lebenswelt,* or lifeworld–a world of practical experience–as a condition of theory and ideas.[12] Even the most abstract thinking is related to the human lifeworld and is thereby limited.[13] One can find a glimmer of this interest in practice in Kant's preoccupation with the realm of practice.[14]

In both American pragmatism and European phenomenology, however differently they developed, the world of the street is pictured as the realm of human experience and problem solving. The lifeworld acts as a limiting factor on the realm of theory. In other words, theory must be derived from the lifeworld as its condition of possibility, its necessary basis, and must be capable of being applied back to the everyday realm of *praxis* to gain its acceptance.

It is also important to realize that the world of the street is both personal and social.[15] Disease and health, sickness and healing are all experienced in both a personal and a social context.

The lifeworld is personal because every experience has some kind of meaning for us. Each experience comes decorated with value. There are no neutral experiences.[16] We are involved as biological organisms in everyday life prior to any reflections we make on this experience. Thus we live and die with basic valuations about experience. Our views of health and disease are among these valuations, as are the thoughts we have about the doctor-patient relationship. Thus a philosophy which focuses on the implications of practical experience must deal with the meanings of everyday life as well as with more theoretical constructs. This effort will become apparent when we examine the concepts of health and disease and the a priori condition of medicine.

The lifeworld is also social. Our experiences take place in a community rooted in time.[17] Axioms of community responsibility, the responsibility of one human being to another, are among those developed in the social context. This is why James focused on the "fringes" of social existence, explaining that over these aspects of human life science has no control.

We have spent a few pages discussing the lifeworld concept because it illustrates the importance of practice in philosophical reflections on medicine. With respect to this practice, Natanson and Straus observe:

> It is within the everyday world that the individual first comes to recognize the signs of disease, and it is within the confines of his naive immediacy that he comes to grasp the meaning and status of what is deemed normal.[18]

The realm of practice triggers our perceptions about our own health. When our usual conditions of life are in the normal state of flux, growth, and decline, we consider ourselves healthy. But when they are interrupted, we begin to wonder. Something is wrong. What is taken for granted no longer is the case. In order to find the meaning of this interruption, we then seek expert help. Thus the lifeworld and the world of theoretical knowledge reflect an epistemological division of labor. Professionals and laymen are distinguished by their degree of involvement in either world: that of theory or that of everyday experience. Both are interrelated. One cannot presume that the ability to name a disorder experienced in the everyday world automatically means that one "knows" more about the disorder than the patient. The patient has a richer, more personal knowledge of the disorder because it is happening to him or her. The physician only has a more theoretical knowledge of the disorder due to training. The relationship between theory and practice means that the personal situation of the patient must be taken into account in any theoretical attempt to explain and dislodge the disease.

The importance of relating theory to practice in a philosophy of medicine cannot be overrated. In recent years Chester Burns and Alasdair MacIntyre have both analyzed the medical enterprise historically in search of norms and an ethics for modern medicine. Both have highlighted the relationship of the profession to canons and norms of the everyday world. With the dissolution of absolute norms, and in the face of the moral pluralism of our times, medicine is left normless. It is a sea with ancient life preservers, so to speak.[19] Theory is left behind by the changing lifeworld. As James says at the end of his *Varieties of Religious Experience,* "Assuredly the real world is of a different temperament–more intricately built than science allows."[20]

The challenge to a philosophy of medicine is to locate and ground its thinking in medical practice, in the everyday experience of medicine. Husserl's challenge is as important for a philosophy of medicine as it is for any other discipline:

> The concrete *Lebenswelt* must be brought into consideration for the final clarification, not only of science, but of all other human activities and their results.[21]

The idea of a lifeworld, or world of practical experience, is important for a philosophy of medicine because medicine is a practical discipline, a discipline of experience in which much theory is theory about practice. Medicine must make correct decisions on behalf of patients. In addition, medicine proceeds by analogical thinking. In medicine, a disease is identified through a syndrome of patterns analogous with each other. And as Buchanan observes, "you never get an abstraction out of this."[22] Theory in medicine is theory about the world of everyday reality, about fundamental human values played out in daily life. Thus, in medicine, reflective reasoning operates along with ordinary, unreflective knowledge. The former moves along with direct experience, connecting as much as possible through analogy. As Buchanan also observes, all the liberal arts are the arts of handling the symbols through which we think in analogous terms.[23] Medicine is no exception.

Methodological Description

The best starting point for medicine, we propose, is the possibility of a cure in the real world of practice. The choice is our attempt to separate what is important from a field of matters of fact. Other starting points have been used, however, and in fairness to their authors, we should mention them.

One could start with the language used in medicine, as Wittgenstein did for philosophy, and discover that language does not refer to objects but to other everyday languages.[24] One may begin with a scientific perception (Husserl used the concept of a mathematical circle) and argue that this concept depends upon prior real world experience in perfecting materials to which the concept refers.[25] One may begin with perception, as did Merleau-Ponty, and discover that the world is already interpreted by the body prior to any articulations and conceptual expressions.[26] Or one may begin with scientific canons of correctness, as did MacIntyre and Gorovitz, and be led to the discovery that medicine deals with a different class of individuals than science, individuals in the nonscientific world of everyday experience.[27] One may begin, as did Dewey, with the physiological organization of the body and derive therefrom the realm of experience.[28] The approaches are almost endless, as are the insights to be derived from them. Science, institutions, concepts, organizations, theories, laws, and philosophy itself all depend upon a logically prior world of experience.

Our understanding of what is important about medicine, and the methodology we adopt, leads us to characterize the philosophy of medicine as a philosophy of practice. We suggest that this philosophy can be described by the following statements:

1. A philosophy of practice is realistic rather than idealistic. The lifeworld is a realm of direct, immediate experience in which the body sorts out illusion from reality because of the immanent presence of objects. The test of ideas is best conducted against this realistic backdrop.

2. While mistakes about reality can be made in the lifeworld, they are less apt to occur than in the realm of theory. Rather than state that the lifeworld is subjective in this respect, it would be more accurate to assert that the "facts" of everyday experience are value-laden. In this way, the facts of the lifeworld, the matters of fact about which Whitehead wrote, are value factors. Thus practice as an origin and end of the philosophy of medicine requires attention to values.

3. An ontology of practice attends to the context or situations in which ideas come forth, including theories about health and disease. Because such an ontology entrusts to the lifeworld the task of correcting theoretical postulates, just as clinical medicine is ruled by the patient's problem, an ontology of practice places limits upon speculative philosophy. The more limited scientific realm of objects and correlates is grounded in the seemingly unlimited web of interrelationships which characterizes human life.

4. An ontology of practice is also pragmatic. As many pages will be devoted to practical applications of the philosophy as to its development. Man is considered to be *homo faber* and *homo symbolicum* logically prior to being *homo rationalis*. While all these functions occur simultaneously in the real world, we consider the practical world to be the logically prior setting in which and out of which ideas are born.

5. While practical ontology places importance on everyday reality, it is not limited to this world. If it were so limited, it would simply be an art of description, an art of capturing the concrete singular. But the search for understanding can be a search for patterns or lasting conditions as well as a search for appreciating the concrete. Having a grasp of the concrete, one may choose to revel in it (art). On the other hand, one may choose to discover the commonalities in the concrete common conditions shared by all mankind which make it possible for a concrete person to emerge.

Based on the point of view in this chapter, then, the philosophy we adopt has at least four important steps. The first step is *describing* what is important about matters of fact. This task helps us to choose a starting point for the philosophy of medicine.

The second step is *thinking at a critical distance* from the reality chosen as important or interesting. We will call this function *radical reflection*. The products of this activity are what are more important and from them what is most important about the set and the starting point. Thus if the starting point is the clinical milieu in which cure takes place, the process of radical reflection will capture the conditions under which this is possible. In simpler terms, the activity of curing will be defined.

The third step we shall call *critical reflection*. This function turns upon the most important feature of medicine and searches for its ground or condition of possibility in the real world of experience. This step will produce an ontology of the body.

The fourth step occupies virtually one-half of the book. We call it *practical reflection,* the attempt to apply the ontology of practice to ethical and policy issues in medicine.

In the remainder of the book, we will employ these four functions of philosophy. First, we will describe what we consider to be important about the clinical relationship constituting the discipline of medicine. We are acutely aware that other thinkers may find this choice less than optimum. For this reason, we develop a dialectic in Chapter Four to indicate the range of opinions about what is important to the medical enterprise and the reasonableness of our choice.

It is also worth noting that what is considered less important for a philosophy of medicine is also what is taken for granted. One should not assume, for example, that Descartes really thought the body and soul were completely distinct. Rather, he seemed to take this for granted. Instead he was interested in how any distinction might be drawn between body and soul. Therefore, what we regard as important should not be considered a rejection of things we take for granted.

To this point, we have used unwieldy terminology. For readability and clarity, we will shorten such phrases as "what is important" and "matters of fact." The products of *description* we shall call "modes" of the clinical relationship. Those features considered more important, the products of *radical reflection,* will be called "forms."[29] The feature we regard as distinguishing medicine from all other disciplines we shall call its "form."

The necessary conditions unearthed by *critical reflection* in Chapter Five we shall call "structures" of medicine. We do not intend to signify by any of these terms some immutable essences of which Idealists are fond. Instead, at the most, these modes and forms are present to a greater or lesser degree throughout the history of Western medicine. They may not exist in other practices of medicine which originate in a different set of cultural assumptions about health and disease.[30] In other words, modes are more likely to change from one era to the next than forms. And forms are more likely to change from one historical epoch to another than structures because the latter, by definition, are lifeworld conditions surrounding the possibility of cure.

Conclusion

The claim has been made that the choice of a philosophical method is not blind or capricious. It is circumscribed by problems highlighted in culture, by the nature of those problems, and by a disciplined focus separating important or interesting features from matters of fact.

The problems posed in this book reflect a concern for medicine. They therefore establish a criterion for choice of a suitable philosophical methodology. Since medicine is largely a discipline of practical experience, as we argue in the next chapter, and arises in an inter-human event we call the clinical interaction, the philosophy chosen must fall into a tradition of analysis characterized as an ontology of practice. Such a philosophy would be capable of describing and categorizing the realms of experience which lead to a cure. Cures and healing take place. They are experienced. How is that possible?

A glance at the more successful philosophical approaches to medicine in the past confirms this realistic stance. Aristotle's realism influenced thinking about medicine through the time of Harvey. Empiricism was clearly chosen over Idealism, with the exception of Descartes and nineteenth-century thought in continental Europe. Perhaps John Locke's view best illustrates this realistic tendency. Himself a physician, Locke created a design to acquire "a historical, plain method," a method of observation and description chiefly dealing with "particular matters of fact."[31] It is in this tradition that we turn next to a description of medicine.

3

What Is Medicine?

Few medical textbooks set out an understanding of what medicine is. Usually they proceed via a rapid overview of clinical judgment or the physician-patient relationship to the detailed description of specific disease entities. This failure to define medicine as a discipline leads to some rather loose construals of medicine: Medicine is what doctors do; medicine is a science practiced humanely;[1] or medicine is an art, embracing all human concerns.

In Chapter Nine we will move beyond a description of medicine as a discipline of craftsmanship by considering it as a profession. In so doing, we will subject this former description to critical analysis.

A definition of medicine is something more than an academic exercise. It is necessary for any critical reflection on the functions and purpose of the profession, the way we educate physicians, what we can expect from them, and how medicine is linked to other cultural manifestations of modern man. If we see medicine primarily as a science, we expect a degree of certitude and fewer mistakes than it can deliver. If we see it primarily as an art, we may accept less precision in exchange for more *Gemütlichkeit*. If we view medicine primarily as a craft, we may find some of its philosophical pretensions at least fatuous, and at worst totally irrelevant.

Clearly, the idea we hold of medicine strongly shapes every facet of the medical enterprise–the educational, the practical, the medico-legal, and the ethical, as well as the social and economic.

It also underlies clinical decisions, the attitudes of physicians, and the image they hold of themselves. The modern distaste for definitions notwithstanding, then, it becomes necessary as an early step in any philosophy of medicine to state what medicine is. For behind every medical behavior there is at least an implied conception of medicine which must be explicated and clarified if we are to speak logically of that behavior.

It is our thesis that medicine is neither solely an art nor solely a science in the modern sense of those terms. Instead we argue that medicine is a distinct intermediate discipline, a *tertium quid,* between art and science but distinct from both of them. In the Aristotelian sense, it is a habit of practical understanding refined and perfected by experience in dealing with patients.

The distinguishing features of medicine are to be found in its modes and form, the essence of which resides in the clinical event. The special character of the relationship between physician and patient, the goals of that relationship, and the ways in which they are affected in the moment of clinical decision set medicine apart from all other related activities, particularly the other helping professions.

The chapter is divided according to the steps indicated in Chapter Two: first, an initial description of medicine; second, a catalog of important features of clinical interaction (modes); third, attention to more important features (forms); fourth, an articulation of the distinguishing feature of medicine (its form). The chapter closes by briefly examining concepts of health and disease and their relationship to psychiatry and religion.

Is Medicine a Unitary Discipline?

This section has a twofold purpose: to offer an initial description of medicine and to establish medicine as a unified discipline.

Description of Medicine

Medicine, unlike philosophy, is capable of a larger measure of descriptive agreement. Almost all observers cite the unique combination of science and art, of theory and practice.

Moreover, a long line of thinkers–some of whom were both

philosophers and physicians, others of whom were trained at medical centers or had relatives who were physicians–have addressed the problem of describing medicine in more detail. This history of philosophy about medicine would include such thinkers as Empedocles, the authors of the Hippocratic corpus, Socrates, Plato, Aristotle, Galen, Avicenna, Maimonides, St. Albert the Great, Hume, Harvey, Bernard, William Osler, E. B. Straus, Scott Buchanan, and a host of others. The next chapter contains a sketch of historical thinking about medicine with a focus on applying theory to practice. At this point, we will extract only a few important points.

The Hippocratic corpus focuses on treatment and prognosis, with somewhat less attention to diagnostic skills.[2] The latter are viewed as derived from, and shaped by, the former. There are two reasons for this focus of Greek medicine as the art of healing. First, Greek medicine, like Greek moral philosophy, was permeated by a notion of well-being. The goal of all disciplines, including medicine, was to establish well-being (*eukrasia*) or happiness (*sophrosynē*). Second, happiness was conceived of as a balance or harmony with nature and self. Physicians were therefore wary of exceeding their task through too extensive intervention, which would have made them guilty of hubris.[3] Man owes his art to an imitation of nature. In healing, he should also work in congruence with the *vis medicatrix naturae,* the healing power of nature. Hence, Democritus can say that by using the principle of harmony or balance, we may attain calm of body–health–and calm of soul–happiness.[4]

Because of the well-developed nature of Greek medicine, Socrates, Plato, and then Aristotle (whose father was a physician) often cite it as an example of an art.[5] One of the first dialogues of Plato, the *Charmides,* presents Socrates arguing about cures, medicine, and temperance.[6] Aristotle cites medicine in the *Poetics,* as exemplifying an analogue of *Catharsis* in poetic argument. Earlier, a Sophist, Gorgias, compared the effects of tragedy to those of purgatives used in medicine.[7] Clearly medicine was seen as an art, and healing as analogous to some of the effects of tragedy.

By the Middle Ages sufficient scientific knowledge was assembled for medicine to be regarded as a practical science or a mechanical art, similar to agriculture.[8] In fact, Avicenna had written a treatise which examined in remarkably clear fashion the division between theory and practice in medicine itself.[9] However, before the rise of modern science and the fascination with positivism, it was sufficient to describe a physician as *vir bonus mendendi peritus,* an expert at good healing.[10]

Given the enormously more complex nature of contemporary medicine, we regard as insufficient the recent attempts to describe medicine as either an art of healing or a science of individuals.[11] While medicine cannot be reduced to physics, chemistry, or biology, it can in part be derived from these sciences. On the other hand, while medicine does not resemble the fine arts in its products, it does share with the arts the characteristic of productive reasoning toward practical ends. For this reason, we regard medicine as the most scientific of the humanities and the most humane of the sciences.[12] It is neither a pure science nor a fine art. Further refinement of this opinion will be necessary.

If one accepts the notion of a profession as a construction, occupation, or discipline which applies the art of handling symbols through which we think, then medicine is a profession.[13] Like all professions, medicine shares in the dual requirements of sufficient skill and commitment to human purpose. The skill required in medicine embodies sufficient theoretical knowledge of the sciences, a creative power of handling symbols, such as concepts of disease, and experience in applying both to individuals. Commitment is a form of altruism essential to medicine if the physician is to place the patient's interest above his own. Later, we will comment in more detail on the special implications of the notion of profession.[14]

Because medicine is a profession which applies skill to curative intent, it is not like a theoretical science, which aims at understanding what is the case. Because medicine demands sufficient biological knowledge for diagnosis and therapy, and furthermore is aimed at restoring a patient to the state of health, it is not like the fine arts, which create new works. We conclude that medicine is therefore a derived discipline, a third class of human enterprises that combines theory and practice in a unique way. Others in the class might be law and education.

Medicine as a Discipline

A philosophy of medicine presumes that medicine is an integral discipline—that is, that statements made about the uniqueness of medicine apply generally to all its branches. If one examines the concept of medicine carefully, one sees that medicine is an analogical profession, one shared by health professionals in various degrees. One way to understand this notion is to classify the participation of health professionals in the discipline of medicine by their proximity to actual touching of the patient or classes of patients.[15]

The question posed by this analogical sharing of medicine on the part of surgery, family practice, internal medicine, nursing, pharmacy, dentistry, medical record librarians, and so on is this: Is there some feature of the discipline that is shared proportionately by all these professions? Can each of the specialties of medicine lay claim to a participation in some identifiable medical enterprise? Is there a distinctive "medical event" common to the branches of medicine? We suggest that the clinical event is the key which unlocks this common feature and sheds light on why medicine is neither art nor science.

At first, the distinctive event constituting medicine as a discipline seems to be restoration of well-being. The argument would run as follows. It is sufficient to describe medicine by citing its goal. The goal is a restoration of well-being, a medical event. The argument is strengthened by indicating how, when medicine fails to produce a cure, it falls back on secondary means to obtain a restoration—either management of a patient's illness or, failing that, at least a reduction of suffering. Each branch of medicine has a role to play in this goal.

However fine this argument appears at first, it confuses the goal of medicine with the discipline. Furthermore, it fails properly to distinguish medicine from religion, psychiatry, psychology, some political actions, and a number of other human enterprises. In fact, all human beings have in some sense the task of healing. In this task is included healing in the broader sense: healing rifts in the community, healing relationships, and so on.

Nor will it do to refine the medical event only to a "cure." Not only would this do an injustice to "caring" and the other forms of clinical management found in medicine, it would also neglect the fact that nature heals itself. Not all cures are specifically medical. Some can be legitimately ascribed to nature, religion, psychiatry, counseling, and the general level of nutrition and health awareness in a population.

Consequently it is not sufficient to describe the medical event, the constitutive activity of medicine in terms of its goal of restoration of well-being. Some other feature is necessary.

A second argument contains more specificity. It runs as follows. Minimally speaking, medicine aims at a restoration which can only be asymptotic to former well-being. Because "well-being" is a cultural and even an individual perception, the medical event is constituted perforce by a customized form of individualized knowledge which includes conceptual tools drawn from a culture. In this view, what distinguishes medicine from other enterprises is its restorative aim, individualized clinical intuitions, and a language about well-being formed from past and present cultural life.[16]

While this description is sufficient to distinguish medicine from physics, it is not wholly satisfactory to separate medicine from counseling, religious advice, or even psychology, all of which have restorative aims, involve individualized knowledge and "clinical" intuitions, and use language formed from culture.

Our suggestion is that a specifically *medical* event is formed by clinical interaction. The rest of the chapter is devoted to clarifying this notion. First, however, a brief digression is required to show how clinical interaction is important to the debate about the scientific and artistic nature of medicine.

Clinical Interaction

Those who attempt to describe medicine as a science must modify their notion to include clinical interaction. The *idée directrice,* guiding idea, as Bernard called it,[17] of medicine is some adequate scientific interpretation of living reality with restorative intent. Thus the principal conceptions of medicine, health, and disease are necessarily related to, and acquire their meaning from, the epistemological features of clinical interaction. Both health and disease are essential conceptions of medicine as a discipline.[18] To the objection that health and disease are definientia only of organ systems, one must counter with the large body of evidence that both concepts are evaluative; that is, they include in their meaning the values of patients, societies, and cultures.[19]

If, indeed, clinical interaction is the modality that constitutes a specifically medical event, then medicine as a discipline falls into the philosophical category of an identifiable relationship.[20] By way of summary and amplification, this section concludes with the following arguments that clinical interaction is the source of the integrity of medicine as a discipline.

The skills and commitment of medicine are aimed at restoration of human beings; the concepts of health and disease are both biological and evaluational. Hence medicine cannot be understood without attention to the clinical relationship. Furthermore, the moral force of medicine derives from and is applied to the necessity for patient care. Thus Otto Gutentag can decry the rise of technology by warning that it "loses sight of an axiomatic foundation of medicine: man cannot be understood only in mechanical terms."[21]

In addition, the moral nature of the medical enterprise does not stem from following rules and guidelines for behavior alone. Instead the moral nature stems from the fact that patient and physician mutually enter into a healing relationship.[22] The healing relationship is the source of the division of labor from which physicians and patients derive rights, duties, privileges, and other forms of approval by society. Practitioners of pure science do not have these obligations and rights.

Finally, the internal organization of medicine–its specialties, levels of care, distinguishing concepts, and the connections between theory and practice all depend upon clinical interaction as a point of reference.

The conclusion of these arguments is that clinical interaction is the material a priori of medicine as a discipline. Such an observation means that, as Aristotle noted, medicine and rhetoric are closely parallel. Both are persuasive tools. Plato also notes this in the *Phaedrus*. Hence our science will be beautiful when its form and content are properly adjusted to the particular nature and situation of the patient.[23] The clinical interaction, then, is persuasive like rhetoric, individualized, and finally a relationship of friendship, as once again Plato explores in the *Lysis:* "The sick man is a friend to the physician" for the sake of a good.[24]

We therefore conclude that clinical interaction establishes medicine as a unitary discipline–one in which the whole is greater than any of its parts.[25] Its proper motive is compassion or friendship, its purpose is an individualized satisfactory state of well-being, and its structure falls into the category of a relationship.

Modes of Medicine

We have tried to show that medicine is a specific kind of relationship. It is now necessary to describe important features of this relationship, bearing in mind the distinction made earlier between importance and matters of fact. The selection of what is important (modes) should not be misconstrued as a comprehensive catalog of all features of medicine. Indeed, as we focus more and more on the clinical relationship, the more specialized and remote subheadings of medicine seem to slip into the background. However, what we predicate of the clinical interaction should remain analogically true of the branches and specialties of medicine not attended to in the following process.

The modes to be discussed are: responsibility, trust, decision orientation, and etiology.

Responsibility

The clinical interaction is the locus of mutual responsibility of a patient and a physician. In the clinical interaction there must be an interpenetration of minds as well as physical contact, because, as Kant showed, the human mind deals with experience in concepts. Both physician and patient "teach" one another in dialogue. However, in the clinical interaction there is an imbalance of scientific knowledge which places the heavier burden of responsibility on the physician.[26]

Clinical interaction, therefore, participates in the social and epistemological division of labor necessary for any civilized society. No one person can survive without dependence on the expertise of another. The responsibilities inherent in an imbalanced relationship flow, therefore, from an ethic of survival in a complex and specialized society. The need for professional skills of knowledge and experience reflects the broader cultural links of the individual to society, individual mores and social rules, desires and stimulations, and knowledge and beliefs.

While the physician is responsible for a skill in an imbalanced relationship, the patient also has responsibilities arising out of the commitment of the physician. Seneca summed up the source of this patient responsibility as follows:

> Why then, are we so much indebted to these men [physicians and teachers]? Not because what they have sold us is worth more than what we paid for it, but because they have contributed something to us personally. . . . Such a man has placed me under an obligation, not so much as a physician, but as a friend.[27]

Mutual responsibility is an essential mode of the clinical relationship because it involves a deeper human and moral obligation than adherence to rules, guidelines, or codes. Instead, it reflects one of the more profound survival necessities of civilization. The need for skill and commitment, guideposts of the medical profession, stems from the imbalanced relationship. Such a relationship also requires trust.

Trust

Trust is a mode of clinical interaction because it cements imbalanced relationships in society.[28] Trust is also necessary because of the curative intent of the physician. This intent is sociological, personal, and objective. The physician's motive is to help the patient become socially useful,[29] personally cured,[30] and objectively free of morbid abnormality.[31] Each of these motives involves the physician in objective givens and subjective interpretations. And each immerses both patient and physician in a mutual bond forged by terror, fear, anxiety, resignation, and patience. In short, both are locked in a human relationship the acuteness of which is rarely encountered in day-to-day life. So much is this the case that trust is reserved in our language to denote the vulnerability of that condition of inequality inherent in being ill. Hence von Lyden used to say to his students that "the first phase of treatment is the act of extending a helping hand to the patient."[32] Medicine is therefore assistance and explanation, skill and commitment, all based on an ethic of trust which, in turn, is based on the ontological and sociological reality of an imbalanced relationship.

Decision Orientation

The tension between medicine as assistance and medicine as explanation is bridged by an experiential judgment. In other words, theory in medicine is always related to the pressure to decide, which is another important mode of clinical interaction. This mode is frequently missed by observers who undertake a critical understanding of medical judgments without experience in the clinical setting. Medicine is decision oriented. Two points need to be made.

The first is that the helping hand extended to the patient is attached to a person committed to his or her well-being. Hence some decision must be made eventually, usually as soon as possible. The problematic aspect of the decision is that it interprets living reality that cannot be easily captured in concepts. That is why musical analogies are often very useful for comparison with medicine. Both are involved in temporal interpretation, and time is a primary category of illness, rather than space. While disease location in the body is important, it cannot compare to the importance of living the natural history of the disease in time.

The second point is that experiential judgment is a kind of empirical-inductive reasoning dominated by the unique style of the physician and the values of the patient. The process is never exactly the same in two patients with the same diagnosis.

Clinical judgment is not precisely inductive, because it is not mere fact hunting. As Medewar observes, following Karl Popper, "unprejudiced observation is a myth."[33] Instead clinical judgment is an imaginative preconception of what the truth might be. Experiential judgment explores the uniqueness of individual patients by circularly setting up hypotheses corrected by negative feedback. Rhetoric, dialectic, and other forms of argumentation are involved in arriving at the right action, as we shall show in Chapter Six.

Etiology

Finally, clinical interaction as a relationship has a multi-etiological mode; that is, as a human enterprise it is analyzable in terms of a number of causes that bear upon it. This bundle of causes is the source of the complexity of clinical interaction and the probable reason why physicians are hesitant to spell out the logic of clinical decision making. We devote a separate chapter to this problem (Chapter Six). At this point, it is sufficient to note a number of the causal factors involved in the clinical interaction.

The curative intention of the patient and the physician governs the clinical interaction as its goal. This curative intention is an end-in-view. It is immediate enough in most cases so that it can function as the objective of the physician-patient relationship. In this way, its acts as a definer of the relationship and a source of judgment about whether or not a good medical decision has been made.

The curative intention as end-in-view is also related to the motive of the relationship. But motives are so varied among patients and physicians that not all can be classed under the curative intent. Some motives on the part of the patient, for example, could include a checkup, fear, cultural attitudes toward a disability, seeking information or even confirmation of suspicious changes in the body, an irritation or disruption of life-style, and so forth. Insofar as the motive is seeking assistance or help, the clinical interaction can become one of curative intent. B. M. Randolph compared this tendency to seek medical assistance to the emotional element in religion. Both are based, in his view, on "a deep-lying instinct in human nature that relief from suffering is an obtainable goal."[34]

The clinical interaction is also influenced by the nature of the complaint, independent of the motive which created the interaction. The history of the patient, the symbolized recounting of that history, the quality of the questions asked by the physician, the level of care demanded by the complaint, and the diagnosed disease are all material factors which distinguish one type of clinical interaction from another. In addition, the number of specialties called on to provide a solution to the problem, and their corresponding division of labor, qualify the kind or mode of clinical interaction and can influence its outcome.

A fourth causal factor in clinical interactions is the distinguishing feature. This feature–that which constitutes the interaction as specifically medical, rather than legal, or educational, or even religious–depends upon the primacy of the body, as we shall argue shortly. Before taking up this question in the next step of our argument, we must note that what is primary in the medical relationship is not reconciliation (which is proper to a religious setting), or coping with emotional disturbance (which would be proper to a psychological counseling interaction), but well-being. In Aristotle and Plato, well-being is *sophrosynē,* happiness, which describes a successful medical event as well as a successful moral life. For this reason, the medical event must be related to morality, a theme we will develop in Chapter Eight.

Conclusion

These four modes–responsibility, trust, decision orientation, and etiology–are the essential ingredients of a medical event. All are tied together and represent categories of importance to the clinical relationship.

Using these four modes, it is possible to describe medicine more specifically than we did earlier in the chapter. Medicine is the cognitive art of applying science and persuasion through a complex human interaction in which a mutually satisfactory state of well-being is sought, and in which the uniqueness of values and disease, and the kind of institution in which care is delivered, determine the nature of the judgments made.

Two personal intentions at least are needed to form a clinical interaction, both with a curative intent, one to seek help and the other to extend it. The link between intentions is the special character of the event. Since it is cognitive (diagnosis), predictive (prognosis), operative (therapeutic), affective (friendship or trust), and cultural (beliefs about man, nature, and society), the clinical interaction establishes medicine as a *tekné iatrikê,* a technique of healing. *Tekné* here means a knowledge of how to act according to what is the case and why it is the case.[35]

The Forms of Medicine

> To know these things well, one must know them in detail, and as this is infinite, our knowledge is necessarily superficial.
>
> *La Rouchefoucauld*

Before proceeding to even greater specificity about what medicine is, it is important to pause and reflect on the weakness and strength of definitions. While definitions have come into disrepute in philosophy, they can still play a legitimate role in the establishment of disciplines. Definitions cannot capture the rich variety of reality, and consequently are less preferred today than analysis of language and categories of description (phenomenology). However, definitions are useful to establish differences between things. In the case of a philosophy of medicine, it is important to establish the set with which it enters into dialogue, before proceeding to analyze the details of the discipline. We are aware of the shortcomings of any definition of medicine, since it perforce leaves out so many characteristics. We hold that it is nevertheless useful to sort out certain central features of this highly complicated discipline.

With this background, we can state the thesis of this section: that the mode which predominates in the medical relationship is clinical judgment; the latter category constitutes a set of more specific forms which serve to set off medicine from other disciplines.

The following are forms, important features of clinical judgment:

1. Judgments combine, in words and ideas, real objects perceived as separate under new hypotheses about how these objects are related. In addition, judgments may relate a body of scientific knowledge to an individual patient or classes of patients. Clinical judgment establishes such linkages, which are necessary to medicine. We call this *individualized knowledge.*

2. Clinical judgment is a discovery of an unforeseen relationship. Claude Bernard declared that a discovery is an unforeseen relationship not confirmed in theory; otherwise it would have been foreseen. The concept of tragic catharsis developed by Aristotle is helpful for understanding the nature of medical discovery. This form is *diagnosis.*

3. Clinical judgment is anticipatory, based on the organization of the body, the environment, past clinical experience, values of the patient, and scientific knowledge. This form is *prognosis.* We have already cited the importance of prognosis for Greek medicine. It is equally important for contemporary medicine, but for different cultural reasons. In the main, prognosis determines the extent of intervention either on the basis of knowledge about disease or patient

needs, or both. In this regard, Gracian declared: "Hope is the great falsifier of truth; let skill guard against this by ensuring that fruition exceeds desire."[36]

4. Clinical judgment is governed by therapeutic necessity. This form is *therapeusis.* Of the three forms, diagnosis, prognosis, and therapeusis, the last is the most important. But why?

First of all, this form comes closest to the motives and curative intent of clinical interaction. What to do for the patient, as shall be seen in Chapter Six, is the epistemological guide for all aspects of the medical event.

Second, help to become well could surely be named as one of the three basic needs of man (the others are moral and economic well-being). Deeply value-immersed, therapeutic necessity also establishes an imbalanced relationship, the source of the modes: responsibility, trust, and decision orientation. In short, therapeusis is the medical form of the four medical modes.

Third, it is a judgment formed both personally, in Polanyi's sense of the term; rationally, in a discursive, scientific sense; and intuitively, in an artistic sense.

It is therefore a notional inductive judgment, the *idée directrice* of Bernard.

The Form of Medicine

What, then, is the distinguishing feature of medicine? A definition of medicine requires a discovery of its form: features which distinguish it from other human activities. Philosophizing on the form of medicine can lead to insights about it as a discipline and the characteristics of man it presupposes (the structures of medicine). We might establish the form of medicine with the following line of argument:

1. Medicine is a person-person, as distinct from a person-thing relation. But many other enterprises are inter-human events, from board meetings to sports.

2. Medicine is an inter-human event of mutual consent. It is a meeting of at least two personal intentions, one seeking help and the other offering it. These intentions create a medical event by effecting a *tekné iatrikê,* a craftsmanship of healing. Although it is

more specific, this statement cannot serve to distinguish medicine from the other helping professions.

3. Medicine is a kind of craftsmanship of healing placed within an imbalanced relationship. The therapeutic intent of the clinical interaction tends to place the patient in a passive role *vis-à-vis* the physician. The latter is expected to acquire and maintain a superior fund of knowledge and skill. Even the diagnostic ability of patients which brought them to the relationship is superseded by a more scientific attempt to categorize the complaint and search for causes. In addition, the imbalance of the relationship can also be analogically noted in the role of medical institutions in education, where a virtual monopoly of decision making on the part of medical education takes place to the exclusion of the interests of society.

If we were to follow the notion of Plato that the clinical interaction is a form of friendship (*philia*), the imbalance described above could be overcome only in an ontological realization by both physician and patient of their mutual share in the human condition. Once again, however, this point of view can be applied to other helping professions, especially law, education, religious counseling, and the like.

4. Medicine is a didactic relationship distinct from law and education by the mutual interpretation of the life of the patient acting to eliminate physical suffering. However, religion and psychiatry also act sometimes in this way.

5. The goal or *telos* of medicine includes motives and ends. The motive for seeking help minimally involves a sign or symptom in the lived body with which one cannot cope; an interruption in the ability to function as a "lived self" (which includes one's historical identity and values); a deviation from one's concept of well-being, a value-laden concept including social function, identity, and interpersonal relationship; or fear in which one seeks confirmation of pathogenesis.

The end minimally involves a personal and organic restoration to a former or better state of perceived health or well-being. Information valued for preventive action against community disease is also sought.

This last statement does distinguish medicine from other helping professions. The key words are "physical" and "organic." Perceptions of illness, the forms of judgment, and the motives and ends of medicine all depend upon working *with and through the body for corporeal ends.* Through touching the body, the physician touches the personal life of the patient. But the curative intent is also corporeal, not spiritual or mental.

The distinguishing feature of medicine, therefore, is that it is a *craftsmanship that involves healing the body with the body.* It is easy for us to forget that Western medicine followed Plato's advice in the *Phaedrus* that medicine cure the body and rhetoric (philosophy) cure the soul.

Health: Body and Soul

As the foregoing discussion makes clear, concepts of health and disease are essential to the form of medicine. Normally any treatise on medicine would highlight these important epistemological tools. We have chosen to wait until this point to raise the issue of health and disease because usually such discussions are rather unclear and confused. The confusion is caused, in turn, by a lack of clarity about the nature of medicine–in particular, its link to psychiatry and religion. This section is designed to remove some of the sources of confusion about health and disease.

The Lived Body and the Lived Self

A philosophical distinction exists between a living body, a lived body, and a lived self. The distinction has been created largely by phenomenology and existentialism in their attempts to bridge the Cartesian duality of body and soul. A lived self is an historical projection of a lived body and describes the activity of symbolic interpretation of one's life by which one ascribes continuity to a set of interpretations about the world.[37] Knowledge gained through this activity is apodictic in that it describes the experience of experiencing, though the content of interpretations may be wrong.

The lived body is that experience of our body which cannot be objectified. Gabriel Marcel developed this notion as a central feature of his philosophy. He says:

> I *am* my body in so far as I succeed in recognizing that this body of mine *cannot,* in the last analysis, be brought down to the level of being this object, *an* object, a something or other.[38]

In this second activity, the lived body becomes a condition of community. Why? Because others are incorporated into the changing relations of the lived body while simultaneously sharing common lifeworld language, values, and situation. Hence the lived body has a role in distinguishing illusion from reality prior to more refined scientific symbolization. In this view, death would represent a break in the shared objectivity of the world.[39]

Finally, a living body describes the activity of the whole organism as the body interprets the world prior to articulations by the lived body. Merleau-Ponty called this realm of perception the "body-subject-in-the-world," arguing that it is an a priori condition of the *lifeworld,* the latter already distinguishing objects from the lived body. In other words, the living body organizes a field of perception on a preconscious level prior to articulations of experience.

In the sections to follow, the philosophical concepts of lived self, lived body, and living body will be used to help clarify the notions of health and disease with a view toward amplifying the discussion of the form, or distinguishing feature, of medicine. A test of the validity of these analytic tools is not intended at this point in the discussion. However, their usefulness will be underscored in the chapter to follow.

Health and Disease

These two concepts are building blocks of medical logic, but this logic is not exclusively scientific. In fact, as Rothschuh indicates, disease is a relational structure between sickness, the sick person, the physician, and society. The ill person enters three relations–one to the self, another to the physician, and still another to society and environment–all of which are governed by the need for help. The physician also enters three relations–one of responsibility to the sick person, another to the disease (what is the case? what to do?), and another to society. Society is also involved with individual good for the patient, the common good, and a relationship of aid, prevention, and research on the causes and effects of disease. Rothschuh therefore defines disease as the presence of a subjective, clinical, or social need for help in persons whose physical, psychic, or psychophysical balance of boundaries in the organism is disrupted.[40]

Health, or well-being, on the other hand, is characterized by the presence of order and balance in the organism and no perceived or actual need for help. This analysis recognizes the primary referent of health and disease as conditions of the body.[41] It is in this perspective that Thomas' conception of health and disease, derived from years of labor in infectious disease and genetics, focuses on the reactions of a living body to invasion. In Thomas' view, health is a kind of boundary established by a living body. Many diseases are pathologically caused by overreactions of the body to specific agents, e.g., rheumatic fever.[42]

However, social perceptions, and perceptions of the lived body and lived selves, also enter into the notions of health and disease. The tension between organic function and social perception within the concepts of health and disease correct overly broad goals for medicine.[43] A disease in the body does not mean that valuational aspects of disease are eliminated. It is in understanding this tension between organic function and social perception that the distinctions borrowed from phenomenology are of help.

First, the living body in the realm of brute, prereflected experience must experience pain and suffering. Some disruption in the organism must be present to establish a preconditional substrate for disease. It is important to note, however, that some diseases are not accompanied immediately by disruption. On the other hand, pain is often not a sufficient motive to seek help.

The second level of the lived body is an experience of experience. E. Straus says:

> To sense pain means to sense oneself at the same time, to find oneself changed in relation to the world, or more exactly, changed in one's somatic communication with the world.[44]

In other words, the lived body forms dis-ease, an experience of disruption. This experience is distinct from scientifically explained disease. Dis-ease is not yet a scientific symptom, but a sign created by the lived body. A sign is not an object, in this sense, but a displacement of meaning between itself and other signs. Dis-ease is a symbol of dis-function or an inability to cope with the everyday.[45] In this realm of the lived body, dis-ease is an interpretation of disruption, an interruption in the ability to cope. Dis-ease is not a symptom but a sign of dysfunction. As such, it is heavily value-laden. Insofar as the subject perceives a need for help based on dysfunction, a clinical relationship is established; a condition of possibility for concepts of health and disease is formed. Both are necessarily related to the medical acts of diagnosis and therapy.

The scientific concepts of health and disease have their origin in the lifeworld, as Wartofsky has argued. Hence these concepts always lead to action for the lived body. Concepts of disease are also therefore intrinsically and extrinsically evaluative. That is, they depend on organic dysfunction, a perceived need for help, and physician intervention.[46] Therefore health and disease are explanatory scientific theories used to describe both organic dysfunction and lifeworld disruption. The goal of medicine is primarily the relief of perceived lived body disruption, not scientific explanation. Cure of the organic dysfunction is a necessary but not a sufficient step toward this goal. Obviously explanation and organic restoration are important, but they are not always possible.

Abstracting from the everyday to the realm of the lived self, both patient and physician are capable of a conceptual or symbolic understanding of health and disease. Here the organic dysfunction and perceived disruption becomes a symptom. With further distancing, disruption takes place, such that patient and physician then refer to the symptom or the disease as an object, an "it."[47]

Yet even this objectification cannot hide the fact that disease is a conceptualization of a disorganization of a patient's whole world, with implications for the patient's self-image and posture as a person.[48] It is for this reason that medicine entertains multiple etiologies for disease, which include psychic, somatic, constitutional and genetic, and social and environmental causes. For the same reason, medicine can also entertain multiple conceptions of well-being, ranging from the homeostatic and metaphysical clinical entities to natural models of disease, the latter ranging, in turn, from ontological to functional.

With the distinctions drawn from phenomenology about health and disease, we are able to further support the contention that medicine is distinct as a discipline because it works in and through the body. An analysis of religion and psychiatry follow as illustrations of the distinction.

Medicine and Religion

Both sin and illness are treated conceptually as a diathesis of personal unity. Presumably the body would be affected by either. Thus St. Clement of Alexandria and St. Gregory of Nyssa, basing their thinking on Plato, argue that the director of souls also cures the passions of the body. Such a director of souls is engaged in a moral *pathematologia,* the science of healing disruption. On the other hand, illness can cause a pathos of a personal nature and affect the spiritual life.[49] Because of the personal conditions of man's psychophysical reality, Bernard warned that "the physician must not forget in his practice the influence of the moral upon the physical."[50]

The close conjunction of the values of health and virtue can cause confusion, as Kass noted, in the nature of medicine. Does medicine aim at moral virtue? The wide scope of clinical anamnesis requires that the patient explain to the physician how he interprets his life; the physician subjects to interpretation all that is seen and heard. Such mutual interpretation touches very closely on the moral order.

These similarities notwithstanding, medicine and religion are truly distinct. Medicine deals with dis-ease through symptoms and organic causes, but religion does not deal primarily with expressions of bodily disorder. Instead, religion views the body and the lived self as expressions of the invisible (the sacral nature of the body).[51] For religion, dis-ease is not detected through the organism per se, but rather through lived body disruptions. The *telos* of religious interactions is not obtained by intervention with and through the body, in consort with nature. Instead religion works on the lived self through the body by action-at-a-distance, utilizing a therapy of the word.[52]

In other words, medicine acts with and through the body to obtain a restoration, while religion seeks to establish reconciliation or unity by appeal to that which is beyond man's control. Religion, psychiatry, and medicine are all realms of mediatorship. But psychiatry and medicine are distinct from religion because the former mediate between man and what is presently or potentially in his control. The conjunction of the three human enterprises lies in the way the body interprets the world. But medicine and psychiatry do not presume an invisible partner in this interpretation, as does religion.

Because man is a psychophysical unity, it is easy to confuse the link between religion and medicine. But the distinction we have made between medicine and religion is clear enough to assert that medical judgment is indeed distinct from ethical or moral judgment.

Medicine and Psychiatry

Recent developments in neuroscience have prompted some psychiatrists to argue that their discipline ought to be abandoned. Those disorders due to organic brain dysfunction, they suggest, ought properly to be turned over to neurosurgery and neurology. All other aspects of coping with life ought to be turned over to counselors and tutors. Although the suggestion is radical, it does highlight an important problem about psychiatry.

Although psychiatry is usually considered a branch of medicine, it shares with religion a primary focus on the lived self, the symbolic integration as a person. As we pointed out in the foregoing section, medicine focuses primarily on perceived needs of the lived body, rather than on the lived self. Thus psychiatry shares with religion the methodology of verbal therapy. Psychiatry is primarily a persuasive art whose therapy consists of understanding, interpretation, and coping. Unlike religion, it does not seek to remove guilt and anxiety; rather, it helps patients to cope. Insofar as psychiatry discovers organic causes of dis-ease, it is medicine.[53]

Another way of looking at psychiatric attention to the lived self as distinct from medicine is to consider the curative intent of psychiatry. While medicine attends to the living body and the lived body, psychiatry aims at constructing a biography with the patient. The psychiatrist helps the patient form a personal identity from which he can construct a possible future. A normal person has a sense of a possible future through experience as a past lived self. Mental illness is primarily a symbolic disorder, not an organic one. Thus Straus argues that the function of analysis is to "help the patient realize his conative and creative possibilities," so that he may discover his own personal myth.[54]

The concept of biography is essential to the distinction between medicine and psychiatry. For psychiatry, the nature of the dis-ease is an interruption of the lived self. The subject finds an inability to cope *precisely* because he lacks a sense of being a lived self, a sense of personal symbolic identity and history. In medicine, on the other hand, the patient seeks help *primarily* because organic pain or suffering interrupts a lived body. The lived self is in reasonably good order and can judge that the lived body has not always been this way. A dis-ease in the lived self is a psychiatric symptom, often without pain in the living body or perceived need in the lived body, because the patient no longer has an intact lived self.

Having noted the way in which psychiatry is distinct from medicine, we should also note the ways in which it is, in fact, a branch of medicine. Although sometimes materially distinct, it shares with medicine the same healing intent and formal methods of working toward that healing in and through the body. Historically part of medicine, and still such through training, psychiatry remains wedded to the body precisely because the body and one's self-image created by corporeal possibilities are intrinsically linked. Despite advances in medicine occasioned by Descartes' rupture of body and soul, psychiatry is that branch of medicine which continually reinforces, indeed presumes, the link between body and mind. Evidence that psychoses have an organic base, the control of manic-depresssives with drugs, and the countless other patterns of mind-body interaction detailed by psychiatry contribute to our understanding of the complex bridge between the body's possibilities, a person's character, the mind, and the environment. In order to reconstruct the lived self, psychiatry, as a branch of medicine, must focus on the body as an object as well.

Medicine as Craftsmanship

We can now conclude justifiably that medicine is a craftsmanship of healing. It is not wholly an art because the body through which and with which it works is the artistic product. The body is also the artist of its own healing. Medicine is not wholly a science because its explanatory function always has a practical healing intent. Its scientific symbols are always related to action for the living and lived body.

Skill or craftsmanship (*tekné*) means that the physician must have experience of the living organism, its pain, suffering, and human condition. Compassion means a shared bodily structure. He must also have skill in relating notional empirical explorations with the values of patients (the lived body), as well as skill in connecting symptoms to the causes and effects of disease.

Unlike science, a craftsmanship of healing must link all functions to an individual. Thus public health measures more closely resemble an applied science than clinical medicine because they apply knowledge to classes of individuals, while the clinical interaction is guided by a *telos* of individuation.

A simplified definition of medicine would therefore be: *a relation of mutual consent to effect individualized well-being by working in, with, and through the body.*

Where,

1. "Relation" is a medical event in which rationalized individuation takes place. "Rationalized individuation" entails the discovery of a necessary analogous relationship between scientific pathogenesis and the individual patient.

2. "Medical event" is the *praxis* of two or more personal intentions, one asking for and the other receiving help through a craftsmanship of healing.

3. "Craftsmanship of healing" consists of an interpretive judgment relating science and experience to specific individuals, mutually motivated by human concern in which an ontology of man is presupposed.

4. The interpretive judgment linking knowledge and care establishes the moral realm of medicine because it interprets and establishes values. Some of these may or may not be ethical.

Since medicine is a relationship, and its concepts of health and disease are established in a clinical setting, is it possible to describe what form the discipline takes in the physician? Such a description would still include an orientation to patients precisely because it would describe a term of a relation: *Medicine as a disciplined body of knowledge is a science respecting the perfection of lived bodies concretized by skill in experiencing and effecting connections between corporeal symptoms and remedies.*

Having established the form of medicine as working with, in, and through the body, we are now able to turn our attention to the structures of medicine, the a priori conditions of human existence that make medicine possible.

4

Critique of Medicine

In the previous chapter we argued that medicine is a unique form of relationship, obtaining its desired effects by working in, with, and through the body. This characterization of medicine as its form is not unique. Fritz Hartman's penetrating discussion of the philosophizing physician, and the need and role of philosophy in medical practice, directly links the primary responsibility of healing the body with the responsibility for moral health as well. The primacy of the body is also highlighted in the Alexandrian commentaries on Galen's *De Sectis,* which influenced the practice of medicine from the time of Galen to the Middle Ages.[1] The commentaries state explicitly: Medicine is an art dealing with human bodies and affecting health.[2] We judge that the form of medicine proposed rests on excellent logical and historical evidence.

A critique applies the critical powers of reason to the form of a discipline. It examines the structures of experience, not the concrete and various matters of experience; it examines the unitary features of a discipline, not its individualities; and it results in an ontology of conditions of possibility. Hence, a critique of the form of medicine, a way of working with the body, will issue in an ontology of the body.

Immanuel Kant first developed the idea of a critical philosophy. His *Critique of Pure Reason* was an attempt to discover the conditions of possibility of synthetic a priori judgments present in the natural sciences. He was impressed by David Hume's position that "causes" are constructs of the mind, "constant conjunctions," with no foundation in reality, as knowledge can only be of discrete experiences. On the other hand, Kant was concerned to preserve both the natural sciences and ethics, which would suffer in Hume's view. What impressed Kant was that the sciences *worked.* Predictions were possible. If causes were constructs of mind, presumably varying from one person to another, then how could science discover regular laws? Asking how synthetic a priori judgments were possible through a critique was therefore tantamount to asking how scientific knowledge was possible.

A critique of medicine as we have defined it presents a certain similarity to Kant's project.[3] However, the kind of critical philosophy suggested herein bears a closer resemblance to Dewey than to Kant. Dewey's theory of criticism was founded on an appreciation of reality gained by analyzing conditions and consequences.[4] We are interested not with how science works but with how medicine works. Although the philosophical basis of medicine has changed as it has become more scientific, it has always presented the interesting philosophical problem of how one can apply theory to practice. More specifically, how can medicine apply theory to a concrete, singular, individual body and produce a cure? A "cure" is a successful medical event. What are the conditions of its possibility?

To be properly treated, the question demands more space than a single chapter would allow. This chapter is, therefore, an initial and somewhat initiative venture, an outline of a more detailed study.

In this chapter, we will present the "critical question" of the individualized application of medical theory as it has been examined by important thinkers about medicine in both classical and modern periods. The procedure will clearly establish the importance of the question. In the next chapter, we will present an ontological critique of medicine as propaedeutic to the entire second section of this work.

The Critical Question

The interplay between medical practice and medical theory is not simply one topic in the epistemology of medicine; it is the fundamental or categorical framework for the construction of such an epistemology.

Marx Wartofsky

By "critical question" we refer to the epistemological problem central to medicine. It can be formulated by asking how theoretical knowledge can be applied to concrete, individual body-persons with therapeutic results. Thus the critical question is an examination of the form of medicine, as we have already suggested.

Prior to an ontological critique of the form, it is helpful to examine how the question was posed in the history of medicine to the present, and what answers, if any, were given.

In the previous chapter, we noted how the Hippocratic corpus focused on prognosis rather than diagnosis. As a consequence, all theory was shaped by practical ends. Generally, the Hippocratic school rejected the fanciful philosophy of the early Greek cosmologists. Hence "What will happen?" and "How can we cure?", not "How does a cure happen?", were viewed as the guiding questions of medicine.[5]

The Classic View

By the time of Socrates, Hippocratic medicine was on a solid footing. Philosophy had also matured, beginning to pay attention to problems of human interaction rather than cosmological ones. The time was ripe for the critical question to emerge. Socrates and Plato first posed the question.

In the *Charmides* Socrates is presented to a young man who has a headache. Socrates has learned of a cure, composed of a leaf and "charm." In retelling how he learned of it, he mentions a Tracian critique of Greek medicine: "and this is the reason why the cure of many diseases is unknown to the physicians of Hellas, because they disregard the whole . . . if the head and body are to be well, you must begin by curing the soul."[6] The rest of the dialogue proceeds about the nature of *sophrosynē,* that unique "rightness" of body and soul which does not exceed the bounds of nature. *Sophrosynē* is considered the aim of all human endeavors, including medicine. The problem is: How does medicine work toward *sophrosynē?* Should it treat the body or the soul?[7]

While the dialogue is inconclusive, some important distinctions are drawn. It is clear that one does not know health from wisdom or *sophrosynē,* but from the art of medicine. Medicine is a science distinct from others in its subject matter of health and disease. A wise man cannot grasp the matter of medicine without being a physician, and wisdom by itself will not produce health.[8]

Considering the meaning of wisdom given in the dialogue, it is also clear that Socrates and Plato regard medicine as a different kind of science. Knowledge of health itself does not produce health. An otherwise knowledgeable person cannot produce health unless he also knows the art of medicine.[9] These initial observations are important for Plato's later thinking on how medicine works. They also illuminate the change in character from early Greek medicine, which was primarily verbal, to medicine at the time of Socrates, which was primarily somatic. Lain-Entralgo believes that Plato was interested in reintroducing verbal dialectic and rhetoric into medicine (the first to convince patients, and the second to persuade them). Medication alone cannot produce *sophrosynē.*[10] Only "apt words" with medication can do so.

It is equally apparent that Socrates and Plato respected medicine as a science too. In Plato's argument that rhetoric ought to cure the soul while medicine should cure the body, Socrates asks if someone with a little knowledge about a cure could claim to be a physician. Phaedrus answers that that person would also have to know to which patients it applies, when, and for how long. Comparing rhetoric and medicine, Socrates later says:

> In both cases there is a nature that we have to determine, the nature of the body in the one, and of the soul in the other, if we mean to be scientific and not content with mere empirical routine.[11]

In the *Philebus,* Plato introduces more clarity in his ascription of medicine as an art. He distinguishes the exact arts (such as numbering and measuring) from empirical arts, which "attain a most unreliable result with a large element of uncertainty."[12] Medicine falls into a category of empirical arts (*tekni*) such as navigation, agriculture, and military science. Aristotle later was fond of comparing medicine to agriculture.

In this view, then, *tekné* can be of two kinds: *mimesis* (imitation of nature), such as painting and music, and *poiesis* (a creative parallel with nature), such as architecture, politics, and medicine. Plato therefore considers medicine an empirical art with enough scientific data to predict some outcomes with a degree of certainty. Plato's final view of the matter contrasts two kinds of physicians: those who offer empirical injunction without an account of the disease (as slaves are treated), and those who take patients into their confidence and go into things thoroughly in a scientific way.[13] In other words, a good physician attempts some rational individualization of diagnosis and therapy by using medical enlightenment, a biography of the patient, and persuasion.

These observations by Plato indicate his considerable struggle to distinguish (or make more precise the distinction between) the discipline of medicine from "wisdom" (which was somewhat consonant with science in Plato). They do not, however, reveal his solution to the problem of how medicine works. They only establish the conditions under which it works best. Yet Plato does have a theory of some importance to offer.

His answer to the question of how medicine works is that the happiness of the whole human race is sealed in love.[14] Couple this view with that found in *Lysis* to the effect that the love of friendship is necessary for a sick body to be cured, and one can say with some certitude that Plato thought healing took place through a *proton philon,* a sort of proto-love between physician and patient for the sake of a good, health.[15]

Aristotle's more advanced conceptions of a science enabled him to be more precise about how medicine cures. Lain-Entralgo quotes Aristotle's view of friendship or *philia* as "one of the most indispensable requirements of life," noting that, like Plato, Aristotle would ground medicine in a relationship of mutual characteristics and friendship, *oikeion.*[16]

Mutual characteristics in nature are an essential step forward in determining how medicine works. It is clear that Aristotle places medicine among the practical or natural sciences, rather than among the theoretical ones. He uses the example of health to illustrate the starting point of natural sciences: that which comes to be. The theoretical sciences start with that which necessarily is.[17] But is the "likeness in nature" only that found in Plato, that both physician and patient share in the process of healing? Evidently not. To pursue this question, one must consult other works of Aristotle.

For Aristotle, the discipline of medicine is the *logos* of health, its formal cause.[18] This means that one cannot define health without reference to the doctor-patient relationship and medical science. Faced with the problem posed by Plato regarding the wise man's knowledge of health versus the art of medical practice, Aristotle notes that all sciences admit of two kinds of proficiency: scientific knowledge of the subject, and educational acquaintance with it such that one could "criticize the method of professed exposition."[19] From this statement, the wise man might appear to have an educated knowledge of the subject, health, but would not have scientific knowledge of it. But this conclusion is clearly not Aristotle's thinking on the topic.

In his *Politics,* Aristotle argues that there are some arts whose products are not judged solely by those who possess the art. To illustrate this point, he cites three kinds of physicians: the ordinary practitioner, a higher class physician, and the "intelligent man who has studied the art."[20] In the last class, Aristotle must have placed himself. Hence the power of judging what is healthy, of having scientific knowledge about health, falls to physicians and intelligent laymen who have studied the art. Aristotle meant this observation to answer the objection that only physicians know health.[21] In this view he departs from Plato because of his more precise idea of scientific knowledge.

In Aristotle's view, scientific knowledge is knowledge of something which cannot be other than it is. It is knowledge of the cause of the fact, as the cause of that fact and no other, and that the fact cannot be other than it is.[22] In the Middle Ages this requirement of science became known as a *propter quid* demonstration. A modern example would be the scientific knowledge regarding bacilli and their role in causing infections. One knows the disease, its cause, and the fact that this bacillus causes this disease. It is clear that this knowledge can be understood by an educated layman.

Aristotle also noted that the more empirical sciences can often demonstrate the fact (demonstration *quia*) without obtaining knowledge of the "reasoned fact," the proximate causes.[23] Thus a physician knows that fever often accompanies a cold, but cannot cite the precise agent of the fever.

From these brief reflections, we can conclude that a cure works when medical science has a *propter quid* demonstration of the cause and medical art knows the proper therapy. This process is made possible from patient to patient by the similarity in human nature shared by physicians and patients.

That medicine is not simply an empirical science is shown by Aristotle's almost constant use of it as an example in his *Rhetoric,* which he defines as an art of persuasion.[24] Argument based on knowledge does not always produce desired results, because some people cannot be fully instructed on the topic. In these cases persuasion is necessary.

Aristotle then explicitly compares medicine and persuasion: "It is not the function of medicine simply to make a man quite healthy, but to put him as far as may be on the road to health; it is possible to give excellent treatment even to those who can never enjoy sound health."[25]

Following the parallel, medicine would persuade a patient toward health by the personal character of the physician (his credibility), the responsiveness of the patient, and the proof or likeliness of what is said.[26] In order to effect this, the physician must be able to reason logically, to understand human character and goodness in their concrete forms, and to understand emotions.

The drama of medicine is therefore highlighted by Aristotle. Both physician and patient, alike in nature, aim for the end of human nature, happiness. One component of this happiness is health, "the excellence of the body; a condition which allows us, while keeping free from disease, to have the use of our bodies."[27]

The physician is a friend insofar as he "shares your pleasure in what is good and your pain in what is unpleasant, for your own sake." Kindness aims at responding to a need for the sake of the needy one. Pity is aroused by deprivations of a good, including afflictions, disease, old age, bodily injuries, and death.[28]

Because persuasion leads to decision, Lain-Entralgo believes Aristotle taught that medicine was like dialectic and rhetoric in that it sought to convince and persuade patients toward health. He also cites the tragic catharsis of Aristotle as having therapeutic value, because it unleased violent emotions and was conducive to decisions, the latter a result of *sophrosynē*.[29]

For Aristotle, then, a cure happens because of causal knowledge, friendship, or likeness in nature, and decisions formed from dialectic, rhetoric, and tragic catharsis. Medicine is indeed a complex discipline embroiled in virtually every aspect of the human condition. As medicine developed more systematically through Galen and toward the Middle Ages, a gradual distinction was drawn between its theory and practice. The theory included physiology, etiology, and semiology, while practice was subdivided into hygiene and therapy. Temkin shows that this distinction was drawn for educational as well as philosophical reasons. Texts in medicine were often taught by "iatrosophists," who were either philosophers of medicine or medical theorists. Handbooks of practical medicine were penned by practicing physicians. During this period, it was practically impossible to teach medicine without being a philosopher.

The second reason for the division between theory and practice rested on more speculative grounds. Medicine was regarded as a *tekné mixté,* an art among other arts, such as rhetoric and philosophy, which was speculative, active, perfective, and possessive. It "mixed" or combined these elements because medicine required its practitioner to consider both the body and its parts as well as to deal with, by intervening for, its health. Thus the commentaries on Galen solved the problem of medicine's mixed character by attributing to Aristotle (incorrectly) the statement that "medicine was philosophy of the bodies and philosophy the medicine of the souls," comparing these two arts as "two sisters."[30]

The Christian era offered a further empirical focus on the proximate causes of disease but added an extra duty for the doctor, that of consoling the dying. Because nature was created by God, it was progressively desacralized. A more interventionist model of medical practice emerged. At the root of medical theory was the notion that there was an internal source of healing, the virtue or power of nature, in turn designed by God.[31]

The Medieval View

By the Middle Ages, medicine was sufficiently developed to allow St. Thomas Aquinas to spend some time on its nature as a discipline. This discussion is helpful in order to gain a clearer grasp of how theory can be applied to individuals.

Aquinas argues that science is knowledge through causes. As with Aristotle before him, it is knowledge not only of fact but of reasoned fact. All sciences gain knowledge by abstracting and separating from concrete and accidental features of their object of study to gain appreciation of general or universal laws. But unlike Aristotle, Aquinas does not feel that physics can abstract from matter which is part of its subject. A science can abstract from concrete individuals, however.[32]

Among the theoretical sciences Aquinas places metaphysics, mathematics, and physics (not our modern physics). As the modern form of physico-mathematical sciences were in their infancy, Aquinas describes them as "intermediate sciences" located between mathematics and physical sciences because their method is different from mathematics, though they share its rules of analysis. Each science has its own unique method of inquiry, an important point for medicine.[33] Mathematics does not demonstrate through final and efficient causes, while intermediate sciences, dealing with matter and human beings, must do so. Additionally, the intermediate sciences use hypotheses and theories, which can explain experimental data but may not necessarily be true.[34]

That being said, where does medicine fall among the intermediate sciences? Two objections are raised in Aquinas' *Division and Methods of the Sciences.* The first is that medicine is an operative science that includes both a speculative and a practical aspect. Since ethics is a similar discipline, medicine ought to be linked with ethics. Second, mechanical arts, like medicine and agriculture, are operative sciences and should not be seen as branches of physics.[35]

Aquinas' answer is that speculative or theoretical sciences deal with things "that cannot be made or done by us," while practical sciences deal with what can be made or done, so that "we can direct the knowledge of them to activity as an end."[36] In this view, medicine is a practical science very much like ethics, because it aims at *recta ratio agibilium,* reasoning correctly about action. In fact, some sciences are called arts because they involve "a work that is a product of reason itself." Medicine is an art, therefore, in the sense that it is "productive reason" involving bodily activity.[37]

Quoting Avicenna,[38] Aquinas further distinguishes the application of "theoretical and practical" in philosophy, art, and medicine. When medicine is so divided, it is not on the basis of its end or goal but on the basis "of whether what is studied is proximate to, or remote from practice. For the whole of medicine is practical, since it is directed to practice. Thus we call that part of medicine practical which teaches the method of healing . . . and that part theoretical which teaches the principles directing a man in his practice."[39] Even though medicine contains theory, it is theory about the right way of acting–i.e., about therapeutic intent–and is not on that account a theoretical science.

In answer to the second objection, Aquinas argues that medicine is not a branch of physics because the curable body is not the subject of medicine (as it might be of biology), but the curable body *"as curable by art."* Art is nature's handmaid in healing . . . for health is brought about through the power of nature with assistance of art.[40] Instead medicine is an intermediate science.

It is clear that Aquinas finds the medical event to take place in the realm of practice, wherein art aids nature in healing. As a consequence, all of medicine is aimed at concrete action on behalf of individuals. It is scientific insofar as it searches for causes; it is an art insofar as it involves productive reason for the sake of bodily activity. In its scientific aspects, medicine abstracts from individuals but not from matter. The individual is known "through the universal nature of man." In this view, scientific knowledge of causes can be abstracted even from one case. In medicine's artistic aspect, knowledge is applied to concrete individuals through bodily activity.[41]

It is well at this point to pause and compare the concepts presented so far with current debate on the nature of medicine. To summarize, Plato argues that the clinical interaction works because of a proto-love of friendship between doctor and patient. Aristotle cites likeness in nature, persuasion, and scientific demonstration. To this Aquinas adds a power of healing in the body, to which medicine is aimed as an art.

Contemporary Views

Although modern medicine and the natural sciences have advanced far beyond their state in the Middle Ages, current debate about medicine and its curative intent focuses on remarkably similar issues. They can be summarized as follows:

1. What is the relation between the theory and practice of medicine?
2. Is medicine a science in the current understanding of the word?
3. Do the concepts of medicine bear evaluative notes? Are they always guided by therapeutic intent?
4. What forms of thinking take place in medicine?
5. Is there a science of individuals?

We can do no more than outline some of the responses to these questions, leaving a more systematic treatment to Chapter Five and a section of Chapter Six.

Marx Wartofsky and Caroline Whitbeck have arrived at similar conclusions about the relation between theory and practice in medicine–namely, that practice and the lifeworld inform all medical judgments. Thus Wartofsky holds that the fundamental entity of medicine is disease and that the locus of medical practice extends to the environment (social, historical, and cultural contexts), which prompts disease. Whitbeck focuses less on social classification, arguing instead that causality in medicine is analyzed in terms of practical knowledge. Thus medicine is based not only on perception but on the ability to manipulate. For different reasons, these two views parallel that of Aquinas on the nature of the theoretical in medicine–namely, that it is theory about practice.[42]

Almost all commentators argue that medicine is a science in the current understanding of science as a body of knowledge about laws of nature using sophisticated techniques of hypothesis formation, including probability. Thus Marjorie Grene lists theses that are part of modern science and applies them to medicine–e.g., that medicine assumes the existence of natural kinds; is concerned with the existence of actually existing kinds; and that concepts such as "healthy" and "normal" include a normative component. However, philosophers of science have difficulty applying the canons of science to medicine and usually, like Whitbeck, modify their view to take into account medical practice.[43]

While it is true that medicine involves scientific knowledge, it is also governed in its methodology by unique patient care needs that call for empirical-inductive thinking about individuals; intuitive, aesthetic, and rational forms of thought; history taking and dialogue; the pressure to decide; and an almost ancient respect for the search for causes, most often abandoned by modern science. We will discuss these aspects unique to the methodology of medicine in the next chapter. Aquinas' distinction regarding intermediate sciences and the practical aim of medicine would be helpful to current discussion.

To the degree that one accepts the pull of practice on the theory of medicine, one cites the evaluative and normative nature of the concepts of disease and health. If medicine is a cognitive art or a practical science, then its epistemological concepts are action-oriented. And insofar as human actions involve values, the concepts of medicine are evaluative.[44]

Finally, the question of how medicine works led Gorovitz and MacIntyre, as previously discussed, to attack Aristotle's notion of a science and to argue that we need a science of individuals. In addition to our criticism already noted–namely, that the normal meaning of science does not apply to individuals–one should also be cautioned that the desire to protect the scientific nature of medicine and still preserve its applications to individuals eventually will lead to a tautology such as "medicine is a science of individuals" and further cloud the language of the philosophy of medicine.[45]

To return to the question of how medicine works, it is interesting to note how concern for Aristotle's *propter quid* demonstration dominated the logic of discovery in medicine. Pietro d'Abano, a physician in the school of medicine at Padua, argued in his *Conciliator differentiarum philosophorum et praecipue medicorum* that medicine was a science by appealing to Aristotle's *propter quid* requirement–namely, that medicine can argue from cause to effect and predict results.

The focus on the logic of discovery, W. A. Wallace believes, can be traced at Padua right through to Galileo and was grounded in the medical school there, the finest in Europe throughout the

Middle Ages. Methodological realism was necessary for medicine to explain the conjunction between causes of disease and the cure effected once the causes were known. Pietro d'Abano defended medicine as a science because it met Aristotle's criteria for demonstrations in the strict sense.[46]

Wartofsky argues that Harvey's discoveries of the circulation of the blood would not have been possible without some understanding of mechanics, hydraulics, and their cultural impact at the time.[47] There is some question about the accuracy of this remark, for Wallace argues from Harvey's texts themselves that they were intended as either an exemplification or a defense of the Aristotelian method in the *Posterior Analytics*. Harvey was also a Paduan, and his interest in the logic of discovery supports Wallace's thesis that this interest stemmed from medical concerns there.[48]

Nevertheless the shift from a religious to a secular society, and the rise of the positive sciences, spelled an end to the answer that medicine works by demonstrations based on a universal, shared human nature. Lain-Entralgo observes that the doctor-patient relationship underwent a corresponding shift away from explanations focusing on necessary natural or theological connections. Instead the relationship was seen in a more functional, voluntarist way. It was seen as grounded not in co-equal natures but in a comradeship of human beings.[49]

The shift from philosophical to empirical explanations was necessitated by a greater focus on the etiology of disease in the seventeenth and eighteenth centuries. Harvey's discovery of the circulation of the blood led to new solutions to problems of life and sickness through chemistry, anatomy, physiology, physics, and pathology. Sydenham, Boerhaave, Hoffmann, and Stahl initiated new ways of clinical teaching. The rise of these sciences and the methodology of scientific proof caused the question of theory and practice to be raised anew, but now in more personal terms.

During the Enlightenment, for example, Zimmerman's *On Experience in the Medical Art* was a classic example. Zimmerman held that experience in medicine was a kind of knowledge bound up in practical duties, less a matter of possessing knowledge than a skill to act correctly. Temkin holds that Zimmerman's position on the link between theory and practice in medicine, combining learning (historical knowledge), the spirit of observation (sensual knowledge), and genius to draw conclusions, was actually a philosophy of the physician rather than a philosophy of medicine. The spirit of observation depends on knowledge of diseases, correct interpretation of symptoms, and prognostic evaluation of the changes in the patient. This is aided by analogy and induction, but cannot entirely be explained by them.[50] Hence, a concern to concretize theoretical knowledge for specific individuals led Zimmerman ultimately to a formulation of intuitionism.

The modern medical concern for discovery was stated most clearly by Claude Bernard in France. As we have already suggested, this concern was motivated by the problem of concretizing scientific knowledge for the individual in the clinical setting. Bernard's insights are worth outlining.

Although Bernard was influenced by the positivism of his day, he is quoted as starting his course with the following caution: "Messieurs, la medécene scientifique que j'ai le devoir de vous enseigner n'existe pas" ("Gentlemen: the scientific medicine to which you aspire does not exist"). He preferred to call medicine a nascent science.[51] Bernard shared with positivists their skepticism about ultimate causes and questions about why things happened. However, he argued that medicine must legitimately seek the proximate causes, the "immediate cause or necessary condition," of disease. Furthermore, he observed that Hume's description of a cause as a constant conjunction was insufficient for medicine. Instead one must also remove the condition to show that the phenomenon will not appear in its absence. One would then have a *nexus* or necessary connection.

The logic of discovery behind this argumentation is also important, for it buttresses our contention that the central problem in a philosophy of medicine is the concretizing of scientific knowledge in and for an individual. Bernard argued that medicine did not proceed purely inductively or purely deductively. In fact, medicine proceeds from an "experimental idea," described as an intuition or feeling about the laws of nature, but where the form is unknown. Experiment and therapeutics put this experimental idea to the test.

A fact, therefore, is an idea that flows from the discovery. Hence, medicine would work a cure if and when the experimental idea is proven a fact through application to individuals.[52]

Michel Foucault develops a contemporary philosophical view of the beginnings of authentic clinical medicine in the mid-eighteenth century. Through textual analysis, he is able to demonstrate the greater specificity occurring in medicine by the mid-nineteenth century. Right after the French Revolution, the style of clinical observation remained largely one of fantasizing. The "experimental idea" of Bernard remained highly imaginative. Approximately one hundred years later, Foucault contends, the style of observation focused more on constant visibility. "Regard" or gaze became a form of rational discourse which made clinical experience possible. Foucault defines this as "a scientifically structured discourse with and about an individual."[53]

Foucault's philosophical observations in this change of perception are exemplified by the change in question from "What is the matter with you?" to "Where does it hurt?" His view is that the change reflects the nonverbal conditions found in a common structure of prearticulated experience, a notion borrowed from Merleau-Ponty:

> Medicine made its appearance as a clinical science in conditions which define, together with its historical possibility, the domain of its experience and the structure of its rationality. These form its concrete *a priori*.[54]

Because of his use of Merleau-Ponty, Foucault's thesis is somewhat hidden by his closely reasoned and philosophical language. Extracting from this, his thesis seems to be that medicine in the eighteenth century neglected the individual in favor of immutable disease entities and Morgagni's pathology of organs. Symptoms were regarded only as signs of these disease entities. Changes wrought by the aftermath of the French Revolution and Condillac's philosophy, which emphasized the link between sign, sense, and intelligence, led to a focus on individuals in their specificity. A probabilistic rather than a fixed interpretation of disease resulted from Bichat's pathology of tissues, which allowed physicians to "gaze," as it were, into the internal structure of the body.

Thus the change from seeing an individual as a sign of a disease entity to seeing an individual as unique and specific results from changing the ground of unity from disease entities to the internal structure of the body. In short, clinical medicine necessarily presupposes, in Foucault's view, an ontological order within the body organizing disease prior to its manifestation. Specific differences among human beings lie in specific ways the organization takes place, leading physicians to more probabilistic modes of explanation. Thus, for Foucault, the source of medical epistemology is not, as in Wartofsky's view, the social manipulations possible in a culture or the imagination as a conjunction between theory and practice, but an ontological order within human bodies.[55]

We have already noted Sournia's critique of modern medicine as more mythological than scientific. He describes diagnosis and therapy as an interplay between objective givens and subjective interpretations laced with mythology and magic. For Sournia, therapy is a collage of approximations.[56] However, it is clear that he wants medicine to be more scientific than it can be. His conclusion is that medicine is still only a form of artisanship depending largely upon the success of the hour. However, the debasement of feeling, intuition, and sensory modes of perception in modern medicine can lead to the same emphasis on disease entities without attention to individuals which Foucault attributes to eighteenth-century medicine. Some forms of the scientific method are inapplicable and unsuitable for human experience.

In a seminal work, Scott Buchanan attempted to preserve the rational content of modern medicine against its elaborate empiricism and antiintellectualism.[57] After exploring the laboratory and the liberal arts used by medicine and establishing their rational content, he proposed that medicine, defined as "seeing the connections between symptoms and remedies," is an integrated science. Because of the unique nature of medicine, Buchanan argued that it ought to be called "physic," a unitary science from which the arts and a philosophy of science might emerge. His program for socialization of medicine is novel, to say the least, for its depends upon prior rational analysis of the sciences and arts which medicine uses, their relation to "physic," the critical study of modes of measurement used, and the construction of a rational science on this basis. From this a truly "social" medicine could evolve because boards could codify and criticize the practice of medicine on the basis of the standards enunciated.[58] In a far less sophisticated way, this is the same aim of current Professional Standards Review Organizations.

The final thinker in this historical sketch must be Pedro Lain-Entralgo, for no other contemporary can match his skill in historical development and philosophical acumen. Lain-Entralgo defines clinical medicine as the art of abundant experience–sensory, intellectual, and affective–of the infirm individual which it describes. Hence medicine is both a scholarly discipline and an intellectual habit concerning profound and systematic knowledge of the nature of man.[59] The intentions of the physician are to produce a cure, to explain the pathology with respect to the clinical sign or symptom and the etiology, and to grasp what the disease is both in itself and as a universal human condition.[60]

The combination of these investigative modes means that the physician tries to discover the necessary link between a scientific concept and its immediate situation in an individual. Medical wisdom therefore becomes a constant restive questioning toward successive tentative solutions to both theoretical and technical problems, with an effort at discovering unity in the midst of diversity.[61] For this reason, Lain-Entralgo concludes that medicine is neither an art nor a science, but a *tekné* of healing.

Our historical sketch has only touched on some of the main thinkers dealing with the way in which medicine cures. It was not intended to be exhaustive, but rather to furnish some of the materials for the systematic treatment which follows. At this point we are able to conclude that:

1. Physicians and philosophers of medicine are concerned about the conceptual validity of explanations offered for disease. These explanations are both etiological and pathological (an attempt at rigorous science) or everyday, the language used in conveying knowledge to the patient.

2. The source of this concern lies in a unique logic of discovery, at the root of which is a process of clinical transaction described as empirical-inductive, an experimental idea, an act of discovering necessary connections.

3. Despite historical variations and changes in culture, and de-

spite positivistic efforts to remove causality from the tools of physicians, medicine continues to search for the necessary connections between symptoms and diseases.

4. Truly scientific knowledge emerges from the clinical interaction such that a physician knows why some therapeutics work for a specific patient.

5. Medicine involves a cognitive art of bodily work which must concretize and individualize its knowledge. Hence it involves elements of art as well as science.

6. The continuing problem for medicine is how scientific knowledge can be extracted from and applied to individuals.

For want of space, we have deliberately passed over a discussion of the enormous influence of Descartes on the less holistic, more reductionistic conceptions of medicine. These conceptions are, in fact, the dominant ones in academic medicine, and they unapologetically equate medicine with experimental science and seek chemical and biological explanations of disease and base their healing efforts solely and exclusively on radical cure.

Cartesianism is, therefore, the unspoken philosophical substratum of much of contemporary medicine—the source of many of its great strengths and equally of its deficiencies. When Descartes mathematicized philosophy, he mathematicized medicine as well. His aim was to create a medicine grounded on infallible demonstrations. The iatrochemists, iatrophysicists, and iatromechanicists who picked up the Cartesian spirit are the intellectual forebears of our contemporary medical reductionists. Gilson carefully delineates the conceptual fallout of the Cartesian mechanicism of the body.[62] It is obvious that a philosophy of medicine based on the modern version of Cartesianism would very likely be assumable under a philosophy of biology and of science. It is the alternative to this philosophy of medicine that this book discusses (see Figure 6-1).

5

Ontology of the Body

The first step in a critique of medicine has been accomplished. We have shown how the epistemological problem of medicine is a search for an explanation of the way the abstract is applied to individuals and extracted from them. In our opinion, the histories of the philosophy of science and medicine demonstrate that explanations of this process have developed from reductionistic and mechanistic models to a complex and richer milieu in the practice of medicine itself. In other words, they have moved closer to the human center of the discipline.[1]

In this chapter, we will address the epistemological problem of medicine from a systematic standpoint, rather than from the descriptive one used in the previous chapter. We will focus on the human body, with which medicine deals as it establishes the human center of medicine. Thus, the role of the practice of medicine and its experience by physicians and patients underlines a continuous entré into the human condition of life itself.

Practical Ontclogy

Although our purpose in the previous chapter was to explore the epistemological problem of medicine, we will here indicate the major areas of current research in the philosophy of medicine by way of introducing the need for a practical ontology. While the four categories of current research bear on the epistemological problem, they do so less directly than the classic and modern views already presented. However, a brief discussion of these views permits the illustration of both themes we intend to cover and points of departure between our method and those of our contemporaries. We discern four major areas of current philosophical research which have a bearing on the practical ontology of medicine: the object of medicine; mind-body issues; clinical judgment; and theory and practice. The last category establishes the moral nature of medicine.[2]

Object of Medicine

Physicians are traditionally less interested in medical ontology than in the practical objects of medicine: curing and caring. As we have seen, this practical object led to classifications of medicine as a technique or craft. Early in the 1100's, for example, Hugh of St. Victor classified medicine as a form of mechanics, a set of disciplines which derived their form from their matter. He meant that the definition of medicine stems from its experience with curing and caring for the body, the person, and the social milieu. It even includes a concern for cultural standards and norms.[3]

Because medicine is a practical theory of human reality, knowledge applied to human ends and purposes,[4] the aim of medicine is to discover knowledge of man. As Steven Levenson notes, "Medical Science becomes Medicine only when it is used to promote health and healing, and thus becomes an intervention into an individual human life."[5] In this intervention science, values, society, and cultures are all intertwined. Thus a concern for curing and caring does entail questions of values, culture, and ontology.

If the object of medicine is seen as curing disease and caring for persons such that they are restored to some quality of life and function, then several important ontological themes result. The first is that science is involved in medicine primarily as a defense of explanatory theories of disease and their application to human life.[6] This pragmatic utilization of science is heightened by a second theme: that medical knowledge and craft are value-laden. Hence a critical concept such as "normal" clearly engages the physician and philosopher in a discussion of personal, social, scientific, and cultural values. Canguilhem concludes, after a survey of positivistic leanings in medicine, that "those who themselves tried most vigorously to give 'normal' only the value of a fact have simply valorized the fact of their need for a limited meaning."[7]

Therefore a physician must combine compassion for the human situation[8]–which is *not* synonymous with learning–with an insight into that situation involving a treatment of the "whole person" and his or her cultural context.[9] This requires an attention to values to achieve results. A practical ontology, such as we propose, can examine these values, the impact of practice on them, and their source in the body as revealing the human condition.

While not asserting that this chapter establishes a philosophy of life, which Yanovsky claims is necessarily propaedeutic to a philosophy of medicine,[10] we do claim that an ontology of the body is the matter which establishes the form of medicine, its source and end of explanatory theory, and the basis of its judgments and axioms.

In this respect, attention to the object of medicine guides our method toward the "human center" of the discipline, a process not found among those who use philosophy of science as their tool to examine medical concepts. While valuable, such examination is usually confined to a realm of abstract and objective concepts, rather than the realm of life in which these concepts arise.

MIND-BODY ISSUES

The advances in neurosurgery, neurology, and the classification of mental diseases have all contributed to a renewed discussion of the relation of mind to body, free will, and medical anthropology. Only the vaguest outline of a new anthropology is possible at this time, however.

But some important features of the debates spawned by this issue are worthy of mention. First, the overpowering dualism of Western civilization continues to divorce the body from the mind and even from the personality.[11] Second, the debate has illustrated the descriptive, evaluative, and normative functions of medical explanations.[12] Third, the debate has given rise to the use of the term "lived body" as a philosophical antipode to its neglect in theories of human consciousness.[13] And finally, the categories of mental diseases, as Engelhardt points out, have more bearing on the integrity of persons than the categories of physical diseases.[14]

We have avoided any suggestion of dualism in our philosophy of medicine. However, as we shall shortly describe it, the ontology of the body in medicine must take into account at least three levels of experiencing the world: the level of objective experience, the level of experience not objectified, and the level of physical survival. The distinctions are unavoidable, but are meant in the Kantian sense of different perceptions of the world by the same unity.[15]

The distinction between body and soul by Descartes, and his attempt to locate the organs in the body through which the soul operates, are still with us today. It is not unfair to claim that Descartes' distinction made possible the enormous gains in anatomy and physiology during the two centuries after its formulation; the body could now be examined as an object of experimentation and observation. However, as the section "Theory and Practice" will show, it is not only objective science which establishes the norms of clinical judgment, but engagement with the forms of life presented by the body.

In this regard, the mind-body problem may, as Spicker suggests, be a nonproblem,[16] a kind of philosophical bromide which neglects current advances in vigorous philosophical research and in the neurosciences. For it appears that the neurosystem is not an organ but an embodiment of the mind.

It is therefore opportune to construct a practical ontology of the body as the human center of medicine prior to any distinctions between mind and body. By doing so, we avoid the distinction as far as possible. We claim that such an ontology can contribute to overriding the distinction for medical practice and can demonstrate the *sine qua non,* the absolute necessity, of the body in any philosophy of man and epistemology of discovery.

Clinical Judgment

Clinical judgment has received philosophical attention in three areas. The first is the scientific aspect of medical judgment, especially those features which may possibly be computerized. These will be discussed in detail in the next chapter. Here it is important to note that a shift from disease entities to diseases as patterns makes computer diagnosis especially practical. This shift in perspective is simultaneously more complex and more realistic.[17]

The second area of research respects the role of art, not only in the development of scientific models of explanation but in the crucial moment of applying science in the clinical decision to human beings. Feinstein notes that the artistic aspects of medicine are not confined to the "bedside manner," as per the usual misconstrual.[18] Clouser and Zucker argue that the real "art" in medicine is precisely the act of linking the general to the particular.[19] Cassell calls this "applying the abstract to the usual."[20] Apart from the details already sketched regarding this problem, we will offer arguments in the next chapter on the artistic status of clinical judgment. However, it is important to note that in the ontology of the body, "application" to and "extraction" from the body occur on more than one level. Ignoring this multiplicity leads to confusion about whether clinical judgment is scientific or artistic.

Third, the moral nature of medicine has been explored through analyses of clinical judgment. Moral issues arise in the conflict between physician as scientist and as healer,[21] the contexts of the practice of medicine,[22] the role of moral and philosophical ideas in framing medical practice,[23] and the profound sense of communal ethics through which the physician is dedicated to the preservation of life.[24] These examples are hardly exhaustive. But they serve to illustrate the fruitfulness of exploring moral issues in medicine from the perspective of clinical judgment. Based on an ontology of the body, a refined exploration of clinical judgment and consequent moral issues is possible.

Theory and Practice

The fourth category of current research in the philosophy of medicine concerns theory and practice—in particular, concepts of health and disease and the moral end of medicine.

From the exploration in the previous chapter, it should come as no surprise that philosophers of medicine have recently become interested in the connection between theory and practice. We have already cited Wartofsky on this point. Findlay, commenting on Hegel's methodological insights, says, "What intelligent activity aims at, however, practical activity achieves, i.e., the complete mastery of *individual* natural reality by rational pattern."[25] This mastery is the guiding motive of medicine in dealing with individuals. Yanovsky considers attention to individuals and the patterning of diseases essential to relieve medicine's excessive dependency on deterministic cause-effect explanatory models.[26]

The impact of the practical nature of explanatory models in medicine on theoretical constructs has also been noted. Romanell has demonstrated Locke's interest in practical ideals in life, profitable knowledge, and his philosophical method of experience and conjecture was derived from his medical background.[27] More to the point of this chapter, Engelhardt has argued that models derive their explanatory force from their applicability to treatment and observed response.[28]

Thus it is not just the scientific ability to match complaints to concepts of health and disease derived from pathology, but the additional consideration of what these concepts do for patients, that is of interest in linking theory to practice. As Mack Lipkin argues, "The practice of medicine is to a large extent what the individual doctor makes it. His ideas of what illness is and how it is caused determine the first steps in his deciding what to do for his patient."[29] Consequently, if health is not just an absence of disease, then judgments about the health of a patient require weighing the complaints against *clinical* norms and the previous standards of function of this *particular* patient.[30] It is at this point that the moral nature of medicine is revealed to its fullest extent, in an ontology of the body of the patient and the physician's approach to this body.

This insight about the link between concepts of health and disease and the patient's actual functioning leads Engelhardt to the conclusion that disease is a relational concept, both normative and descriptive.[31] A judgment of what is "normal" rests on a *technique* of establishing or restoring the normal in patients. The normal cannot be reduced to a single form of physiological knowledge because it rests in part on man's action on his environment. Kant recognized this clearly.[32]

For the same reason, Canguilhem concludes his assay of theories of normality in medicine with this observation: "It is life itself, and not medical judgment, which makes the biological normal a concept of value and not a concept of statistical reality."[33] Life is fundamentally not an object of study but a struggle which engages both physician and patient in the realm of sheer physical survival.[34] We discuss this feature of the ontology of the body by exploring the wisdom of the body and its role in cures.[35]

The profound connection between theory and practice can supply a missing component in theories about the link between science and ethics. If both the latter are viewed as limited and perspectival, and, as Kuhn suggests, are developed by researchers interpreting their communities' view of the world, then no clear connection between science and ethics can be drawn.[36] But if both science and ethics can be drawn from the particulars of the body and the anatomy of persons found in a practical ontology of medicine, then the moral end of medicine can contribute to the moral ends of science and society. We have set out for ourselves no less a task than this.

Conditions of Possibility of Clinical Interaction

In Chapter Three we described the form of medicine as a clinical interaction working in, with, and through the body. The ontological critique of medicine focuses on this form and asks what the necessary conditions of possibility are for clinical interaction to work. Thus, the critique handles the capacities of action found in medicine. Guiding this critique is the critical question developed in Chapter Four: How is it possible for medicine to apply theory to an individual living body?

One should note that the conditions of possibility established herein are conditions of a *reality* experienced in an effective medical setting of healing. Cures take place. How is it possible? Such a critique leaves aside ineffective medical events as well as some of the complex aspects of care which are part of modern medicine (e.g., preventive, community, crisis, experimentation, and so on). However, insofar as these participate in medicine as we have defined it, what is established applies to them as well.

In order to simplify language, we will call the necessary conditions of possibility "structures" of medicine. Furthermore, we will treat these structures under the logically distinct categories of the scientific realm (world of the lived self), everyday realm (world of the lived body), and survival realm (world of the living body).[37] Reflections on an anthropology based on the body conclude the section and the chapter.

While the distinction between these three realms of perception is borrowed from philosophy, it has been suggested by the dialectic developed in the first section of the chapter. If the clue to establishing the normal in medicine derives from both the realm of scientific models of disease and the life of patients in their social milieu, then at least these two realms should be included in the ontological examination of the conditions of possibility of cures. However, the explanatory force of the models also requires direct engagement with the physical survival of the body independent of its social milieu. Thus an "originary" or primal realm of the individual physical characteristics of the body must also come under ontological purview.

The terms "lived self," "lived body," and "living body," although previously introduced, may still cause some confusion. They should be viewed as a shorthand for complex human characteristics. First, "lived self" refers to the objective catalog of characteristics human beings create and present to the world as their personality. These are the public aspects of a human personality. Second, "lived body" refers to the experience of being a body which cannot be objectified. This experience is conditioned by continuous interaction in a world of physical objects and other persons. But the objectification of these experiences into a personality in civilized society always leaves a residue of nonexpressed and nonobjectified material. It is for this reason that as social animals and as individuals, we constantly search for more and more adequate expressions of human life in the scientific world. No object, word, symbol, category, or social structure in that world is safe from tampering with its meaning caused by its inadequacy in the everyday world of experience. Finally, "living body" refers to the ontologically prior realm of individual survival as a physical organism, ingesting, interpreting, and modifying its environment in the struggle and defense of its own existence.

Two additional points are necessary before continuing. The three worlds of human experience are distinguishable from the whole that is human life only by the fact that their actions have different ends: the creation and preservation of meaning in symbols, the creation and preservation of experience, and the creation and growth of life itself, respectively. A second point is this: Our use of these distinctions is motivated by a desire to clarify somewhat a decidedly complex process of curing patients. We have already noted that the ability to classify a disease (the scientific realm) does not mean that greater knowledge of the personal impact of the disease than that of the patient is present (the everyday realm). Further, if the process of diagnosis and theory is confined to the realm of scientific probity and the social milieu of the patient, no real engagement with the moral center of medicine (the commitment to the survival of life despite its race, class, social standing, or personality) occurs. Unless the physician engages the patient toe to toe as a biological entity, the entré to the human condition is neglected. It is this very entré that makes medicine such a satisfying profession. It is demanded by a profession to treat the whole patient.

Thus we have no intention of trying to defend the three categories used as philosophical verities. Rather, they are used as convenient shorthand expressions for clarifying realms of clinical interaction such that, after the treatment of clinical judgment in the next chapter, we can move on to practical applications of this ontological question.

The Structures of Medicine

The Scientific Realm

In order for a cure to take place, clinical judgment must be a complex interaction which, at root, links scientific knowledge with individual human beings. At the very least, this structure implies that:

1. Human bodies are capable of creating scientific (and/or conceptual) formulations about the causes of disease. Three further implications are derived from this one.

a. Human bodies are capable of objectifying themselves in symbols. What is objectified we have called the "lived self," when applied to the entire life or biography of an individual.[38] The difference between human and other animal bodies seems to lie in the ability to symbolize, to create a record of experience *outside* of our bodies.

The capacity to objectify the body also allows the body to objectify parts, or even diseases. Thus Cassell, cited earlier, observed clinically that patients objectified and depersonalized their illnesses by referring to illness as an "it."[39]

What is noteworthy about objectifying is that it demands a common language and a world of common objects. One cannot describe oneself without referring to analogies of experience of objects in a common language. Thus Kant argues that permanence of the ego (the sense of being "I") does not live in substantial identity or in the flow of inner experience. Instead personal identity depends on the existence of objects in space outside of the ego.

What is objectified, therefore, is *not* unique. To objectify oneself as a lived self or person, or to objectify disease categories and etiological agents, is to enter the world of common characteristics. Uniqueness lies instead in the historical, space-time configuration of the "capacity to objectify but not totally"–that is, the lived body.[40]

Hence one condition of a successful cure is that the general knowledge of science matches in reality objectifications of common characteristics of bodies. When a body objectifies its disease and a physician compares this with general classifications of diseases common to human bodies, the search for scientific explanation takes place. One of the motives of a physician, as noted by Lain-Entralgo, is to explain the etiology of the disease and to understand its pathology as a general condition of human experience.

Because the world of common objects and the objectified lived self are the results of a capacity to objectify on the part of lived bodies which cannot be objectified, scientific explanation of disease is not the only, or even the major, task of medicine.

b. A second implication of objectifying and explaining causes of disease is that the etiological agents are real. Bernard noted that Hume's description of causality as constant conjunction is insufficient to explain the real, experienced effect of agents on the body, or the real effects on the body of therapy used to minimize or delete the agents.

The search for proximate causes of disease by medicine is a search for objectively existing agencies which act upon and within the body. Another condition of a cure, therefore, is a scientific knowledge of real causes.[41] The requirements of medical knowledge include a knowledge of a cause, prediction of the effects of its agency, and knowledge that this cause is specific for *this* disease.

These requirements parallel the requirements of Aristotle for *propter quid* or essential demonstrations, which establish a science. To object that medicine does not always or even often know the cause of a disease is only to recognize that medicine is science in the making.

c. A third implication of objectifying the causes of disease is the specificity of medicine. The history of medicine is the history of a search for more and more specific causes and treatments.[42] Thus "cancer" is discovered to be of various types which may not even be related in structure or process. The search for specific causes leads medicine from external agents, such as environment or bacteria, to actual reactive processes in the body. In a profound sense, then, all diseases are caused by self-destructive processes within the body.

The implication of specificity leads to the unique methodology of medicine. As will be discussed in the next chapter, the process of diagnosis is aimed at specificity for the sake of action. Physical and laboratory diagnosis is a process of narrowing the range of possibility by comparing a specific body with normal values. The process is governed by the nature of the interaction, a requirement to reach a decision on behalf of the body in need. Hence the method of medicine is not the same as that of the other physical sciences, which have no requirement to act on behalf of a body in need.[43]

Also, the greater the specificity, the less medicine acts like a science and the more it acts like an art. For as specificity increases, the uniqueness of a body as an individual also increases. The pressure to decide, or the therapeutic imperative, gradually leads to evaluative connotations of the disease for the particular patient. These value coordinates, in turn, influence the mode and extent of therapy.

2. A second feature of the structure of a cure is that clinical judgments differ from those in pure science in that they are governed by individualization. Clinical judgments must be a complex process of perceiving individual uniqueness in the midst of common objectivities.

Consequently clinical judgment must also include modes of convincing and persuading patients about appropriate actions, features which Aristotle called dialectic and rhetoric. The specificity of medicine leads it from the realm of scientific thought to the realm of the everyday world, the realm of the lived body.

If disease is primarily a self-destructive process of a body, then the art of medicine produces cures by working in, through, and with that body. If one accepts Aristotle's definition of an art as a cognitive discipline which produces either a work or action, then the "work" of medicine is an action in conjunction with the body. In this sense, rehabilitation depends upon the extent of individualization. Individualization, in turn, depends upon the physician's discovery and utilization of the wisdom of the body.[44] The response of each patient to therapy cannot be predicted scientifically.

The extent to which individualization is possible is one source of the distinction between primary, secondary, and tertiary care. If the lived self is the historical result of the ability to symbolize, then as active bodily engagement is diminished, so too is the lived self. Thus the body is treated more as an object in tertiary care, where the lived self is diminished or even threatened, whereas the lived self is more actively engaged in primary care. Treatment in primary care can more actively utilize the wisdom of the body than the more interventionist care in tertiary settings.

Because a living organism is a system which takes advantage of favorable opportunities, the wisdom of the body includes an anticipatory note.[45] It is by this preconscious organization of itself for maximum effectiveness that living matter, even a cell, is distinguished from inanimate matter. Hence the physician's response to specificity and the possibility of a cure must ultimately be grounded in a unique organization of matter which we have called the living body.

The structure of a cure must therefore imply that medicine be multi-etiologic. Clinical judgment involves a search for real causes; a comparison of categories reflecting normal values with an individual body in need of help; the values of the patient as a lived self; the world of common objects; responsibility arising from an imbalance of knowledge in the relationship; trust; and a share in the experience of a living body.

To speak more systematically, the structure of medicine implies a discovery of real relationships between causes of health and disease and the effects of these causes on individuals. The material a priori of medicine is the individual body, which is both the work of medicine and the artist of its own healing. Being a body in the clinical relationship means being alive (the living body), experiencing experience (the lived body), and symbolizing historical identity (the lived self).

The motives of the physician must therefore include scientific explanations of disease; more specific understanding of illness as it interrupts the lived body; and a perception born out of the wisdom of the body to guide therapy and cure.

Constitutively speaking, medicine is an intuitive act that recognizes specificity. This recognition is acquired through skill in perceiving analogous relationships that occur in applications of scientific knowledge to specific health problems. Solutions and rehabilitation depend on mutually satisfactory decisions about therapy. Because the concept of disease is normative on the scientific level, evaluative on the level of the lived body, and structurally linked to the wisdom of the body on the level of the living body, medicine must epistemologically include values. It is at all levels a moral enterprise, where "moral enterprise" means action involving values.

As a result of the above reflections, it should be clear that coherence is an insufficient condition of medical theory. Medical theory must include norms for action and proven applicability. Medicine therefore does not conform to the canons of correctness found in the physical sciences, as Gorovitz and MacIntyre have argued.[46]

Because the structure of a cure implies specificity about the wisdom of individual bodies, it should also be clear that grounding in the everyday world of *praxis*[47] is also an insufficient theory of medicine (Whitbeck, Wartofsky). While it is true that medical concepts are grounded in *praxis,* it does not follow that all concepts are culturally relative or proceed merely from the everyday world.[48] The theory and *praxis* of medicine are both grounded in the specificity of *this* living body.

3. Therefore, the third feature of the structure of a cure is that the threefold aspect of clinical judgment–diagnosis, prognosis, and therapy–depends upon reference to a body.

Diagnosis not only compares scientific classes of disease to symptoms of the lived self but is also guided by the unique historical configuration presented by the lived body. It must create a dialogue with this body to ascertain the nature of the disease.

Prognosis not only links the disease with similar patterns of disease, and not only attends to the scientific record of probabilities, but must also be governed by the values of the lived body and the insight into the wisdom of this particular body in hopes of rehabilitation and restoration.

Clinical judgment is governed by therapeutic necessity because the medical event is constituted by a need for physical help, health being one of the foundational needs of man. Therapeutic necessity is the ground of the legal and moral nature of clinical interaction. Because it is impossible to understand any person, much less any group of persons, all at once and entirely, therapy cannot be viewed as scientifically predictable and secure. And because the values of patients and society enter into all stages of the clinical interaction, therapy is inherently value-laden. If medicine is guided by therapeutic necessity,[49] even in its theory, then medicine in its totality is a value-laden enterprise.

Therefore therapy depends on the biography of the lived self, the dialogue between the physician and the interpreted and uninterpreted signs of the body, and the wisdom of the body. Therapy aids in the appreciation of instinct and dialogue as components of human life.

The Everyday Realm

The condition of possibility that scientific concepts can be applied to a lived self with beneficial effects is that both scientific concepts and the lived self are grounded in the real world of everyday reality. This world contains the capacity to objectify as the uniqueness of individuals. At the very least this structure implies the following:

1. There is a shared world of real objects and a commonality of language by which the process of objectifying is given objective standing. Things and realities are recognized as other—that is, as connected with the lived body without being united to it.

2. Physician and patient must share in the experience of being a lived body. This experience is a recognition, as Marcel pointed

out, that in the last analysis my body cannot be made into an object, where an object is connected as other to me, but not united. An individual is his or her body.

3. A cure implies not only a scientific explanation of disease but a real effect on and in the lived body with all its values. On this level, the physician must have an experience of disease—a disruption of the lived body—and an imaginative preconception of what the truth might be to guide the scientific classification process.

4. The therapeutic process must be guided by the possibility of perceiving the patient as a lived body, a subject rather than an object.

5. The patient, as well as the physician, must have the possibility of making "notional judgments," everyday, gradual syntheses of empirical value experiences. For this constitutes the uniqueness of living bodies—namely, that they exist in space and time and create their own histories as a consequence. Because the cure must be satisfactory and rehabilitative, it must be grounded in a cultural and individual value system created by lived bodies. Accordingly, the physician is guided by the *praxis* of the everyday world in diagnostic and therapeutic decisions.

6. The everyday world of *praxis* cannot be viewed as an absolute reality captured by scientific concepts. As Ernest Cassirer observes in this regard:

> It would be a naive sort of dogmatism to assume that there exists an absolute reality of things which is the same for all living beings. Reality is not a unique and homogenous thing; it is immensely diversified, having as many different schemes and patterns as there are different organisms. Every organism is, so to speak, a monadic being. It has a world of its own because it has an experience of its own.[50]

We have made other observations about the relation between the realm of science and the realm of the everyday, between theory and *praxis,* in the preceding section.

Survival Realm: Structures of the Living Body

The ability to cure requires specificity. But the requirements of specificity include clinical entities in a scientific sense and the individualities of patients. However, in order for a cure to take place, the clinical interaction must include another factor: some common structures of living organisms. This is the realm of the wisdom of the body discussed above. The condition of possibility of cure, therefore, is that bodies organize themselves in a common manner, although the extent and degree varies from one to the next. At the very least, this structure implies:

First, that the body creates the world of its perception and is the object of its own creation. Scott Buchanan illustrates this point: "The human body . . . becomes a most marvelous work of natural art. It is an artist fabricating tissues, organs, fluids and gases out of raw materials . . . it is the product of its own art."[51] The uniqueness of the body is its own "wisdom," its pattern of artistic achievement.

Second, the body is immediate to itself. It is there and needs no scientific justification or proof. The living body is an a priori to the actions of the lived body which distinguishes objective and subjective. The body is experienced as a centered unity.[52]

Third, the origin of seeking and offering help as the condition of the medical event lies in the compassion of living bodies. A direct awareness of pain is conveyed by the body to other bodies without intervening language. The insight into concrete singulars required for a cure depends on this compassion, which might be described as a prearticulated shared awareness of bodies regarding the human condition. This awareness grounds medicine in tragedy and gave rise to the myth of Aescupulus, a myth of the wounded healer. In a very real sense, one must "suffer with" in order to heal.

Fourth, bodies have a common capacity and structure. Otherwise, general medical concepts could not be applied beneficially, since they are derived from therapeutic experience and necessity. *A cure cannot take place without common bodily processes.* All bodies are homogeneous in that they subject their parts to a whole activity. All bodies inhabit and adjust to their environment. All bodies subordinate their activities to an end in view.[53]

Thus a unitary substrate of life and experience exists in the "bionomic order" of the body which unifies all causal factors necessary for a cure.[54] It is our view that the reality of cures in medicine establishes the reality of the human body as composed of its own unique wisdom and a common bionomic order with other bodies. It is further our view that medical theory and practice are applied to and derived from the wisdom and bionomic order of bodies. Since theory and practice in medicine are part of a moral enterprise, a possibility exists to ground medical ethics in a philosophy of medicine, rather than in older ethical theories or in cultural relativism. This enterprise is the subject of Chapter Eight.

Bodies interact with other bodies in arrangements. These arrangements are not capricious, because they rest on common structures of living bodies. On the other hand, the reality of each living body is unique, because it arranges itself according to its own wisdom.

The source and origin of the everyday and scientific realms is bodies interpreting themselves and the world. Thus facts are already values. Thus medicine as a science is forced by the body it helps heal to be medicine as an art.

The primal experience of the body must be present in medical interactions in order that scientific explanations have a common base. In this way, "it hurts here" is understood by the physician in a direct, compassionate way as body while simultaneously understood in an indirect way through the disruptive effects on the practical world of the lived body and the interruptive effects on the lived self through scientific conceptions of pain. But without the direct experience of "hurting," and its implications for the wisdom of the body, the structure of specificity will be absent from the clinical relationship.

Put another way, medicine refers to its own collective body of theories, to the everyday world of values and disease, but primarily to the individual body, both in its universal organic processes and in its unique selective wisdom.

Ontology of the Body: Toward an Anthropology

The conditions of possibility of medicine themselves have conditions of possibility. Because of the structure of medicine, its specificity, is related to a real event, a cure, specificity is a real occurrence in human affairs. Therefore an ontology based on the body is possible and would constitute the outline of a philosophical anthropology.[55] The topic deserves more extensive treatment than can be devoted to it here. We will simply note some of the implications for an anthropology based on a philosophy of medicine developed so far.

The fact that living organisms not only react to but also shape their world establishes what we have called a bionomic order. Logically prior to individual experience, but in reality concurrent with it, is an organization of reality by a living being.[56] Among the organizations of the world is the active selection of what is best for the organism, which we have called the wisdom of the body. Hence the living body proto-selects health as a desirable goal and considers it obtainable. In this fundamental sense, health is a perduring value of living bodies if "value" is defined as that which is judged both obtainable and desirable, i.e., a good.

These observations are important not only to describe the structure of medicine, but to ground the reality of cures in what are common *living* organization patterns and specific organization patterns individual bodies adopt. Hence the next chapter will explore clinical judgment, the epistemological heart of medical practice, from the standpoint of these conditions of possibility.

The conditions of possibility of a medical event also point to the possibility of an ethics based on the value of health and an ontology of living bodies. Since medicine cannot fully explain itself by understanding the body in purely mechanical terms, neither can human life be so explained. Furthermore, the ancient conjunctions of values and medicine are shown to have their roots in the common and unique functions of living bodies. Thus if a modified natural law theory were suggested by the structure of medicine, such a theory of commonalities would have to be tempered by attention to specificity. In other words, the structure of medicine, its condition of possibility, reveals that as absolute statements may be made regarding commonalities, these must be relativized somehow by the specificity and uniqueness of living bodies. It is for this ontological reason that etiology is more scientific than prognosis and therapy. Similarly, if health is a foundational value, an ethic of medicine must simultaneously consider both individual and social good, as both are rooted in the living body.

Since both health and illness presuppose a personal unity based on biological organization and historical identity, medicine suggests that individuality and personhood are activities of the body.[57] Thus personal identity, as many realists such as John Dewey have argued, is a symbolization of the body. In this symbolization, medicine presupposes the perfectibility of man, a condition it shares with ethics.

Finally, sorrow and death are part of the tragic condition of man. They are not transcended by medicine so much as made bearable. In this consists the nobility of medicine and its connection to the arts.

6

The Anatomy of Clinical Judgments

For it is uneducated not to have an eye for when it is necessary to look for proof and when this is not necessary.

Aristotle[1]

Introduction

In 1916 Richard Cabot, one of the most celebrated American diagnosticians, labeled his attempts to anatomize the process of differential diagnosis "a very dangerous topic–dangerous to the reputation of physicians for wisdom. . . . Physicians are naturally reluctant on such matters, slow to put their thoughts to paper, and very suspicious of any attempts to tabulate their methods of reasoning."[2]

Sixty years later, most clinicians remain reluctant to detail the process of clinical diagnosis and more than a little suspicious of those who do. Many still take refuge in the "art" and its exclusive mysteries, to resist formalization of their mental operations. In recent years, the "dangerous" subject has been boldly attacked by a few clinicians with unusual facility in the language of logic and statistics so that dissection of the tangle of science, art, and conjecture is now well underway.[3] They have been joined by statisticians, engineers, psychologists, and philosophers who are bringing the more

This chapter is based on a paper presented at the Fifth Trans-Disciplinary Symposium on Philosophy and Medicine: "Clinical Judgment," University of California School of Medicine, 14–16 April 1977. Now published as "Anatomy of Clinical Judgments" *Philosophy and Medicine,* Volume VI, D. Reidel Publishing Co., The Netherlands, pp. 169–94.

sophisticated techniques of their disciplines to bear on this important and complex question.

Physicians and philosophers have puzzled for a long time over the nature of the physician's enterprise. Its dissection began with the Hippocratic physicians, who first insisted on the primacy of observations of patients, refined by reason. They thus made medicine a natural science, separating it from both philosophy and religion, with which it had so long been intimately associated.[4]

Intuitive, hieratic, artistic, and even magical elements of the physician's enterprise were not so easily removed, however. Celsus, the Roman Hippocrates, spoke of medicine as an *ars coniecturalis,* conjectural art; William Osler, the modern Hippocrates, deemed it ". . . a science of uncertainty and an art of probability." Medicine has yet to become a science comparable in method and explanatory power with the laboratory sciences–though this is the expressed aim of some of our contemporary thinkers. We will deal with their position in a moment.

The puzzlement continues today in the growing tension between the scientific-actuarial and the artist-intuitionist models of clinical judgment.[5] Each view tries earnestly to understand, and thus to improve, the clinical enterprise. One seeks to transform the conjectural elements into respectable science by formal analysis in terms of probabilistic logic or decision theory. Meanwhile, the other declares the nuances of clinical judgment to be an art, insusceptible to formal analysis and improvable only by cultivation as one cultivates painting, music, or sculpture.

This chapter undertakes nothing so pretentious as the resolution of what seems to be a polemically seductive polarity in viewpoints. It takes the view that clinical decisions can be made more rigorous logically without reducing everything to algorithm and regression equations. While much of the process remains opaque and insusceptible to extant methods of formal analysis, this need not forever be the case.

Much of the polarization between explanations of clinical judgment seems avoidable if two significant features which have been neglected are sufficiently taken into account. First is the overriding fact that the whole process is ordained to a specific practical end–a right action for a particular patient–and that this end must modulate each step leading to it in important ways. A value screen is thus, in a way, cast over the entire sequence. Second is the fact that no unitary explanation or logical method can encompass the several different reasoning modes and several kinds of evidence acceptable in responding to the different kinds of questions the clinician must answer.

The description of clinical judgment offered must therefore take into account medicine's search for classifications in which an individual becomes a class instance. It must also include explanations of the real existence of causes and conditions of disease, the inductive process or "psychic shuttle" in which the physician forms hypotheses and tests conclusions, and the value screen governing the therapeutic intent of the process.

The aim of this chapter is *not* to countermand the general utility of scientific actuarial formulations or to offer in their stead a benignant eclecticism which allows equal place to the explicable and inexplicable–i.e., to the "science" and the "art" of clinical judgment. Rather, it hopes to locate more precisely the several reasoning modes useful at each of the sequential and simultaneous steps which eventuate ultimately in a clinical action. This localization constitutes the anatomy of clinical judgment, an essential foundation for further formalization of the process.

The complete process is a multistep, end-oriented concatenation of decisions demanding different types of reasons and reasonings which will justify a particular course of action for a particular patient, given that patient's existential situation at the time of the decision. Each step is shot through with uncertainties, some eradicable, some not. Selection of the "right" action requires optimization of these uncertainty states.

Inasmuch as the nature of the uncertainties varies, the logical instruments used to achieve a decisive judgment will vary also. Thus, the methods of deductive and inductive reasoning, of dialectic, ethics, and rhetoric are each appropriate to some step. These classic modes of persuasion and decision are all found in the medical enterprise. Prudent and judicious action, rather than a true statement of scientific law, is the end to which the whole is directed. Thus logical or epistemic modes of scientific evidence in the modern sense cannot suffice to cover all aspects of medical judgment.

Customarily, discussion of clinical judgment ends at the establishment of the most probable diagnosis, or at best at the selection of a treatment. The third step–whether the treatment selected ought to be instituted, how, when, under what conditions–is usually not formally analyzed. Yet, one cannot speak legitimately of clinical judgment without seeing the whole process, particularly the way the end conditions the steps that precede it.[6]

Four questions must be examined to sustain these assertions:

1. What is the character of the end of clinical judgment?
2. What questions must be answered in attaining that end?
3. How does the end project itself on each step–i.e., what kinds of reasons does it require?
4. What are the theoretical and practical implications of the proposed view of clinical judgment?

The answers bear, to some extent, on the difficult problem of a general theory of medicine. Such a theory must account for the full range of medical activity–seeking general laws of disease and treatment, but also taking specific actions in the interest of specific patients. Science, art, and right decisions infuse the several operations. But medicine justifies itself uniquely as medicine–as opposed to medicine as clinical or basic science, or as the art of performing medical acts–when it ends in a decision to act for, and in behalf of, a human who seeks to be healed.[7] To the extent that it identifies features which distinguish medicine from other human activities, the analysis of clinical judgment can contribute to the emerging structure of a theory of medicine.

Modes of Clinical Judgment

What Is the End of Clinical Reasoning?

When a patient consults a physician, he or she does so with one specific purpose in mind: to be healed, to be restored and made whole, i.e., to be relieved of some noxious element in physical or emotional life which the patient defines as dis-ease–a distortion of the accustomed perception of what is a satisfactory life. Usually some event has occurred–pain, lack of appetite, fatigue, trauma, a lump, spitting blood–some sign or symptom which exceeds a certain highly personalized threshold of tolerance in such fashion as to compromise, obstruct, or discolor the person's perception of the self and his or her health. At the point when this perception leads to the *need* to be healed, the person becomes a *patient*. This transition has two existential connotations crucial to this discussion. Becoming a patient is to become one who suffers (*Patior, pati*) and simultaneously one to whom something is done, a recipient as distinguished from an agent (O.E.D.).[8] The patient, then, is a suffering person who enlists the physician's aid in regaining a former state or a more optimal one.

It is important to interject here that the term "patient" does not necessarily imply a passive restoration in which the physician is the sole agent. The patient ideally also participates in the restoration. He or she is seen as bearing a burden of illness which requires some action or decision mutually arrived at for cure to take place. The patient can yield this moral agency to the physician only by direct mandate. Only in the rarest circumstances will the physician legitimately be the patient's moral agent.[9]

The end of the medical encounter, and the process of clinical judgment through which it is achieved, then, is restoration and healing. Some corrective, remedial, or preventive action is directed at what the doctor and the patient each perceive as a diminution of the patients' wholeness. The end is not a diagnosis, a scientific truth, testing a hypothesis, or evaluating a treatment, though the knowledge derived therefrom informs these processes in making the decision to act.

This point is important in distinguishing clinical medicine from an empirical science. Although the inductive process in modern science parallels the process of forming tentative hypotheses in medicine and the overlapping subject matter in these sciences, the decision to act colors not only the application of information but its very formation.

The clinical decision comes at the end of a chain of deductive and inductive inferences, serially modified by recourse to "facts" and observations–which themselves are usually, to some degree, uncertain. Truth and certitude are, therefore, almost always problematic. Out of the uncertain conclusions of earlier syllogisms, a decision to act must be taken which has a different character from the conclusions that precede it. The conclusions of the earlier reasoning chains become premises for further reasoning. This is the normal condition of scientific reasoning–a cumulative and progressive series of hypotheses and conclusions, always open to further recourse to fact and experiment.

Each clinical decision is, however, a terminal and unique event in that it cannot remain forever open and it is not universalizable. It must close on the selection of one or a series of remedial actions–or none. The action chosen must be the *right* one for this patient. That is to say, it must be as congruent as possible with his or her particular clinical context, values, and sense of what is "worthwhile" or "good." What the physician and the patient seek together is a judicious decision, one which optimizes as many benefits and minimizes as many risks as the situation will allow. The definition of risk is highly personal, and it turns on the patient's estimate of a danger "worth" running. The end is, therefore, not a general statement of the probabilities but a specific statement of what a particular patient *should* do.

If it is true that the end of medicine is a specific statement about what particular patients should do, then the end of medicine is irretrievably *personal*. This end cannot be overemphasized. A clearer conception of the end of medicine can aid recognition of the goals of the health care system as well as the criteria of good clinical decision making. The criteria of a right or good decision lie not in its certitude, rigor, logical or mathematical soundness, though the probability of a judicious action is enhanced greatly when these qualities inhere in the prior conclusion on which it is built. These qualities must be secured wherever possible, but they are not sufficient for a "right" decision. They can, on the view we are propounding, be displaced or modulated by the more complex criteria of a decision "good" for this patient: What among the many things that *can* be done *ought* to be done?

Clearly, value considerations and moral issues–for both the patient and the physician–can color the selection of the facts and reasons which justify placing one diagnosis over another, the justifications accepted for taking action, and the degree to which the physician persuades or the patient assents to the final decision. The end must, therefore, be understood in all its fullness, because it projects itself so forcefully on the entire sequence.

The primary end of clinical judgment–a right healing action for a particular patient–imposes an atmosphere of prudence on the whole process. To borrow a concept from Aquinas: Truth, for the practical intellect, is rightness with respect to human deeds, those dependent upon human will and intention. It thus differs from the truth of science, which is a certain conformity with the reality it seeks to explain, and art, with the product it wishes to produce.

It is the end of medical judgment which also gives authenticity to the profession a physician makes–to use his or her knowledge and skill to "heal," according to the fullness of meaning of the word for the patient. Not to keep that end paramount is to make an inauthentic–indeed, an immoral–profession. Medicine as medicine is, then, more than a clinical or basic science applied to individual cases. It is a particularized knowledge of prudent healing actions, dependent upon scientific methods and art but not synonymous with them.

Whatever formal analysis one favors–traditional syllogistics, the logic of probabilities, Bayesian conditional probabilities, decision analysis theory, information-processing models, or judicial algorithms–it must account for the modulation and shaping imposed by the end. This would be so even if a high degree of certitude were possible at every step. Usually, however, we deal with varying "degrees of belief," and the judicious choice of actions becomes an even more critical and sensitive activity, difficult to formalize and formularize.

What Questions Must Be Addressed and with What Reasoning Modes?

When a person becomes a patient in the sense we have defined that state, a whole series of questions becomes crucial for him or her as a knowing and valuing being. What is wrong? Is it serious? What will it mean to me? Can it be cured, and by what means? Is the cure worthwhile? What will it cost? What *should* I do? These and corollary questions must be addressed if the process of clinical judgment is to be a complete and authentic medical judgment. They are reducible to three *generic* questions: *What can be wrong? What can be done? What should be done for this patient?* (Fig. 1) Let us

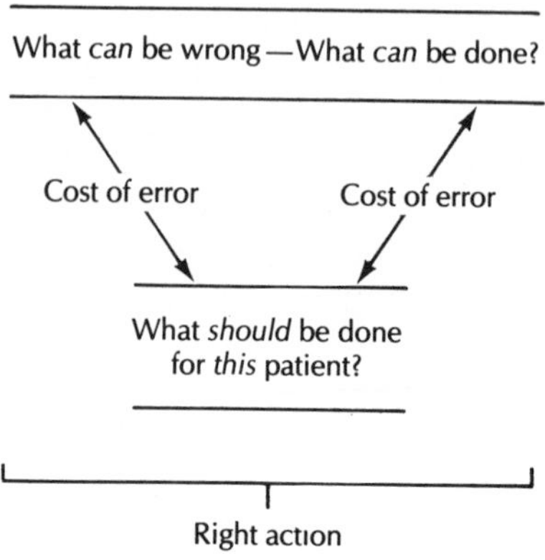

look briefly at each question to see the kinds of reasoning relevant to it and what kinds of justifications are acceptable. In the following analysis, we have distinguished three generic classes of questions which all occur simultaneously or at least feed into one another in real life. Thus, to underline the way in which each of the categories of questions is tied to the others, we have designed circularity into the schema of Figures 2, 3, and 4. It is especially important to retain the conception that the end enters into each step of the process of clinical judgment, although we can discuss its role only in a discrete portion of the chapter.

A. What Can Be Wrong?

This is the diagnostic and classificatory question–the first part of the process and the one which has received the most vigorous theoretical examination. Given the signs and symptoms presented by this patient, what classificatory patterns fit best? Of the possible patterns, which is most probable, and with what degree of certainty?

This part of the process most closely fits the scientific paradigm and under ideal conditions can yield a diagnostic conclusion with a high degree of certitude–i.e., the error rate approaches zero. The conditions for such certitude must be stringent, however. The input data of signs and symptoms must be reliably observed, standardized, and specified; the classificatory patterns must be equally reliably determined; the probabilities of different combinations of signs and symptoms must be derived from sufficient numbers and combinations of sets and subsets of signs and symptoms; laboratory and other ancillary data must be sensitive, accurate, specific, and precise. The rules of deductive or probabilistic logic must be followed rigorously.

In addition, a highly specific and sharply discriminating test is required–such as a biopsy, a fiber endoscopy, an angiography, or an enzymatic or immunological determination. Where all these conditions are met, *diagnostic closure* can be obtained. This means that all essential criteria for a diagnosis have been met. The diagnosis could even meet the test of scientific "elegance" if it is arrived at with an economy of steps.

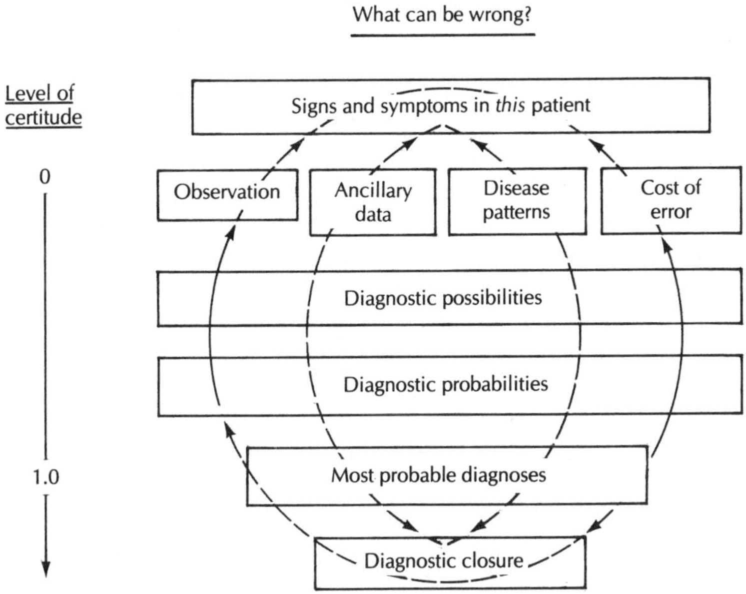

These rigorous conditions are only rarely satisfied in clinical reality. Bedside data are notoriously unstandardized and poorly quantified;[10] laboratory tests vary widely in sensitivity, specificity, reliability, and accuracy.[11] "Almost all data on the general incidence and prevalence of disease are inaccurate."[12] Considerable evidence and argumentation exist that even the concepts of "health" and "disease," and the categories in which we place the latter, are determined by and circumscribed in a context of values which would rule out absolute scientific rigor. Even less secure are estimates of the cost or error of a clinical act, so that the hopes of decision theorists to assign a numerical value to every nodal point in a decision tree are even less secure.[13] Finally, probability statements say something about the population of individuals sharing some common characteristic, but they are weakest in their description of the actual state of any individual in that population. Since clinical medicine deals with individuals, decision theory must also take into account the specificity of individual bodies–a difficult if not impossible task.

Thus, even when the rules of probabilistic logic are rigorously applied, the diagnostic conclusions are still open to question. More often than not, they are tentative "working" diagnoses and have more the quality of opinions than of scientific judgments.[14] Adding more empirical data may as easily compound an error as move the conclusion closer to the asymptote of a true statement. At some point, adding more tests adds only marginally to certitude, if at all.

Differential diagnosis consists, then, in the selection of some diagnoses as more probable, or more justifying of an action, than others. At some point, every diagnosis must proceed without further recourse to empirical input. The strength of the case for each diagnostic claim must be assessable and put in some order of priority against the others. Why, for example, is this chest pain due to angina pectoris and not to the fifty or more other kinds of chest pain? The selection must be made when all the empirical data are in, and further appeals to the empirical are either impossible or insufficient to bring us any closer to diagnostic closure. This part of the differential diagnostic process is not synonymous with application of the laws of statistical probability. Indeed, a critique of the statistical argument as one among other arguments is itself requisite.

The process of differential diagnosis is really most akin to the process of classic dialectic.[15] Each diagnostic possibility can be seen as a "claim"; the strength of arguments for and against each claim is evaluated; each position is clarified and set against its opposite; and the inherent logical probity of each is delineated. Dialectical discourse, properly conducted, becomes an internal soliloquy in which the clinician examines personal conclusions critically or tests them externally against colleagues or consultants. No new truths are discovered this way, and the dialectical end of an appeal to experience is possible. The process is, therefore, not "scientific" in either the classic or modern sense of science.

Differential diagnosis is usually addressed as synonymous with an assessment of relative probabilities. Yet part of the dialectical procedure is to examine the probity of the statistical method itself. When the facts are not determinative, we must establish which diagnostic claim has the strongest logical position. This is more akin to arguing a case in court than it is to proving a scientific hypothesis. The whole effort is to make one diagnosis sufficiently more cogent than the others so that it becomes a defensible basis for decisive action.

The dialectical process is especially important in science, where it has been shown that psychologically the tendency is to prove rather than disprove one hypothesis.[16] New possibilities are often uncovered only by disproving an existing hypothesis entirely. Dialectical discourse assures an adversarial stance which challenges the tendency to settle too easily for a merely "workable" hypothesis.

The traditional clinico-pathological conference was primarily an exercise in clinical dialectic. It has fallen into disrepute, yet it remains an invaluable way to teach the process of internal soliloquizing, which enables the diagnostician to examine his or her own reasoning critically when the possibility of adding more observations and tests no longer exists. Contemporary pedagogical opinion to the contrary, the dialectical discourse of a clinico-pathological exercise more closely approximates the clinical conditions of differential diagnosis than the scientific model of serial hypothesis testing.

In answering the first of the triad of questions that make up a clinical judgment, several different kinds of reasoning, and reasons, must be employed. To understand the pathophysiology of clinical manifestations, to define and apply a classificatory schema, "scientific" reasons are appropriate. To make general statements of probability for populations, statistical logic is needed. In differential diagnosis the rules of dialectic are the most pertinent. Uncertainty pervades every step of the diagnostic process, from its epistemological assumptions to its logical operations. Each of several reasoning modes is suited to optimizing different forms of uncertainty. In the next section we shall see how the practical end modifies each of these modes at every step.

B. What Can Be Done?

This is the therapeutic question. Once some decision has been made about the nature of the patient's problem, what kinds of actions could be taken to remove or ameliorate the probable disorder?

Here again, the process is in part, and under certain stringent conditions, scientific in character. When there is a verifiable data base on the course of the untreated disease, and its modification by drugs, surgery, diet, or other measure, the conditions for a scientific decision can be fulfilled. Equally indispensable is quantifiable and precise information about effectiveness and toxicity, since these must be weighed against each other before the decision is made. Under these conditions, closure on a therapeutic action can approach certitude. As certitude is approached, medicine more clearly involves causality.[17]

The therapeutic decision is easy to make when there is a spe-

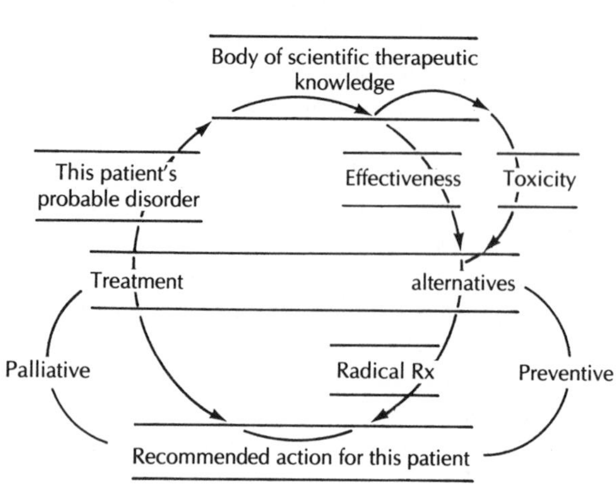

cific and highly effective treatment which demonstrably alters the natural history of the disease. Penicillin for pneumococcal pneumonia, isoniazide and PAS for tuberculous meningitis, vitamin B_{12} for pernicious anemia, and abdominal surgery for ruptured peptic ulcer are examples. In these instances, the action recommended can be scientifically validated, and it will, in most instances, take precedence over other considerations. The recommended procedure then becomes synonymous with right actions, and little choice is open to patient or physician, though the patient may in extreme circumstances reject even this kind of advice–e.g., refusal of therapy for religious reasons by Christian Scientists.

Unfortunately, to a much larger degree than in diagnostic decisions, genuinely scientific information in therapeutics is scanty. The many pitfalls of therapeutic trials have been the subject of a vast literature. They are generally acknowledged to be among the most difficult experiments to design, control, carry out, and interpret. Even for logical reasons, the randomized clinical trial has come under fire recently.[18] Especially problematic are the large number of therapeutic maneuvers which are not *radical*–i.e., they do not eradicate the causal agent or the offending process. Their benefits, if any, are marginal, and the ratio of risk to benefit often vacillates widely. One has only to recall the sad history of anticoagulants in myocardial infarction, the recent national dilemma about influenza vaccination, or the belated appreciation of the long-term vascular effects of oral contraceptives or antidiabetic agents.

Today, we must often decide whether to recommend complex, expensive, palliative procedures with unpleasant and dangerous side effects–as in chemotherapy for cancer. Data on effectiveness and toxicity are usually available in these circumstances, but the questions are of a different order: Is the discomfort worthwhile for this patient? Is length of life more important to him or her than its quality? These kinds of questions must rest firmly on scientific data, but that is only the foundation for a discussion permeated by the physician's and the patient's value systems. Actually, the more severe the illness, the greater the clarity of choice between values. The situation of choices for treatment of cancer is paradigmatical for all therapeutic decisions.

The therapeutic and prognostic domains may well be, as Feinstein (1967) opines, the truly unique elements of clinical "science." They are also the least secure scientifically. We simply lack the long-term observations of carefully selected patients in sufficient numbers to warrant secure prognostications about the course of a specific disease in a particular patient. It may be that long-term observations of specificity will never be enough to scientifically circumscribe therapeutics and prognostics. It was for this reason that we postulated a "wisdom of the body" with which the experienced clinician must grapple as the source of individuality. Without such data, it is impossible to ground the effectiveness of any agent scientifically unless it is so radically effective that a few cases will suffice. If untreated, mortality is 100 percent. Any change will indicate effectiveness, as it does in treating subacute bacterial endocarditis or tuberculous meningitis with specific antibiotics.

The choice of what action to recommend involves far more questions of value than diagnosis. The closer we come to the end of the process of clinical judgment–the right action–the less useful and less available is the scientific model. Reasoning becomes, in smaller part, scientific and probabilistic, and in larger part, dialectical–arguing one alternative against another without recourse to new factual data.

C. What Should Be Done for This Patient?

Once it is decided what the probable diagnosis is, and what treatment can be expected to be most effective and least harmful, the final question in clinical judgment is, *should* the treatment be used with this patient, and what alternatives can be offered? The right action–the best one for a given patient–is not always synonymous with the logically or scientifically deduced action. The amount and kind of information needed to secure a diagnosis may be quite different from that needed for decisive action. It is the task of the last stage of clinical judgment to make these distinctions with as much precision as possible.

Decisive action frequently involves the counterposition of what is good scientifically, what the physician *thinks* is good, and what the patient will accept as good. Scientific, personal, and professional values intersect each other and can be in conflict. The scientific evidence and the probability statements about diagnosis, prognosis,

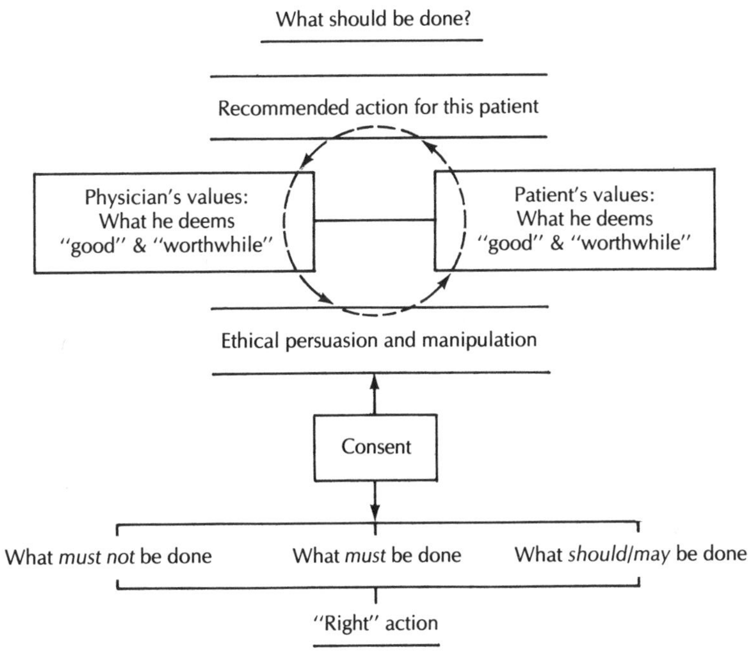

and treatment become arguments for or against a choice of alternatives–to do nothing, or, if something is to be done, what must be done, what may be done, and what should be done.

If, for example, the patient exhibits the minimal criteria for an acute abdomen, signs of intracranial pressure, or a stab wound of the heart, an operation *must* take place; with severe blood loss, bacterial endocarditis, tuberculous meningitis, or diabetic coma proper, medical therapy *must* be instituted. On the other hand, a nonstrangulated hernia, symptomatic gall stones, or mildly symptomatic benign prostatic hypertrophy are things that *should be* treated but may not be in the *must* category. Finally, hemorrhoids, varicose veins, or lipomata *may be* removed surgically; or mild hypertension, a cold, or sinusitis *may be* treated, but need not be.

When it comes to making the *right* decision–the *judicious* one for this patient–the categories of *must not, must, should,* and *may* can all shift, depending upon myriad factors in the patient's life situation and his or her notion of what seems worthwhile. In the more obvious situation–such as a Jehovah's Witness rejecting transfusion or a Christian Scientist rejecting surgery–the shift is to the *must not* category regardless of the canons of good science alone. In the more usual case, the categories into which a recommendation falls may shift several times in the course of the illness.

For one person, a lipoma, acne, or a sebacious cyst is something to be ignored; for another, it is a horrid blemish, so emotionally disabling that it demands removal. For this person, *may* becomes *must*. For an elderly man or woman, chemotherapy for disseminated cancer may mean a few months more of life, less pleasantly lived. For this patient, a *should* or *may* becomes a *must not*. For another person, the few extra months to do some essential things may make the rigor of treatment worthwhile. For still another, mild depression, anxiety, or headache is tolerable, and can be tolerated without resort to daily medications. To another, as the twenty-four million Americans who daily take mood modifiers will attest, even slight anxiety must be treated.[19]

The movement of persons among imperative shifts sets before us the lesson that medicine must look to trans-medical explanations for its justification. Imperative shifts from person to person show that therapy and prognosis depend upon the values of patients to a greater extent than diagnosis. Decisions to do what is right for particular patients, therefore, are unpredictable in a class because they vary from patient to patient. A discussion of "rightness" must, by consequence, include social and personal values.

In making the "right" decision for an individual patient, then, personal, social, economic, and psychological characteristics of the patient must be weighed. They clearly may modify, or even nullify, the scientifically cogent or logically consistent answers to the questions, What can be wrong? What can be done? Here, where we are closest to the end, the *telos,* of the whole process, scientific modes of reasoning and scientific reasons are least pertinent, and indeed, must be submitted to drastic revision in consideration of the patient's value choices.

The reasoning at this stage is mainly dialectical, ethical, and rhetorical. Physician and patient together must clarify the relationship of one recommendation with its opposite and weigh the reasons for each action. The ethical nature of the discourse at this point is obvious. Conflicts in the obligation of patient and physician to each other must be resolved before a "right" action can be settled upon. Where these conflicts are fundamental, the medical relationship may even be severed by either party, to be resumed with another physician.

Once the ethical and logical possibility and "strength" of arguments for one action over another are assessed by dialectic, then the reasoning becomes "rhetorical"–in the classic sense of artful persuasion, of relating a dialectically established decision to prudent action, generating belief of another kind from scientific or logical cogency, belief that this particular action should be taken in preference to all others.[20]

We enter here the delicate realm of how much persuasion is ethically defensible, how vigorously the physician should pursue a personal priority system. Does he or she believe that the scientifically recommended action must take priority? Is he or she a therapeutic enthusiast who prefers to "do something" rather than nothing? Does he or she think people should be "strong" and ignore a minor infirmity?

Likewise, the patient can use artful persuasion to modify the physician's scientific or dialectically secured recommendation to gain an action more congenial to a personal view of what is good. The patient's vulnerability can easily tip the resolution of conflict in the physician's favor. But these are subtle influences, as well, which can significantly shape the physician's final judgment. We will discuss the vulnerability of the patient in this regard in Chapter Eight.

The last question in the sequence then–what should be done?–the capstone question, which completes the whole structure, is the most prickly. Scientific and semiscientific conclusions of varying degrees of certitude are examined under a light strongly tinged with moral hues. The accessibility of the questions to scientific modes of reasoning declines, as does the degree of certitude, as we move from determining what *is* wrong, to what *can* be done, to what *should* be done. The optimization of several kinds of uncertainty remains a central concern even when the conclusions are scientifically defensible.

The intermingling of several modes of reasoning—clinical scientific, probabilistic, dialectical, rhetorical, and ethical—does not suggest immunity from explicit statements or deprecation of attempts to secure truly scientific conclusions. But it is warrant for setting limits on the utility of any of the current explanatory models—scientific, probabilistic, Bayesian, judicial simulation, decision analysis, inference, information, or catastrophe theories. Perhaps the fullest explication will come from some combination of these new theories and more classic modes of reasoning.

Projection of the End of Right Action on the Process of Clinical Judgment

We have seen that clinical judgment requires confrontation with three generic questions which end in a specific decisive action for a particular patient. Several interdependent reasoning modes are requisite and suitable to each question, and no one question is entirely isolatable from the others. We now turn briefly to a more specific delineation of how the end of right action projects itself upon the way the questions are answered. Accordingly, we might label this discussion "clinical prudence"—or medicine viewed as a virtue.

Whenever possible, the clinician will try to achieve diagnostic closure—i.e., to satisfy all the stringent criteria for certitude in locating the patient precisely in a classificatory schema. This is the admirable aim of scientific medicine, the ideal taught in academic settings. The more it is achieved, the better foundation there will be for the decision to act.

Many clinical realities can upset the orderly processes of diagnostic reasoning: the urgency of the patient's condition; the absence of a diagnostic set or algorithm which fits the presenting signs and symptoms closely enough; lack of specific tests to discriminate among probable diagnoses; incomplete or inconclusive probability estimates; limitations on data selection related to cost or geographic locale; unreliability of the patient as historian; and the dilemma of weighing the probability of a serious versus nonserious, and treatable versus nontreatable disorder, when none of these possibilities is definitely excludable.

Experienced clinicians deal with these commonly occurring inevitabilities with interpretative schemata, which enable them to act prudently on inadequate information and incomplete evidence. These schemata can be loosely regarded as rules of clinical prudence, empirically derived but certainly not mysterious sources of inspiration. We can examine a few of these (Fig. 5).

For one thing, the clinician thinks not so much of meeting the criteria for diagnostic closure but of how much evidence is "enough" to take an optimizing action. Diagnostic closure in streptococcal pharyngitis, for example, might demand a sore throat, plus cervical adenopathy, tonsilar exudate, and positive culture for Beta hemolytic streptococcus. The physician is justified in giving a specific treatment with penicillin on any combination of these signs and symptoms and positive culture. But he or she usually acts presumptively–taking a culture, treating, and awaiting the culture to determine whether to continue or discontinue penicillin. If the patient, however, lives in a family or school in which streptococcal illness is frequent or currently present, the most minimal clinical signs may justify treatment even without culture.

Acute abdominal pain is another example. It may result from a wide variety of conditions all of which can present similar signs and symptoms. Examples are: ruptured peptic ulcer, appendicitis, twisted

Figure 5: Some rules for clinical prudence

1. Act to optimize as many benefits, minimize as many risks as possible.
2. The serious and treatable *must* not be missed; the nonserious and nontreatable *may* be missed.
3. Use the clinical Ockham's razor: Don't multiply causes, diseases, tests, or treatments without justifiable necessity.
4. "Rest" the case for any diagnosis or treatment with reluctance.
5. Clinical skepticism is the only guard against the tyranny of the "established" diagnosis, or ancillary data, and the findings of colleagues (lab, x-ray, etc.).
6. Maintain a high index of suspicion for uncommon manifestations of the common.
7. "Hoofbeats don't mean zebras" unless zebras are in the vicinity.
8. When the data are in, continuing debate is the safeguard against error.
9. Recognize your own clinical style, prejudices, and beliefs about what is good for patients.
10. Be wary of hunches, intuitions, E.S.P. Gamble with your own fate, not the patient's.

ovarian cyst, strangulated internal hernia, mesenteric adenities, pancreatitis, and cholecystitis. Some of these conditions require immediate surgery, some delayed surgery, some no surgery, and in some, surgery is positively dangerous. The surgeon looks not for a definitive diagnosis but for the least signs of acute abdomen–spasm and rebound–which justify laparotomy. Only in this way can he or she assure that the treatable lesion is not missed. Each surgeon is allowed a certain number of normal appendices or negative explorations, provided he or she has *no* cases in which life-saving surgery is missed.

In every branch of medicine, there are disorders for which specific and dramatic treatments or genuine cures exist. They must not be missed. They shape the diagnostic process often out of proportion to their probability in a given case or in the general population. Some, such as pheochromocytoma, are rare; others, such as parathyroid adenoma, are relatively rare. Some, such as malaria, actinomycosis, or blastomycosis, are rare only in a particular locale. Still others were once common in our own society but retain their importance though found only infrequently; these include late manifestation syphilis, smallpox, leprosy, and diphtheria. No disease ever seems to have been completely eradicated.

The clinician's attention, therefore, may not be focused on getting all the information needed to fill out the most probable classificatory set in its entirety. Rather, more emphasis is placed on the information needed to take decisive action or to rule out the conditions which, in the interest of the patient's safety, must not be missed. The clinician must find justification for his or her actions, therefore, in terms of what is right and prudent for the patient. If a serious treatable disease cannot be adequately ruled out, therapeutic trial may be used as a diagnostic maneuver. In other words, specific treatment is undertaken for the serious disorder, and a diagnosis is arrived at indirectly by observing the effect. Such a course of action may be taken justifiably even if the probability of a less serious, nontreatable disease is much higher.

A corollary principle, which to some extent balances the search for the treatable and serious, is the admonition, "Don't look for zebras when you hear hoofbeats." This is a precaution against accepting the rare and esoteric even if the symptom complex is suggestive. Obviously, one cannot justify missing the more common, or losing the more unusual, manifestations of a common disorder in the search for the curable but esoteric. Of course, on the African plain, hoofbeats do mean zebras and not palomino ponies or quarter horses.

Equally influential is the clinician's Ockham's razor: "Plurality of causes and diseases is not to be assumed without necessity." Clinicians, particularly in the clinico-pathological conference, are conditioned to seek unitary explanations of signs and symptoms. This is another of the organizing principles which become part of the projective schema used by clinicians to select, screen, and weigh data and to justify their decision. The same advice is salutary in therapeutics: The rule of therapeutic parsimony states that treatments must not be multiplied without necessity.

Another rule of prudence is the cultivation of a "high index of suspicion"–another quasi-rational way to cope with uncertainties and avoid missing something. Clinicians who follow this rule are unusually sensitive to the most minimal criteria for a diagnosis. They use that sensitivity to open up previously unsuspected possibilities or to challenge what appears to be a more firmly established diagnosis.

Indeed, the most dangerous ground for clinical judgment is often not in making a new diagnosis but in maintaining an index of suspicion high enough to challenge what appears to be an established diagnosis. Physicians, like all humans, tend to rest their cases if no contrary position challenges it. They become locked into or even enamored of the patient's classification, which can render them unresponsive to the most obvious signals of a new disorder or an original diagnostic mistake. The more prestigious the original diagnostician or institution and/or the more respect one has for the colleague who made the diagnosis, the more seductive is this error.

Skepticism is, as Santayana so mordantly said, the "chastity of the intellect." An indispensable attribute of the prudent clinician is an untiring skepticism about every aspect of a diagnosis or treatment. Perhaps the greatest failing of the contemporary clinician is an overadulation for laboratory and x-ray data fed in by specialists, whose techniques grow more arcane and also more potent daily. Far too often, a right action is justified by the uncritical acceptance of a chemical determination, a biopsy, or an x-ray examination.

We do not intend to provide here a complete primer of clinical prudence. These few principles derived from experience illustrate how the intensity of the clinician's concentration on the end–a good decision for the patient–provides a projective schema which shapes every step of the process.[21]

Projective schemata are, of course, individualized and personalized. They summate what a particular physician holds to be "good" medicine. Which rules of thumb are selected, why, and how, are fascinating questions still very much open to logical and psychological examination. A whole series of attitudes of mind, logical and epistemological assumptions, are combined to make up a clinician's diagnostic and therapeutic "style," just as genuinely as the way words and phrases are used to make up a writer's style. The clinician's "style" is really a statement of the reasons he or she will accept as justification for a particular action, for setting aside certain probabilities, or for earnestly persuading a patient to take one course rather than another, equally earnestly propounded by a colleague.

Are these not the elements of the "art" of medicine, and are they not closed to precise analysis, the way the style of Horace or Camus is closed? We think not. We agree with Claude Bernard's warning against sole reliance on clinical instinct and clinical sense:

> Everyone knows in fact that habit may give a kind of empirical knowledge of things sufficient to guide practitioners, even though they may not always be able to account for it at first. But what I blame is willfully staying in this empirical state and not trying to get out of it.[22]

Each clinician's rules of prudence need more precise statement. Many are held in common by all good clinicians. Their utility or fallacy can and must be better studied. Most theoreticians have concentrated on the *normative* aspects of clinical judgment. We need to know more about the descriptive nature of the process: Who uses what justifications, and how do they benefit or imperil the outcome for the patient? How much difference in mortality, disability, side effects, and costs is there between a good and a poor decision maker?

Some physicians are therapeutic enthusiasts. They treat more often than not; they require less justification for using a medication than parsimonious therapists, who insist on demonstrable evidence of effectiveness and frown on the use of placebos or chemical coping for minor disorders. How much of "style" is simply peer conformity, personal intolerance of ambiguity, an obsessive compulsion to "prove" the diagnosis or to satisfy some idealized notion of what constitutes clinical "science"? Much of the cost of medical care, and even its outcome and satisfaction for the patient, can turn on how the clinician plays the "game" of clinical judgment.

The psychological components in different reasoning styles are coming under closer investigation.[23] We also need more extensive empirical descriptions of the reasoning habits of good and bad clinicians. What is the effect on outcome of different habits of reasoning? Which habits are crucial, which incidental, and which positively deleterious? In this era of concern for the quality of care, answers to these questions cannot be avoided for very long.

There remain, to be sure, certain features of clinical judgment which for the moment seem closed to explicit analysis. Clinicians have their undeniable moments of sudden insight and discovery. Some clinicians are more consistently accurate in their insights than others. What does happen at that precise moment when the clinician decides that there is enough information to make a diagnosis or take a decisive action? When does a set of signs and symptoms suddenly assemble themselves into a new classificatory pattern? When do a patient's clinical features suddenly fit a previously described pattern? When is the precise datum which will answer a puzzling question suddenly identified?

There is no reason to suspect that clinical diagnosis is unique in this regard. The phenomena of "insight" and "discovery" are common to both scientific and nonscientific endeavors. Polanyi and Lonergan have attempted to describe the deep epistemological structures and relationships which permit the leap from the obvious and the known to the previously unknown. Polanyi holds that scientific knowledge is never wholly explicit but resides in tacit understanding which provides the belief that makes thinking about a truth possible. Lonergan links belief to immanently generated knowledge. Polanyi's "discovery" and Lonergan's "insight" are likened by their authors to the "Eureka" of Archimedes.[24]

To what extent these epistemological notions can account for the obscure features of clinical reasoning is problematic. What must be avoided is the easy appeal to some special illumination peculiar to clinicians. Zimmerman's appeal to "genius," discussed in Chapter Five, is a case in point. To resort to terms such as "art" or "intuition" is to impede explication of a socially significant process. Whatever name we use to subsume the indefinable elements in the process, the effort to explicate them further is a moral as well as an intellectual responsibility. Understanding the process is, therefore, a moral pressure for the physician.

This warning against subjectivism is consistent with a major thesis of this chapter–that the nature of the end projects itself on the steps leading up to it. Everything in medicine ultimately is judged by its end–the healing of a patient–even those steps we think most immune to prelogical or subjective interpretation, such as pattern definition and recognition. In defining a disease pattern, for example, we must choose among an infinite set of properties–signs, symptoms, tests, etc. That resultant pattern is useful only if it includes a finite and manageable number of characteristics. In making the finite selection we apply a test of utility, related to the purpose of the pattern definition. That purpose is making a right decision for a particular patient.

In pattern recognition, the selection is similarly shaped by the end. We seek sufficient congruence with the pattern characteristic of the more serious or the more treatable disorder. We select in favor of patterns which optimize the decision for the patient even though they may be less defensible by the rules of logic or probability.

Statisticians, logicians, and engineers can help the clinician to apply criteria of validity to the character selected and to manipulate the sets once they are defined. But these aids are of limited use without definition of the purpose for which the classificatory set is to be used. Sokal, a pioneer in mathematical taxonomy, recognizes that in medicine we may limit ourselves to fewer characters than might be taxonomically desirable because we want those most pertinent to decisive action for a patient.[25]

Projective schemata shaped to the practical end of decision making are, to a significant degree, subjective. But they do not provide a warrant for a wholly subjectivist interpretation of clinical judgments. The schemata can themselves become objects of critical scrutiny. We can in fact often judge whether a clinical diagnosis, treatment, or decision is the right one by the outcome for the patient. The test of reality is always there in medicine, sharpening and correcting the projective schema and the values assigned in each of the more formal inferential steps. It is as Ernan McMullin said of the interpretive schemata of science, which contemporary philosophers of science have adduced to counter the ultra-objectivism of logical positivism:

> But what must be emphasized is that the skills of interpretation that help bridge the gap between the formalism of inference and the subjectivism of sheer personal assertion are themselves continually responsive to the demands of the objective order.[26]

In medicine we have more immediate and dramatic verificatory possibilities than in many other sciences (death, recovery, disability, complication, dissatisfaction). We can aim realistically, therefore, to reduce to a minimum the residuum of indefinable elements in each step of the process of arriving at clinical action. This applies even to the more subtle nuances in style which distinguish superior from merely average clinicians.

Some Theoretical and Practical Implications

Clinical judgment is what physicians use that most clearly distinguishes their enterprise from other human activities. If there is to be a theory of medicine, therefore, an understanding of clinical judgment must be a central element—though certainly not the whole of such a theory. At the very least, a theory of medicine would also include the role of the patient in the clinical relationship, the role of society, concepts of health and disease, and the role of values.

This chapter has argued two major theses which bear on a theory of medicine: (1) that clinical judgment is justified and defined by its end–a decisive action for a human in distress, and (2) that different kinds of reasons, and reasonings, are appropriate to the formulation of a right end.

There are several important implications for a theory of medicine, or at least its prolegomenon as well as medical education. Only two of these will be examined briefly: (1) Is medicine a science, an art, a virtue, or all three? (2) What information should a physician have?

MEDICINE–SCIENCE, ART, OR VIRTUE?

Sober has summarized the arguments on both sides of the art-science controversy.[27] He firmly identifies clinical reasoning with scientific reasoning. Given the view we have proposed, significant parts of the process unquestionably do fit both the classic and modern descriptions of a science.

In contrast to the paucity of theories of medicine, philosophers of science have until very recently been confident that they understood the nature of science. Beginning with Francis Bacon, and drawing on the methodology of Galileo, Newton, and Descartes, a canon of scientific activity has evolved. That canon contains three elements: a method, a body of knowledge built up by that method, and a post facto explanation of reality based on generalizable laws which relate the facts acquired by the scientific method to each other. Though there is a fairly frequent tendency to identify science exclusively with one or the other of these three elements, most scientists would agree that some measure of all three is intrinsic to their activity.

This traditional canon has been solidified by the logical empiricists of the twentieth century. It still dominates the scientists' perception of their own activity, if not the philosophers'. Of late, however, this canon has come under new criticism. Philosophers and historians of science have in recent years moved to broaden the concept of science to include historical, social, and psychological determinants. One example is Thomas Kuhn's debatable but interesting hypothesis that much of the "paradigm" for science is influenced by the nonrational and that paradigms may shift suddenly in logically incommensurable ways.[28] Another example is Stephen Toulmin's view that ". . . scientific methodology itself needs to be developed rather on a 'common law' model, by the collection and restatement of precedents: the logician cannot simply bring the tablets of the law down to the scientist from his axiomatic Sinai."[29] In far less moderate terms, Paul Feyerabend has attacked the very *notion* of method in science, arguing for an "epistemological anarchy."[30] He rejects any fixed scientific methodology that claims to evaluate hypotheses, pointing to the effectiveness of many "counter rules" in the history of scientific thought.

This controversy among the philosophers and historians of science has as yet made little impression on the physicians who see medicine primarily as "biomedical" science. They adhere to a notion of science which seems certain to be, in part, conceptually disarticulated. The theory of medicine has lagged seriously behind the theory of the other sciences. Instead of attempting to fashion a philosophy of medicine out of what is distinctive about its enterprise, many have equated it with "science," and with a notion of science linked to a traditional canon. That canon now seems a bit naive, or at least less than absolute. It links medicine to a concept of science already left behind by contemporary physics. But medicine and biology have characteristically lagged behind and have mistakenly placed their faith in an outmoded notion of physics.

Where the current critiques of science will lead is problematic, though greatly significant for our conception of medicine. Toulmin—properly, we believe—sees these critiques as part of the recurrent oscillation between the ideas of form and function. The outcome he predicts is a refurbished view of science, with some loosening and expansion of the traditional canons but not in so epistemologically radical a fashion as Feyerabend suggests. We can expect, then, some revision in those parts of medicine we call "scientific." It is hoped that a more rigorous pursuit of the theory of medicine will clarify its identity with, and its distinctions from, whatever new conception of science emerges, and not so belatedly as has been the case thus far.

For the present, at least, the dominant view among those who see medicine as science is the traditional one: Medicine is science, they argue, because it uses scientific method, inductive logic, data verified by a method, and theories based on data so obtained. How much of medical activity actually squares even with this traditional view?

Deductive, inductive, and retroductive inference are used to evaluate, interpret, and explain clinical observations.[31] Hypotheses are tested by further observation, experiment, and measurement, and reliability, accuracy, and standardization of data are sought, if not always achieved. These criteria of the scientific method are most clearly pursued in making the diagnosis and selecting and evaluating treatments. Medicine is even more convincingly a science when it seeks explanations of clinical phenomena in theories and mechanisms of disease. Medicine, then, fits Einstein's definition of science as:

> . . . the century-old endeavour to bring together by means of systematic thought, the perceptible phenomena of this world into as thoroughgoing an association as possible. To put it boldly, it is the attempt at the posterior reconstruction of existence by the process of conceptualization.[32]

But the principal aim of medicine, its distinguishing feature, is not the explanation of clinical phenomena, useful as this may be in raising the clinician's enterprise above empiricism and technicism. Explanations, in Einstein's sense, are the proper business of the sciences basic to medicine, but they are not synonymous with medicine. Medicine exists as medicine only when it engages in the full range of activities which constitute clinical judgment and which lead to decisive action in the interest of a particular patient.

In its complete expression as medicine, the clinician's enterprise embraces nonscientific as well as scientific reasons and justifications. This chapter alludes to the dialectical nature of differential diagnosis, the ethical construction in deciding what is "good" for a patient, and the rhetorical dimensions in the mutual persuasion essential to a decision taken jointly by patient and physician. The latter two are skills traditionally imparted by the liberal arts and humanities.[33] They may be exercised in medicine on data validated by the scientific method. While dependent upon the reliability of these data, medicine is not identical with the means whereby they are validated.

Is medicine, then, in any sense an art? Not as the term is used in the current art-science controversy. We have argued that clinical judgments must not be assigned to realms of the intuitive and ineffable, which find their source in a presumed special intellectual light possessed by clinicians. We would prefer to reserve the word "art" in medicine for the perfection of the things done by the physician–the craftsmanship without which the decisions taken would be improperly, unsafely, or clumsily done. The art of medicine lies in the degree of perfection each clinician exhibits in history taking, physical examination, performance of manipulative techniques such as surgery, and various diagnostic maneuvers–the work done.

Medicine *as* medicine is a process aimed at an *action* taken in the interest of a specific patient. Its chief aim is not discovery of the laws of nature. The end of medicine, its justifying principle, is, in the final analysis, a moral one: the "good" of a person seeking help. The choice of what ought to be done turns on questions of value, morality, and interpersonal dynamics. These questions can be studied scientifically, to be sure, but they cannot be defined by scientific considerations alone.

A large part of the physician's specific activity, as defined above, depends upon skills outside the traditional scientific paradigm. Whenever the physician resorts to experience or empirical data, he or she must use the scientific canon, but once the data are in, the physician's internal dialogue conforms more closely to the canons of the liberal arts. This does not mean that these canons are not susceptible to explicit analysis, but only that any unitary theory of medicine which identifies it exclusively with science is doomed to failure.

The work done must not consist of mindless activities. They are a *tekné* in the classic sense–knowing what to do, how to do it, and why one does it. While we did not consciously set out to use classic philosophy in interpreting the medical enterprise, we found that the thinking of Aristotle and Aquinas on the components of *tekné* was remarkably clear and suitable for application to clinical judgment and the medical relationship. Art and *tekné* were synonymous in Aristotle. Both involved reasoning: ". . . art is identical with a state of capacity to make, involving a true course of reasoning."[34] Aquinas, extending the Aristotelian notion, called art a *recta ratio factibilium,* thus distinguishing it from science, a *recta ratio speculabilium,* and prudence, a *recta ratio agibilium.* That is to say the undeviating determination of the work to be done (art) is distinguished from the undeviating determination of what is to be known (science) and the undeviating determination of the act to be done (prudence).[35] All three forms of *tekné* are disciplined activity.

If we carry this distinction a trifle further, medicine becomes not only science and art but also the virtue of practical wisdom—". . . a true and reasoned state of capacity to act with regard to the things that are good or bad for man."[36] Aquinas expanded the Aristotelian concept somewhat. He argued that while art provides the capacity to reproduce a good work, it does not assure that the product will be used for a good end. That remains to the virtue of prudence: "Consequently, prudence which is right reason about things to be done, requires that a man be rightly disposed with regards to ends."[37]

In this sense, then, medicine is both art and virtue. It is art since it is certainly concerned with the perfection of what it does—with the skills needed to make logically secure clinical decisions and to do the procedures decided upon. But it is also a virtue since it must make right choices about the ends and purposes for which the decisions and actions are produced. Medicine must not only perform well but also act well. It must choose what should be done to heal a particular whose good is the true end of the whole activity.

A quick scan of the many meanings of the word "art" in the *Oxford English Dictionary* illustrates how various are the modern transformations of the ancient meaning of the term. "Art" may now encompass the fine or liberal arts, any skill whatever, perfection of workmanship, studied conduct, and even wile and trickiness. When used in the art-science controversy, art is presumed to include a variety of elements not ordinarily explicable by science—the skill and judgment of the superior diagnostician, the affective humanism of the understanding physician, the bedside manner, "Aesculapean power," or simply the capacity to inspire confidence and trust. "Art" has become the rallying cry for all who are uncomfortable with the effort to make the physician's mental operation explicable in mathematical or logical terms—or to formalize it in a computer program.

As with the concept of science, parts of the medical enterprise are consistent with some part of these many notions of art, but others are not. In no case will the whole of medical activity fit under any one, or even the sum, of the varying connotations of "art." This is so even of clinical judgment, which some would delineate almost entirely as an art–insusceptible to explicit analysis.

Medicine is, then, all three–science, art, and virtue synergistically and integrally united in the clinician's daily activities. Hence the description of medicine as a mixed *tekné* must do until new categories of disciplines are formed. To disarticulate one member of this triad from the others is to dismember medicine–the essential feature of which is the special relationship each holds to the other. When this happens, one becomes a scientist, an artist, or a practitioner, but not a physician. Clearly, any unitarian formalization of the clinician's activity is bound to be misleading and defines part of what constitutes medicine but not the whole of it.

What Should a Physician Know?

One of us has explored elsewhere the many meanings of the term "medical humanism"–which can so easily become a slogan for whatever version of intellectual or practical activities we wish to justify.[38] Here it is only necessary to reiterate that medical humanism is both a cognitive and a compassionate response to the person of the patient. It embraces humanism as a set of cognitive skills largely derived from the humanities, and these are integral to the conception of medicine as science, art, and virtue. Humane medicine–indeed, moral medicine–requires that the physician understand the distinctions between these intellectual and practical activities; the kinds of reasons each may adduce; their limitations when applied to each others' realms; the different sources of their methodology; and the different subject matter appropriate to each.

If there is any merit in these proposals, they should be reflected in what it is physicians are expected to know. If medicine is a science, an art, and a virtue (in the classic sense), medical students will need a more explicit education in the nonscientific components of clinical judgment. The skills required for sound dialectical, ethical, and rhetorical reasoning modes must be more explicitly incorporated into professional education–especially in the clinical contexts within which decisions for patients are being made. The liberal arts and the humanities, even though they might have been presented in premedical studies, need vigorous refurbishment in medical education, where it will become more obvious to students that they *need* the liberal attitudes of mind to function fully as physicians.

The liberal arts have a legitimate place in medicine, not as gentle accoutrements and genteel embellishments of the medical "art," or even to make the physician an educated person. Rather, they are as essential to fulfilling the clinician's responsibility for prudent and right decisions as the skills and knowledge of the sciences basic to medicine.

These are very good reasons for reinfusing the liberal arts into medical education in addition to, but not necessarily to replace, the liberal education in the universities. Premedical education is shallowly rooted for a variety of reasons. The pressure for admission to medical school converts nonscientific subjects into obstacles to be endured rather than essentials for an educated life. Similarly, the humanities themselves may have become too specialized to fulfill their functions as instruments of the liberal arts. For this reason, one of us has developed an "Ethical Work-Up," a process by which students can clearly learn the discipline of ethical reasoning without the requirement of becoming specialists in ethics.[39] If the humanities are to aid medicine, much more attention will have to be paid to the process of disciplined thought present in these subjects, and less to their content.

Appreciation of the humanities may come more slowly than in the sciences—usually only after young physicians have had some experience of the moral nature of so many of their decisions. Then the intellectual constraints of a life dedicated to professional studies are only belatedly perceived. For all these reasons, the liberal arts and the humanities are today being taught as part of a medical education in a significant number of schools.[40]

The full implications of the anatomy of clinical judgment for the philosophy of medicine cannot be examined further in this chapter. Clearly a theory of medicine must account for this, the physician's most characteristic activity. Hippocrates was partially right to make medicine a natural science; Celsus to call it a conjectural art, and Osler a science of uncertainty. Any theory of medicine must accommodate all these elements, and in the special way demanded by the need to make specific decisions for particular patients. A theory of right thinking, right doing, and right acting must then be integrated. The theory of medicine must also be shaped by the end to which all medical activity points–a right healing action–for that is what defines medicine uniquely.

> It is a simple fact but almost universally ignored in modern thought that when one loses sight of the end of one's thought and action, the thought and action waver between fanaticism and futility.[41]

Conclusion

It is well to pause in the process of our argument to note a critical distinction between morality and ethics. Throughout this chapter, we have referred to medicine as a moral enterprise. It is a moral enterprise because its end, making right decisions about patients with those patients, involves values. This is not to claim, however, that every medical decision is ethical simply because it is aimed at making right decisions. The ethical component of medicine enters as one moves beyond medicine into a philosophy of medicine which attends, in part, to examining judgments about which right decisions were good.

Thus we are not claiming that the medical enterprise must completely rely upon ethics for an outline of the good. The interior process of clinical judgment, depending as it does on numerous disciplines, is guided by the end of making correct judgments on behalf of patients. When this process is correctly followed and the patient participates fully, the clinical judgment made is "right." But not all right decisions are good, even though every good decision must be right. A critique of the good is the proper domain of ethics. Hence ethics enters medicine and is used by medicine for a reasoned critique of right decisions insofar as they are ethically good.

In short, clinical judgments are both medical and inherently moral. Their probity does not depend upon ethics or a trans-medical discipline. However, discussions of good or bad clinical judgments may also involve an ethical component, in which case ethics is used by medicine to critique itself. The answer to the question, why should medicine do no harm–i.e., aim at the good? is attempted in Chapter Eight.

II

Applications to Moral Agency: Individual Ethics

7

Discretionary Space in Professional Judgment

A central problem in technological societies is the judicious containment of the expert. Can we benefit from his special knowledge without becoming subservient to it? This dilemma is especially clear in the ambivalent images of the physician in contemporary society. At times, he is the revered benefactor; at others, a threat to human values. Both images grow out of the enhanced powers over life, death, and the future of the species conferred by scientific advances upon the physician.

We are today witnessing drastic revisions in the way physicians relate to patients, hospitals, and the community. What these relationships will be in the next century is problematic. But it is certain that the character of medicine, at least its social character, is undergoing profound alteration. Just as the rise in empirical sciences created a quantum leap in our knowledge about the world, so too a rise in the social forces surrounding clinical judgment today may alter the nature of medicine itself. While we do not think the present situation changes the character of medicine as a clinical relationship, we do see some signs, explored in this chapter, which may alter the logic of judgments made within this relationship. If medi-

Portions of this chapter were delivered as a paper at the Fogarty International Center, November 1976. This chapter is also a revised version based on "The Expansion and Contraction of 'Discretionary Space'," Department of Health, Education and Welfare Publication No. (NIH)77-1288, *Priorities for the Use of Resources in Medicine,* 1976.

cine cannot entirely be classed as a science, then its mode of reasoning cannot be completely scrutinized and controlled through institutional and political policy. Yet the use of a pluralistic value system and the social impact of medicine call for some rational controls.

We must use a thematic notion to help unravel the interplay of sociocultural, economic, and political forces converging on the physician's social position today. Because of the array of possible alternatives, we propose the idea of discretionary space as a leitmotiv.

By "discretionary space" we refer to the degree of latitude in decision-making society accords its experts–those with special knowledge and skill to meet human needs. We permit them, in certain circumstances, to determine the nature of our needs, how they should be met, and to a considerable degree what is good for us. The breadth of this decision-making space is proportional to the uncertainty and the ambiguity of the tasks rather than their complexity. It is narrowest in the technical fields, where manuals and routines define the course to be followed–even in emergencies. It is widest in the professions such as law, education, and medicine, where value choices and discretion are integral to the personal nature of the decision to be made.

Our central thesis is this: A very wide latitude in discretionary space and a relative inviolability have defined the traditional relationships of physicians to society. It is this latitude, under the impact of today's cultural and political forces, which will reshape these relationships in the future. To advance this thesis will require examination of the following matters:

1. The sociohistorical determinants of discretionary space.
2. The forces tending to narrow that space today.
3. Their current impact on the physician's relationship to patients, other health professions, hospitals, and the community.
4. Their impact on the image of the physician in the twenty-first century.

Sociohistorical Origins of Discretionary Space

Modern physicians and primitive medicine men derive their special social position from the fact that they are necessary mediators between men and the forces of nature which can cause disease. Each is accorded a measure of freedom in decision making, because each in his way commands knowledge which helps explain illness and assess what measures are required in a particular patient to mollify, reverse, or eradicate its causes.

There is a very significant difference, however, in the social matrix within which the medicine man and the modern physician exercise their discretionary latitude. The medicine man is bound in a tightly defined nexus of prescribed rituals of divination, chant, trance, dance, or whatever measures have been handed down to him in the mysteries attendant on his own initiation rites. He deviates from those rituals at peril to himself and his patient. The constraints within which he operates are preset and unchangeable. While he tells his society what is right or wrong, he does so within a commonly held value system which he shares and interprets on behalf of all. His discretionary space is very limited.

The modern physician makes his decisions within a space far less specifically prescribed by social mandate. Indeed, since the Hippocratic era, his discretionary space has become virtually open-ended. In the treatise *On Ancient Medicine,* the Hippocratic physician insisted on freedom from magico-religious and even philosophical constraints.[1] Observation, reason, and moral considerations became the bases for his actions. The exciting thing about reason based on observation was its promise of new knowledge, and thus the expansion of human capabilities. As a result, a wide variety of theories of medicine and therapeutics emerged in the Hellenic and Roman world. They replaced the carefully standardized modes of treatment to which the medicine man–priest had been previously confined.

The utility of discretionary space was obvious. Society granted the physician this latitude to gain the benefits of the freedom which reason, in place of myth and magic, conferred on the doctor. The profession was permitted to challenge accepted theory, to devise new treatments, and even to experiment. Technical authority was established so that the physician might judge what was best for his patient, not just what ritual he might apply. Indeed, "Do no harm," as a moral claim on medical activities, is necessarily linked to a freedom to make clinical judgments.

Greek medicine therefore defined for itself a moral framework which made the patient-physician relationship a private affair. The physician became a benign, paternalistic figure who still retained his old hieratic as well as his new rational capabilities. He determined what was good for his patient and disclosed only so much of his reasons or his art as he thought appropriate. He assumed moral as well as technical authority, declaring his relationship with the patient a sacred precinct–guarded by confidentiality and not to be intruded upon by anyone beyond the patient or his family.[2]

This Hippocratic image, combining moral and technical authority paternalistically applied, has shaped the physician's image for the last 2,500 years. It remained essentially unchallenged until very recent times. Progressive infusions of experimental science have enhanced the physician's powers beyond all expectations. The physician is still something of a magician and a mediator with mysterious forces, like the medicine man, but with a profound difference: Even the ends and purposes to which his new powers are put rest largely in his hands. He is free of the intricate social-religious structures that confined the methods and purposes of primitive medicine.

In the mid-twentieth century, the long process of secularization and rationalization of medicine came to such fruition that the physician now has impressive control over procreation, life, death, and human behavior. His actions are changing demography and economics and challenging mankind's oldest values and taboos. Endowed with an ever-wider discretionary space, and assuming moral as well as technical authority, medicine can mold human life to goals and purposes without the societal controls of previous eras.

The capabilities, actual and possible, of contemporary medicine have now forced society to the realization that the authoritarian, autonomous Hippocratic image, with its almost unlimited freedom for decision making is no longer tenable. The conviction has grown steadily that the traditional discretionary latitude of the physician must be critically examined and contained. Ackerknecht, comparing primitive and modern medicine, put the matter bluntly: "While it [medicine] once taught society what is right and wrong, society now has to tell it what is right or wrong."[3]

Forces Leading to Containment of Medicine

The process of narrowing the autonomy and discretionary latitude of the medical profession is already well underway. The forces generating this momentum, over the last decade particularly, are too well known to require anything but brief mention. Their confluence in the late sixties came at the same time that the dangers, as well as the promise, of medical progress were becoming most evident. The effect on the physician's relationships to individuals and society has already been profound.

First, there is the fact of increasing education of the general public, together with the widespread popularization of medical news in the media. More people now understand the achievements, but also the more remote social impact, of every aspect of medical science and practice.

Second, the assertion of civil rights in democratic countries has encouraged increasing interest in the rights of self-determination for every citizen and public participation in decisions which affect the general welfare. The democratic ideal has also challenged the claims of any group, professional or otherwise, to special privileges.

Third, abuse of power, economic insensitivity, and overzealous pursuit of self-interest in institutions and professions–medicine included–have been frequent enough to evoke public cynicism, and calls for regulatory mechanisms have become frequent and powerful.

Fourth, engineering and physics had already produced an atomic bomb, demonstrating for all time that experts could make the most awesome decisions for all mankind without forewarning and certainly without public participation. An about-face occurred in the public's trust in science.

Fifth, health had become, next to defense, the largest single category of expenditure in many nations. Allocation of resources in a constricted economy within health, and between health and other social needs, is now a critical issue.

Sixth, the homogeneity of moral values which characterized the nation for so long has given way to a pluralistic and largely relativistic value system. Under such circumstances, no person or institution, not even the physician, could presume to make moral decisions for another. This problem is so intimately tied to professionals as moral agents that we devote a separate chapter (Chapter Nine) to its analysis.

Seventh, the intermingling of values with technical decisions created conflicts of interest among society's experts. Increasingly, it has become clear that it is in the public interest to disentangle these two kinds of questions. The patient's encounter with the physician exemplifies an especially sensitive intersection of value systems, in which the physician's technical expertise is both a benefit and a threat.

Finally, the move to limit the physician's discretionary space has become confused by the parallel "medicalization" of a whole host of human problems not usually included in the medical domain.[4] The tensions created by the contradictory thrust of those paradoxes will occupy us a little later.

Impact of These Forces on Physician Relationships

The interaction and mutual reinforcement of these forces have already caused serious constrictions in the autonomy of medicine at every level of decision making. They are transforming the way physicians relate to individual patients, other health professionals, hospitals, society, and even other physicians.

Relationship with Patients

The traditional stance of benevolent authoritarianism in the patient-physician encounter is increasingly under scrutiny and challenge. More patients want full disclosure of the therapeutic alternatives. Legal opinion is unanimous in requiring informed consent not only in experimental procedures but in the ordinary therapeutic encounter. The patient's "Bill of Rights" demands that the patient be informed of what is to be done and what the outcome and dangers might be. He must also be given the opportunity to reject treatment.

A sharp separation of the moral and technical agency of the physician is developing. Indeed, the suggestion has been made that physicians should make their values and beliefs on key issues known in advance.[5] In this way, the patient can more properly exercise his own moral agency.

Increasingly, the physician-patient relationship is being opened to scrutiny by the law. Its "sacred" character is no longer inviolate, especially if the patient's desire for partnership and preservation of his values are to be secured. Even the ancient right to confidentiality can be compromised when the public interest demands. Ethical libertarians assert that the only difference between patient and physician is an information gap. Once this is filled, the patient can make his own choices.[6] They strongly deny any sacral character to the relationship and unequivocally abide no paternalistic modulation of what the patient can know. The physician's major responsibility is to close the information gap.

The current search for a more humanistic basis for professional ethics centers on the vulnerability of the sick person to the loss of his moral agency in medical decisions, a point taken up in the next chapter. Closing the gap in power and information between physician and patient to the fullest extent possible would seem to be a moral obligation of the physician. The physician-patient relationship is taking on the quality of Buber's "I-Thou" relationship, with the decision coming from understanding between persons rather than being made by one for the other.

Relationships with Other Health Professionals

In addition to sharing authority and decision making with the patient, the physician in the last decade has also been compelled to share authority and functions with other health professionals. We need mention only a few examples: the expanded role of the nurse as family nurse practitioner and child health specialist; the appearance of the physician's assistant, in both primary care and specialized medicine; the emergence of the clinical pharmacist; and the increasing independence of medical technologists, physical therapists, occupational therapists, medical administrators, and others in the allied health fields.

The concept of the health and medical care team has been greatly expanded in an effort to make optimal use of all available health manpower. While the physician has, in general, been the captain of the team, even that primacy is being challenged in the interests of improvement of patient care and the importance of joint decision making. Chapter Eleven examines the moral implications of this team health care role.

Health care teams are still a functional reality only in a limited way, but already they indicate the need for an alteration in traditional decision-making processes. They raise ethical and moral questions about the assignment and distribution of responsibility for collective medical actions.[7]

Such previously privileged functions as the history and physical examination, supervision of medication regimens, the education and instruction of the patient, the suturing of lacerations, and the like are being performed by health professionals other than physicians.

This expansion has been particularly noticed in the neglected fields of primary care, preventive medicine, care of the chronically ill, and patient education. The emergence of health care teams has added another measure of restraint on the autonomous position of the physician, whose real dependence upon the function and the cooperation of other health professionals has weakened his absolute hegemony. The discretionary space which the physician occupies has not only narrowed but is becoming more crowded, as other health professionals demonstrate their capabilities in meeting specified needs of patients and of society.

Relationship to Hospitals

Over the past one hundred years, the increasing technical complexity of medicine has made it essential to establish the hospital as the physician's workshop and laboratory. There he could concentrate expensive equipment, have access to operating rooms, anesthesia, nursing, pathology, and all the other services which make scientific medicine possible. Whereas in earlier times in Europe and in the early history of the United States, the hospital was reserved for the destitute, the hopelessly ill, and the dying, it became in more modern times the place for cure and the necessary locus for the performance of the most complex medical procedures.

Until a few decades ago, the physician dominated the institutional life of the hospital. He was frequently responsible for its planning, establishment, operation and, in many cases, financing.

Physicians became hospital directors, were dominant figures on boards and executive committees, and in general established the medical model as the criterion for decision making. Under this aegis, standards of quality control and peer review were established and practiced with varying diligence. But the prerogatives of the individual physician, and particularly the inviolability of his decisions with reference to a specific patient, were preciously guarded.

The last few years have seen a remarkable change in the institutional situation of the physician. The administration of hospitals has been transferred to laymen trained specifically as medical administrators and managers of complex institutions; boards of directors tend to exclude physicians entirely, or add them only in small numbers. A whole tier of nonphysician middle managers has emerged who are responsible for the management and coordination of all the services physicians use in a hospital.

Even more directly limiting the physician's discretionary space has been the appearance of a series of institutional measures to insure control of the quality of care. Tissue committees, formulary committees, pharmacy and therapeutics committees, credential committees, utilization reviews, medical audits, admission and discharge clearances, requirements for continuing education, and a variety of other measures all place the physician's decisions clearly within a monitored context in which institutional goals and policies can override individual physician prerogative.

At the same time, communities and boards of trustees have begun to take more seriously the issue of accountability. Boards of directors have tentatively begun to assert their legal, moral, and social responsibility, not only for the fiscal soundness of the institution but also for the quality of professional care provided within its walls. Legal decisions have spelled out the fiscal and legal responsibility of board members for the actions of all who perform within the hospital–physicians as well as all other staff members.

Now a moral dimension to accountability is beginning to appear. Abortion, euthanasia, informed consent, and the many other ethical issues consequent upon medical progress have raised the question of moral responsibility of trustees for protecting the personal values and quality of participation of those who are treated therein. The hospital is, in effect, becoming not simply an administrative and fiscal agent but also a moral agent, a point we discuss in Chapter Eleven in the section "Social Ethics."

Relationship to the Community

The changed relationships to patients, to other professionals, and to the hospital are all occurring within a matrix of political and economic forces whose impact is felt in every aspect of medical practice today. This is the era of consumerism. Members of the community are demanding some voice in how the costs of medical care are generated, how resources are allocated, and how efficiently institutions are managed. The hospital and its board of directors, in addition to requiring accountability of those who work within the institution, must also themselves be accountable increasingly to the public and to a multitudinous host of external regulatory agencies.

It would be inappropriate here to enumerate the large number of federal, state, and local regulatory agencies covering every aspect of hospital operation which have emerged over the past several decades. There are in some states about one hundred fifty agencies regulating some facet of hospital operation. One need only refer to requirements for certificates of need for building hospitals, review of costs and hospital rates by insurance and cost commissions in the state, and the whole apparatus of PSRO legislation to demonstrate how much the discretionary space of the hospital as an institution has been narrowed. This in turn, of course, has of necessity had a very significant impact on the decision-making latitude of the physicians who operate within the hospital.

The history of health planning legislation since 1966 has moved toward progressive translation of the locus of resource allocation from the physician and the hospital to external agencies. Here we can mention Regional Medical Programs, Comprehensive Health Planning, HMO legislation, and the most recent HSA legislation—PL93–641, whose effects are yet to be fully comprehended. It is significant, however, to point out that PL93–641 has spelled out ten goals for the nation's health care system. Ostensibly it is these goals against which hospitals, other health care agencies, and physicians and other health workers will ultimately be judged for their social relevance.[8] We have here an explicit determination of priorities and goals for the Western health care system.

One need add to this only the requirements of a variety of third-party payers, the role of voluntary health agencies, and the increasing emphasis on mandatory continuing education to appreciate the fullness of the extent to which the physician's every activity has become regulated and circumscribed in a way only vaguely imagined two decades ago and totally unimagined one hundred years ago.

The net effect of these regulatory trends is to transform the self-regulating, elite, traditional image of the physician into that of a functionary in a quasi-public utility. In this model, he becomes a necessary technical expert who provides the factual base for policy decisions. He is accorded no special authority in selecting goals, priorities, or alternatives. In fact, the medical model itself is under attack as a means of meeting society's major health needs. Lalonde's careful analysis of the health needs of Canadians, and the more polemical assaults of Illich and Carlson, attest to the growing conviction that medical care and a nation's health are not synonymous and may even be antithetical.[9] Like all experts, the physician is suspected of propagating self-interest when he prescribes for the larger social and health needs of the nation.

The Twenty-First-Century Physician—The Emergent Image

Every one of the physician's most cherished sociocultural relationships has been drastically altered over the last decade. There has not been sufficient time to absorb their full significance for society and the physician. Any attempt to do so is perilous, since the change in the physician's image cannot be interpreted in isolation from the dynamics of new ideas and values now sweeping our society.[10] The weakness of prophetic undertakings notwithstanding, some modest look at implications is unavoidable unless we expect to abandon any hope of anticipating difficulties and adapting consciously to them.

There is no doubt that the force responsible for the profound metamorphosis of the physician's image will continue to operate. More startling technical feats can be expected as medicine continues to pursue high technology, and this means that the drive to limit discretionary space will continue.

Society therefore will have to grapple more directly with the extraordinarily difficult problem of judicious containment of its experts, physicians among them. We must continue to take advantage of the benefits of biomedical capabilities without yielding to any profession the determination of purposes and values in their individual and social application. If discretionary latitude is too severely narrowed, the good of society can be severely compromised. Already there are signs of unwillingness to depart from standardized diagnostic and therapeutic regimens; testing of new pharmacologic agents has been materially slowed by federal regulation; fear of malpractice suits leads to indiscriminate use of laboratory tests in anticipation of cross-examination by a hostile lawyer; even those minor modifications of a standard regimen which every mature clinician undertakes to individualize care can be inhibited. Where is the boundary between judicious containment which will protect the patient and society against the potential tyranny of the expert, and injudicious containment which reduces professional to technical decision making?

There is least danger in limiting physician discretionary latitude in his relationships with society as a whole, a little more in his relationships with the hospital, and the most in his dealing with the individual patient. As we have shown, the essence of medicine is its concentration on particularities–on the uniqueness of each patient encounter. The move to patient participation and respect for the patient's value system is healthy. A more adult relationship will result based on mutual respect for the truly inviolate realm of personal moral choices. More and better disclosure of technical details should enhance rather than hamper the physician's decisional prerogatives. Nonetheless, the exercise of clinical judgment is too easily stifled. It is a precious commodity of the experienced clinician–too often alluded to, too rarely present, yet indispensable when the accepted regimen must be modified, abandoned, or replaced.

Too close monitoring of every facet of patient care, or requiring records of every utterance or maneuver, can consume precious time and energy. We need, instead, to know better what selective indicators of quality, and what key assurances of patient consent, we should monitor. A certain measure of trust is essential in anything so delicate as clinical medicine. But it must be earned, and it must be assured by some system of monitoring, hopefully one which does not assume noncompliance at the outset.

Sharing of authority and responsibility between the physician and other health professionals, and diminishing his pristine primacy, introduces new problems. The simplicity and clarity inherent in one source of information and decision making is necessarily lost. The patient can become even more completely lost in the shuffle and shuttling of functions among health team members. Who is responsible for preserving the patient's humanity and sanity?

While the development of the health team is an undoubted necessity, its size must be controlled and the distribution of responsibility more clearly defined in advance. The number of types of health professionals can be reduced by consolidation of functions and removal of overlapping activities. We need a new ethical code which embraces all health professions and emphasizes the corporate ethical obligations each of us sustains when he acts as part of a collectivity. An argument for the normative nature of that code is found in Chapter Nine of this book.

There is no likelihood that we can obviate these difficult and tendentious issues by a romantic return to the old Hippocratic image. Nor will it suffice to teach again what is so vaguely described as "the art of medicine." The image of the physician has been transformed irrevocably, and the most sensitive indicator of that change is the degree of freedom he is allowed for decision making. The individual patient deserves a more democratic partnership, one in which he may choose between alternatives based on his own definition of health and the good life. The hospital must meet its responsibility for accountability and for assuring the authenticity of institutional goals by more closely monitoring both technical and moral decisions. The community should have the major responsibility for all the larger issues of what constitutes the major social goal of medicine; which goals take priority; how they are justly distributed among citizens; and how much shall be spent on high technology, how much on research, and how much on meeting less dramatic but more voluminous primary care needs.

Society, however, is imposing a confusing and contradictory set of obligations on medicine, producing a dilemma which must soon be resolved. On the one hand, regulation of the physician's decisions is expanding at every level; on the other, we are "medicalizing" every human problem: alcoholism, crime, family and marital relationships, learning disabilities in children, auto accidents, prevention, dietary misbehavior, smoking cessation, drug abuse, job satisfaction, leisure, and so on. Obviously, the technical achievements of modern medicine raise hopes that mankind's oldest problems can be similarly alleviated. But that expectation is not consistent with the equally strong desire to contain medicine–a move inspired by those outside medicine who fear its unlimited hegemony, and those within it who do not see these new areas as legitimate medical concerns.

It seems certain, too, that a profession operating within a restricted discretionary space may attract the less independent, less enterprising, albeit safer practitioners. Is this an unmixed blessing? Or is the answer to educate large numbers of physicians who will operate within clearly defined decisional boundaries, and a very small number who are allowed to exert wide discretion? If so, do we not create another even more dangerous elite corps–those officially mandated for wider latitude in decision making?

Some have begun to call for the physician to assume a role of advocacy for the patient and for alleviating the public health deficiencies and social injustices of the nation. How consistent is the role of advocate with the parallel demand to limit the physician's freedom of decision, especially in value questions? Being a patient advocate will require an even more sensitive assessment of what is good for the patient and society. The physician's definition of what is good may not be at all consistent with society's definition. Establishing a normative medical ethics is therefore even more critical today than in the past. This practical task is the subject of the remaining chapters.

The demythologizing of medicine and the erosion of its hieratic image are not without their dangers. The capacity of the physician to convince, and even to cure–especially with the disorders of emotional or self-limited nature–are often dependent upon the exhibition of "Aesculapean" power. This is especially so with patients who for reasons of cultural orientation or educational deficiency cannot, or prefer not, to enter into a decision-making partnership with the doctor. In the long run, it is preferable to reduce the hieratic role, to secularize and rationalize it. This will continue to be the dominant trend. But what about the interim?

We cannot escape the conclusion that the physician will never again be the sole decision maker, the priestly bearer of technical and moral authority, the dominant figure in all his relationships that he was even twenty years ago. What seems to be occurring is a rather curious return to a sociocultural image very much like, and yet very much different from, that of the primitive medicine man—alike in the sense that the physician is still seen as a mediator with mysterious forces which his knowledge can control (natural causes now, rather than demons). Also, he is being deprived of the discretionary space he gained when medicine separated itself from religion and philosophy. Like the medicine man, the physician today is being firmly located in a more rigid, preset social framework designed to contain his not inconsiderable powers. Interestingly, too, the tendency to medicalize a larger sector of human problems also brings the modern doctor closer to his primitive counterpart. As Sigerist points out, the medicine man had a far more pervasive set of responsibilities than the modern physician. Not only disease but also weather, crops, human fertility, and victory in battle were all under his aegis.[11]

The next quarter century will see the finer details of the physician's image sculpted by the forces of technological and social change. Some of the contradictory elements now present in the doctor's changing relationships with patients, hospitals, other health professionals, and the community will be resolved.

If we had lived in the Hippocratic era, it would have been difficult to anticipate the full effect of the secularization and rationalization of medicine then occurring. We should be charitably excused now from too fine a rendition of the image of the twenty-first-century physician. One thing scientific medicine does not yet claim is the gift of social prophecy.

8

Philosophy of Medicine and Medical Ethics

Medical ethics has always been an integral part of medicine.[1] In the past two decades, however, medical ethics took an unusual turn: It came to be most vigorously propounded by those outside of medicine and independently of the traditional medical codes. The first hesitant steps were largely those of the perceptive theologians who were anxious to correlate medicine's growing technological prowess with sectarian religious morality. Some very valuable beginnings were made by theologians such as Ramsey and Fletcher in the late 1950's. But only in the last decade have the youthful vigor and comprehensive range of interests of a reinvigorated discipline become fully apparent.

Today, over two hundred articles a month appear, authored by theologians, philosophers, ethicists, lawyers, physicians, anthropologists, historians, sociologists, and many others. So rapid an outburst of activity was bound to run two current risks of significant proportions: uneven quality and too early specialization.[2] As a result, some articles consist of largely ungrounded assertions;[3] others are mere collections of woesome, top-of-the-head remarks by otherwise creditable scholars.[4]

These dangers are part of the intellectual development of any new discipline. Maturation, however, requires a degree of conceptual sophistication which is just beginning to appear in medical ethics. If medical ethics is to grow as a discipline, we hold that it must be founded at some point in the understanding of the nature of medicine and in the ontology which makes medicine possible. In addition, it must depend upon an axiology, a system of values about man, presupposed by medicine and the source of the justifications of its actions.

Our analysis of medical ethics is more classically constructed than the dominant views of contemporary philosophers and ethicists generally permit. We consider inadequate and insufficient the views that medical ethics analyzes the language and meaning of propositions only, that it simply applies previously formulated theories to medical problems, or that it need not be problem solving. We consider a metaphysical framework essential for medical ethics, and we discuss this framework in this chapter under three headings: medical ethics and the nature of medicine, medicine and values, and finally, the ontology of medical ethics. The chapter concludes with critical reflections on the limits of the principles formulated.

Medical Ethics and the Nature of Medicine

What medicine actually is, is important for a proper medical ethics–one which is something more than a set of assertions, or an analysis of the meanings of ethical discourse about medical matters. It is important, at this juncture, that we review briefly and then amplify our argument about the nature of medicine.

Civilization is ultimately an organized effort of men to secure the good ends of human life. In some sense, then, all disciplines should aim at these ends, whether or not their method is teleological. Human activity without definable ends is fruitless and eventually self-destructive. Government, for example, should secure those rights which will bring about the ends proper to most humans. Education, as Dewey saw, should give men the capacity for continued growth toward certain ends.

However, all human disciplines do not possess a methodology capable of formulating the proper ends of a good human life. This is particularly true of modern science and technology, to which so many turn today because of their disaffection with religion and the humanities. As a result, we seem to lack the cultural wisdom to formulate moral policy without appealing to ends so vacuous as to be unobtainable, or so specific as to be acceptable only to a very few.

Among the many reasons for our moral dilemmas, two are particularly critical. The first is the notion that science is a body of value-free propositions and that valuing is, hence, a subjective enterprise. The second is the influence of technology, which tends to subordinate values to institutions and techniques.

The notion that science is a body of value-free propositions, essentially indicative and linked logically, leads inevitably to scientism. The result is the idea that valuing is subjective and relative, and therefore largely a capricious activity. In this view, the ends of human society are not a proper subject for any discipline which claims to be scientific. If medicine claims to be such a science, then its activities would not seem to involve values. The ethical implications of medical acts would be reduced to gratuitous applications of moral theory to specific clinical problems.

In its pristine form, this position leads to judgments that the only problems appropriate to medicine are scientific problems. The treatment of chronic alcoholism, for example, would be seen as a chemical and metabolic problem. The social, ethical, and economic determinants would be outside the perimeters of this conception of medicine. In a weaker form, this view considers medicine as a value-free science, but would admit that medicine embodies values when it is applied to specific patients. In both views, value and ethics are external and relative to medical theory. Medicine itself is unable to reveal any knowledge or judgment about the ends and aims of human life. Merely to cite the vast range of irreconcilable positions among ethicists suffices to convince us of the futility of any attempt to define the proper ends of a culture and of medicine itself in the absence of some ontological or axiological ordering principles.

The implications of this philosophical deficiency are by no means trivial. If values and ethics are extrinsic to the medical enterprise, then human investigation, for example, would be legitimized chiefly as a necessity for the scientific advance of medicine. Any imposition of ethical guidelines would be seen as an unwelcome extrinsic pressure inimical to the free pursuit of knowledge, which is a good in itself.

The second critical reason for our moral uncertainties about the ends of human life is the overweening influence of technology. Since the Second World War, the accomplishments of technology have been so impressive that technology is an ideology which defines the conditions of earthly salvation rather than an instrument of human purpose. What *can* be done is confused with what *should* be done. The techniques essential to survival assume more importance than the persons they are intended to serve. The same is true of social institutions, which become self-justifying and self-replicative. As Hans Jonas has so astutely observed, in a technological society, ends and means are reversed. Theory becomes practice, and one technique calls for the creation of newer technologies, rapidly outdating the old ones.[5]

We can see these influences clearly in medicine. For one example, the practice of specialized medicine is virtually impossible without linkage to highly complex institutions. For another, new techniques such as the CAT scanner are developed from older technologies, and already are spawning a newer and more advanced generation of more complex scanners. Specialization and new techniques thus proliferate almost independently of costs and needs, and particularly without conscious reflection on which of the ends and uses of medicine should take precedence.

If, in the context of a value-free science and a technological value system, medical ethics is merely the application of past ethical theories, it quickly becomes dissociated from the real situation of medicine as we have tried to define it in this book. However craftsmanlike its arguments, medical ethics so construed ceases to be helpful and may even be a perverse influence. It is the intuitive appreciation of such a possibility that has given birth to the ethical backlash.[6]

We hold against all of this the view that medicine is not merely a science, and therefore not a value-free science. Instead, we have argued that medicine belongs primarily to the category of relationships; that more specifically, it is a relationship of healing prompted by need, which works in, with, and through the body. Medicine is not a science of individuals, therefore, as has been proposed, but a science of practice, comprising a set of principles which govern the act of healing. Medicine is a *tekné iatrikê,* a combination of knowledge and skill. To be helpful in deciding what is good or right for a given patient, medicine must be grounded, therefore, in the relationship of healing.

This view of what medicine is eventuates in a more positive, less relativistic view of what medical ethics is. We believe it is possible in a technological society to formulate proper ends for medicine which might govern medical ethics. To do this, we would ground medical ethics in a restricted set of aims for medicine and a theory of right action and rational decision making.

We have already delineated a restricted aim for medicine in our discussion of what medicine is (Chapter Three) and provided it with a theory of rational and right decision making in our discussion of the anatomy of clinical judgment (Chapter Six). It remains in the concluding sections of this chapter to provide a restricted aim and a theory of right action for medical ethics as well–both, however, grounded firmly in our prior understanding of what we think medicine is.

If medicine, as we have argued, is not a value-free science, then it is not a value-free theory applied to individual cases. Instead, it is a value-laden theory of practice governed at all points by the patient's need for help with disease. Similarly, medical ethics is not a body of ethical theory applied to medical transactions but an intrinsic part of medicine itself.[7] Its argumentation is, therefore, based on values perceived within the medical relationship and not external or relative to it. The quality of ethical decision making is increased in proportion to the understanding of the medical event which infuses it. If ethics, in general, is a conversation between competing value systems, then medical ethics is a conversation between competing value systems in the doctor-patient relationship.

Medical ethics is, accordingly, a symbiotic discipline embracing both medicine and ethics. To identify what values are in conflict–a necessary first step for ethics–one needs reliable and concrete clinical details on which to place a value. But the clinical situation involves a calculus of complex, interacting variables all governed by and reflecting the patient's need: prognosis, therapy, family situation, life-style, and finances, as well as disease theories and religious beliefs. Medical ethics, thus, has the same relationship to values that medicine has to the range of clinical variables.

If this parallel is true, then the more clearly and fully we understand the calculus of clinical variables, the more we increase the probability of clearly identifying, and properly setting, some priority on values. Ethical and clinical judgments become synergistic but retain their identity and are not fused with each other. Both the calculus of clinical variables and the values they embody are called forth by the patient's need for help. Hence, both medicine and medical ethics are justifiable only if they are ordained by the mandate to help.

It is in this sense that medicine becomes a moral enterprise because intrinsically it involves decisions which are value-laden. This is not the case for medicine when, as basic or clinical science, it seeks understanding of causes and mechanisms of disease or treatments without reference to immediate help for a particular patient, here and now, present.

Ethics or morality arises in the context of turmoil, inner conflict, or opposition.[8] This basic opposition rarely takes the form of right versus wrong, good versus evil. More often it arises between two apparent but mutually exclusive goods. To speak of "moral conflict" is therefore redundant. Yet one can speak of ethics in terms of conflict. In the process of ethical decision making, the following questions quickly emerge: What is the conflict? How can the conflict be resolved? Why is this resolution chosen and not another?

At the core of moral conflict are values, and the moral problematic is a problematic of values. In the conflict, values present themselves as confused as well as conflicting. Therefore, added to the problem of conflicting values is the prior problem of accurately recording the values present or possible in a given situation.

Thus, ethical decision making partially involves both identifying values presented as confused and putting conflicting values into a priority relationship. This is an important point. Ethicists are often tempted to leap to a resolution of conflict, ignoring the fact that values may be questionable or unclear in certain cases. In order to arrive at a moral decision of the nature "X is better than Y in this case," one must not only resolve the conflict between X and Y but first clearly identify X and Y as significant or relevant values in the medical situation.

Thus, the morally problematic situation can be described as a calculus. In the moral process one begins with confused values, the lower limit of the calculus, and moves through value clarification and priority setting to some value choice. This is the upper limit of the calculus of values. Furthermore, the upper limit is always asymptotic to a clear value conflict, as one can never reach an absolutely clear conflict of values. Some confusion always remains in the medical situation. Therefore, the upper limit can only be approximated.

Just as morality might be described as a process or calculus of moving from a confused situation through value identification, clarification, priority setting, and judgment, so too can the process of clinical judgment. The calculus of medicine moves from one extreme, in which the situation is a confused and jumbled complex of human and medical factors, to the other extreme, in which the human factors are precipitated out and analyzed separately. Concomitantly, the medical facts are measured, validated, and explained through physiological, pathological, or biochemical constructs. These constructs seek a scientific and etiological explanation of the body's disease.

Even though there is movement to incorporate human factors in the process of diagnosis, prognosis, and therapy, the range and relationship of all the variables in the clinical situation are governed by a patient's need for help with a specific bodily disease or malfunction. Hence, the human factors may be separated out during the initial process of getting to the root of the problem. However, the human factors must be reintegrated at some point because they contribute to the disease and its healing. There can never be a pure science of medicine *qua* medicine divorced from human values, because at every juncture values are part of the problem and the solution.

All of this is to say that identifying the *problem* in medicine cannot be separated from identifying the *conflict* in ethics. This is not to say that medicine, in its search for causes of disease, is automatically ethical. But it is to assert that medicine is automatically moral, for it deals with human values. If the medical situation is clarified, so too is the value conflict: hence, our assertion that medical ethics is a symbiotic discipline intimately linked with clinical medicine and sharing its goal of help for a particular patient.

The role ethics plays in the process of moral decision making is to critically examine the goods which are ranked in priority in such a decision. The distinction between moral decision making and ethics will become clearer in the pages to follow.

Medicine and Values

The next step in our thesis is to elaborate more fully the connection of medicine and values. This thesis is that medical ethics must rest on an understanding of medicine and ontology.

It is commonplace to state that medicine involves values. Burns and Engelhardt, for example, argue that the core of medicine is a body of issues which concern the value and purpose of man:

> Science and technology presuppose value judgments, issues of purpose. Just as much as facts enable purposes to be accomplished, purposes cause facts to cohere in terms of expectations and meanings. We gather the world around us in terms of what is markedly the case with the central concepts of medicine: health and disease. . . . They sketch the limits and values of the human condition.[9]

It should be clear, from the foregoing part of this chapter, that the purpose of man can be revealed partly from the values which arise in the medical relationship. As this relationship changes in intensity and from institution to institution, the values involved also change. As John Dewey once remarked: "Values are exposed to the contingencies of existence."[10] Hence the need for a critical examination of values, an ethics, is brought forward. But before dealing with that issue, we must examine a prior question: Exactly how does medicine involve values? We suggest three ways: in the fact that medicine is a *tekné mixté* of healing; in that its cognitive aspects reflect values; and in that it is a virtue.

By stating that medicine is a *tekné iatrikê,* we suggested that it combines knowledge and skill about healing. Hence medicine must be a cognitive art aimed at the purpose of healing. As such, it falls into a class of arts such as teaching, law, and ethics in which care is directed to the person, rather than those cognitive arts in which care is directed to techniques and machines, such as engineering.

All cognitive arts share the following characteristics: their theory is a structure of principles about practice; their search is for the right way of making decisions; and their enterprise is intrinsically linked to human purpose. The cognitive arts are distinct from the fine arts in that the product is not a thing–a musical work, a ballet performance, a piece of sculpture–which has a life apart from the artist, but a human action of the practitioner in conjunction with persons in need. Additionally, medicine is governed by a pressure to decide more intense than in teaching, which it shares with law and ethics.

Because the cognitive arts are aimed at decisions about human purposes, their theory is, perforce, value-laden. Thus medicine's concepts and theories are governed by the therapeutic intention: what is best for *this* patient. Even nontherapeutic research implies an altruism on the part of subjects by which, with their consent, they express what is best for them in terms of the human condition and a possible therapeutic outcome for future generations. If it is true, as we take it, that ethics involves values, then medicine as a cognitive art is linked somehow to ethics.

But how, precisely, are the two related? More specifically, is medicine automatically ethical? Is a good medical decision, by that fact, an ethically good decision? To answer this difficult question, one must turn to the cognitive aspects of medicine as an art and the nature of values.

We have described, in Chapter Six, how the decision-making process in medicine is ruled by a heuristic of making right decisions about particular patients. Any act which applies knowledge to persons involves values and consequently falls into the moral realm. By "moral realm" we mean the theater of human actions that involve values as the drama of signification or meaning. This definition creates confusion about the connection of law, medicine, education, and politics with ethics.

Moreover, because the cognitive realm of medicine is composed of theory about practice–i.e., about making right decisions–its cognitive features also fall into the moral realm. But the operative term in this discussion is "right." What is meant by "right"? Does it mean "correct," or does it mean "good"?

This question is all-important. If the right decision is governed by canons of scientific correctness, then medicine is distinct from ethics. If "right" decisions mean "good" ones, then medicine would be a form of ethics itself, unless further distinctions can be made about "goods," for these are properly the subject of ethics.

MacIntyre and Gorovitz have proven to our satisfaction that medicine cannot be governed by canons of scientific correctness because medicine must deal with individuals.[11] Furthermore, development of the conditions of possibility of cures and the nature of clinical judgment also reveals that a "right decision" does not mean conformity with scientific canons, but rather with the living body, the lived body, and the lived self. In other words, the "right decision" in medicine involves the unique wisdom of an individual body, the body as a class instance of living bodies, and the values of the lived body and the lived self. Scientific knowledge of disease, in other words, is indeed one component, but a value-laden component, of the medical event. A right decision may or may not involve such scientific knowledge. The therapeutic intent of medicine for the cancer patient is in no way diminished by medicine's inability to explain the exact causal event in cancer.

Therefore, the "right" decision in medicine must mean a "good" decision, not just a correct one. And a good decision involves some ethical dimension. But if every decision in medicine is moral–i.e., involves values–is every one ethical? An affirmative answer without qualifications would presume that all values are goods, and that all goods are ethical, and that by "ethical" is meant a good moral action. Such a position reflects a terminology confusion, not uncommon when dealing with "values," "goods," "moral," and "ethical."

By "moral" we mean any action involving values. No judgment or comparison of values is implied in describing medicine as a moral enterprise. Such a description merely states that every feature of medicine is value-laden. By "ethical" we mean a disciplined study of values and action which includes a theory of value language and/or the procedures used to distinguish good and evil, as well as criteria for establishing hierarchies of goods. If one followed these somewhat standard usages, the pragmatic aims of medicine would, in theory, be distinct from their ethical force. This is certainly the point of Kant's distinction between ethical axioms and utilitarian purpose.

However, the picture in medicine is clouded by the fact that its aim is not entirely pragmatic or utilitarian, but is actually a good, a healing, a perfection of human nature. The place of values in the purposes of medicine, therefore, will determine the degree to which a good medical decision will also be a good ethical decision. Insofar as medicine is a "habit of the mind," in Aristotle's sense, and respects the good inherent in the process of healing, then it can be viewed as a virtue, as pointed out in Chapter Six. Medicine is a virtue because health is good. It should be noted, however, that our discussion does not embrace all relationships which heal, for this would involve us in an ethics of a series of relationships which heal. Instead we are limiting the discussion to the form of medicine previously discussed, and hence to an ethics for medical practice. Note Chapter Nine, wherein we delineate further the healing context of the patient-physician relationship.

This point can also be examined from the standpoint of values, a brief development of which will shed light on the axiology of medicine and pave the way for discussion of the role of ontology in medical ethics.

Value theory is relatively new in the history of ethics, although implied in the metaphysics of Plato and Aristotle. Originally "value" meant the cost or price of an object. The common meaning of "value" is still that of a property of objects which possess beauty, goodness, or utility. Parker, Hilliard, and Rice reject this use as meaningless, while Lewis and Pepper appeal to this usage to develop their theories.[12] John Dewey focused on the verb form, arguing that "valuing" was a mode of any motion toward an end in view. In view of Dewey's usage of experience as a primary category of interaction between organism and environment, valuing would be a mode of experience in which one moved toward either appraised values or prizings (unreflected values).

Noting for the moment that medicine is a movement toward an end, its actions on behalf of patients, as well as its desire to understand disease processes, would both be forms of valuing. Valuing does imply an ethical dimension because the enterprise is capable of being judged as more or less good according to norms or principles proposed by ethics. But because the good of health is the end in view, and is itself a value in the substantive sense of the word, the norms of medical ethics should be grounded in an axiology of health.

If we accept a definition of "value" as a property of objects capable of having action directed toward them, a property of attitudes directed toward such objects, and a property of the interaction itself, we can see that health fulfills all three features of values.[13] Health is capable of having actions directed toward it; it is descriptive of the attitudes human beings have about their bodies; and it cements the bond of interchange between physician and patient.

While it is fairly clear that health is a value, it is not as clear that it is a norm of medical ethics insofar as it is a value.

In any process of ordering values in some relationship, some principle of selection, an evaluative comparison is presupposed. The evaluating factor lies at the root of judgment that X is better than Y in this case. Now it is clear, from our discussions in the previous three chapters, that the normative concept of health is the evaluative factor in medicine. Hence health is the norm of an ethically good decision in medicine.

Following Lee's argument that an object has intrinsic value when the positive evaluating factor is part of the actual transaction or value contexture,[14] health can be seen as an intrinsic value of organisms which is not only a condition of the positive *medical* event but also of the positive *ethical* event. But because health is basically a way of coping with the environment, the principle that *it is good to be healthy* functions as a moral absolute. That is, health is normative to medicine and medical ethics; it is a value which takes precedence over others.

In saying this, we must note that we are not referring to any particular interpretation of health. Such interpretations are far too various and conflicting to designate any of them as an absolute. Health is absolute only in its most generic sense as a good intrinsic to being a living body; health as a particularized statement of what constitutes that good cannot safely be absolutized. The body must select health as a prime value logically prior to selecting any particular interpretation of it. Health, in short, is an originary need of the body logically prior to its specific conceptualizations.

However, living bodies are part of a space-time framework and are embedded in a cultural matrix. They formulate symbolic representations of themselves and their culture. The value of health can therefore be extrinsic and systemic as well as intrinsic.[15] That is, health can be defined in terms of coping relationships in a particular space-time configuration (extrinsic) as well as in, and by, a system of institutions, boards, government bodies, and so on. Consequently the specific content of the norm is blurred and causes confusion. One might make different ethical and medical decisions about Karen Quinlan, for example, based on whether one held a biological view of health as a human need, or a World Health Organization definition of health as complete physical, mental, and social well-being.

If this line of reasoning has any merit, then the primary ethical question is synonymous with the primary medical question: What is good for this patient? In other words, what is that which contributes to this organism's health? If a medical decision is made on behalf of the patient with the highest quality of biological, personal, cultural, and scientific attention to health as defined by the patient's need, then the decision is ethical.

So far, we have presented a thesis that medical ethics must be helpful because it must relate to the nature of medicine as an interaction of need, and that medical ethics and medicine are both grounded in an axiology of values by reason of the cognitive aspects of medical practice. The latter discussion revealed that medicine is not linked extrinsically to values, but intrinsically through the need of a living body judged as a value. This need is health, which is a mode of coping with the environment. To be ethical, the moral enterprise of medicine must be governed by the norm of *health as value*.

Because health is a value of living bodies as instances of a class, the rights to it can truly be asserted to be a legitimate end of a good human life, to be secured by civilization through political processes. A disruption of this end causes confusion about the nature of medicine, which is either subverted and contained for immoral purposes (as when physicians are coerced to aid in political torture) or aggrandized into a new secular religion requiring it to heal all the wounds of society.

The Ontology of Medical Ethics

If the norm for judging among values in medicine rests upon the conditions of possibility of medicine itself, then medical ethics should be grounded in an ontology. But because medicine is also a moral enterprise, the ontology revealed by medicine includes a value-ontology, or an axiology. We have already shown that medicine is inherently a study of the human condition in that it concerns not only physical and psychological parameters but the complete range of experience and values. A "cure" must also be a "care for the whole," since the living body is so organized that the functions of parts relate to the functions of wholes. Medical ethics must deal with the value-pragmatism of medicine itself. An ethic of experimentation, for example, must also *necessarily* include the fiduciary role of the investigator proper to clinical relationships.[16]

We have seen that the primary meaning of health is grounded in a condition of the living body, and that the norm for medical ethics is also grounded in that living body. Furthermore, we have shown how the conditions of possibility for an effective medical event include ontological insights about the nature of man. In this final part of the chapter, it would be well to sort out those ontological presuppositions which are part of a system of values and restate them as axioms for medical ethics.

The apparent inability to resolve our medical-moral dilemmas stems from a lack of a meaningful view of human nature. Our behavior is not independent of the theories of human behavior we adopt. It is our concern that moral values not be posed in ignorance, or open defiance, of the biological realities of human nature. While the concept of human nature has been dropped by modern philosophy, we have argued that a residue of that concept is necessarily presupposed as an ontological condition of the possibility that cures take place. All medicine is built on the assumption that living bodies are organized in similar ways and organize the world through common objects. Thus they will have predictable responses to specific medical interventions. Furthermore, the specificity of individual living bodies requires that individual interpretations of health be respected *within* the absolute of health as value. This point will become important for one component of the professional code to be developed in the next chapter.

We have not argued according to the lines of the naturalistic fallacy that science itself, or even medicine itself, can determine values which are right or wrong. But we have argued that "it is good to be healthy" is a valuing norm governing both medical ethics and medicine that rests upon a prior law of the nature of living bodies. To neglect this law is to run the peril of destroying the natural base of human societies.

At the very least, modern medicine presents humankind with new options, some predictability about the outcomes of the options chosen, and some comprehension of the biological impact of differing values chosen such that the value of health can be linked to a system of other values. But what are some of the values which are necessary conditions of medicine? And how do these aid in the process of decision making?

The first and primary value is that it is good to be healthy. This is a basic need of living bodies, logically prior to its value for persons. Inasmuch as this value determines the nature of the clinical relationship, it grounds a most ancient medical-ethical axiom in the function of the living body. That axiom is the Hippocratic one, "To help or at least to do no harm."[17] As this rule appears in the corpus, it seems merely to be a sober command to carry out the art of medicine. But considerable evidence also exists to suggest that it was a popular rule of thumb for citizens in Greece regarding the moral duties of citizenship.

Actually the axiom rests on the duties of physicians in the clinical relationship. However, since both physician and patient are locked in the human condition, the duty itself flows from the intrinsic need of a living body for help in restoring itself to health. The response of the physician is not merely contractual or duty filled, but also biological; it exists between two living organisms that take health to be an absolute value. Thus, the axiom to do no harm has a base in the real human condition as well as in the nature of medicine itself. To violate it is not only to violate the nature of medicine but one of the very conditions of its possibility.

The second principle of medicine is that individuals have intrinsic value. This value is an ontological condition of possibility for the movement of medical decision making toward concretizing for individuals, what we have called rationalized individuation. Such a value-principle leads to an axiom as well: Care must be taken for the susceptible individual.

Logically prior care must deal with the uniqueness of an individual living body, what we have called the wisdom of the body. Thus the physician is obligated to deal with organic disease, with a view toward tailoring therapy to *this* individual. Normally this axiom is violated only when some common good seems to take precedence over individualization. Such a clash in values is one of the dangers present in medical education or when physicians are also agents of institutions with broader goals. This prominent mode of the practice of modern medicine is addressed in Chapter 10. Because ethics deals only with what is generally to be done, we would suggest that the health professional has an obligation to individuals which precedes attention to the common good. Our third axiom will also serve as a qualifier of this point.

A second implication of the axiom in question focuses on vulnerability. Because the individual seeks help in an arena of little or no personal expertise, and as care focuses more intensely on threatened organic systems, the obligation of physicians for the patient's values correspondingly increases. Once again, it is the body of the patient that grounds this obligation, not merely social and legal structures. For the body of the patient is placed in the "hands" of the physician in a total response of trust. The body is probed and violated in closer proximity and more intimately than is usually permitted even to those the patient loves. Thus the axiom of care for the vulnerable individual is the ground for an ethics of trust, love, or, as Ramsey prefers to call it, a covenantal relationship between doctor and patient. It should be emphasized again that the ground of the axiom moves beyond comradeship, contract, or legal and cultural expectations to the nature of the living body in need.

It should also be noted that attempts to resolve medical-ethical issues, such as abortion, on the basis of a definition of a person as self-conscious neglect the roots of both medicine and medical ethics in the *living organism in need.* To argue, based on such a definition, that abortion and euthanasia are good ethical actions is to miss the point of medicine and its ontological condition of possibility.

The third value-principle of medicine is that the intrinsic value of individuals also includes their representation as a class-instance of human bodies. The value of the individual is both unique and common to all living bodies. This value-principle is derived from the condition of possibility that cures take place. Not only is therapy to be tailored to the uniqueness of each body, but the entire transaction presupposes common structures in living bodies. The class-instance value-principle leads to the following axiom: The common good of living bodies is a form of altruism expressing the common characteristics of individual living bodies.

Put another way, the common good as it affects medicine should not clash with the common structures of living bodies. However, the common good is an abstraction of biologically based functions which are collected *as a value*—that is, expressed from the altruism of individuals who benefit only insofar as they are instances of a class. Hence, as we have already noted, even nontherapeutic medical research carries with it obligations to do no harm. But the altruism of both physician and patient, grounded in their common human condition, can determine that the benefit or nonharm can apply to class-instance rather than to the uniqueness of the individual living body.

While the above considerations are not exhaustive, they do form the conclusion of the thesis proposed—namely, that medical ethics should be grounded in the nature of medicine, and, though a philosophy of medicine, in the ontological basis of medicine itself: the living human body. The test for apt ethical decisions in medicine lies in the effects on a living body, either as an individual with values or as a class instance of common bodily structures. Because bodies are also symbolic, ethical axioms are relative in their formulations—that is, relative to different situations and conditions—while simultaneously being absolute in their ground: the ontological basis of medicine.

The Limits of Axioms

The argument posed in this chapter was that medical ethics is intrinsically linked to medical practice through the norm of health as value. Furthermore, the living body in need ontologically grounds three principles of ethics which can lead to axioms of nonharm, protection of vulnerability, and benefit as class-instance. Other axioms can be developed from these principles as well. As we shall show in the following chapters, professional norms can also be created from the axioms.

However, it is important to restate in another way both the extent and the limits of a normative medical ethics. This will be done from the standpoint of the moral center of the medical enterprise and the role of the good in medicine. For this amplification, it is assumed that one understands the distinction between prescriptive and descriptive ethical norms.

If, as we have argued, medicine involves values, then medicine is a moral enterprise. Development of this point revealed that the moral nature of medicine stems from health, which is valued as a good by the living body. The principles of medical ethics, therefore, are absolute insofar as the foundational value upon which they rest–health as a good–is taken as primary in the realm of the lived body and the lived self. These principles are descriptive, and not prescriptive, in that they command no action in themselves.

However, the principles are relative to cultural interpretation in at least two ways. First, the principles are couched in language that can mean different things to a community of persons in different ages and cultures. Different scientific concepts of health and disease, and different interpretations of degrees of disruption in everyday life, are but two examples of this relativism.[18] The second way in which the principles are relative is in the ranking of foundational goods. Health is only one of a number of primary goods sought by human beings, even by that aspect of them we have called the living body. As the primary ontological condition of medicine is the biological "desire" of the body to seek what is for its own good, this search leads human beings not only toward health but also toward happiness, friendships, pleasures, sufficient economic means, and a host of other secondary goods which enable one to survive with dignity. Hence, the principles enunciated are relative to an individual and social ranking or hierarchy of goods. Conflicts among these goods may lead individuals to neglect health in favor of pleasure, or to deemphasize health in order to work to earn a living.

These considerations prompt two corollaries. The first is that the limited aims of medicine vary in importance with the ranking of values attached to the physician-patient relationship. The second is that the principles and axioms developed earlier in the chapter acquire normative force when health and healing are ranked as primary by both physicians and patients.

If values can be understood, in part, to mean aims judged good and obtainable by persons, then it is clear that values are ranked differently from day to day, from situation to situation, from cultural epoch to cultural epoch. This observation in no way negates the fact that some values appear in every ranking, though their relative position changes. These values, among them health, appear in each cultural and individual assessment of important values.

Because persons change the relative ranking of values, a clash often emerges between the values of patients and those of the health profession. In fact, ethical considerations often involve a clash between the value of health professed by medicine and other values professed by the patient, institutions, or even the government.

Traditionally, health has been viewed by philosophers as conditional, that is, as a value which allows a person or a society to attain freedom and movement.[19] Most persons still view health in this light. They do not rank health among the primary values of their lives. However, when persons become ill, health does move from a conditional ranking to a primary and even an absolute ranking.[20] The degree to which persons do change the ranking of health is the degree to which they adhere to the professed value of medicine, healing.[21]

Given this discussion, it is important to note that ethics can respect only characteristic situations because the values which enter its discussion and argumentation shift in relative ranking depending upon culture or personal disposition.[22] It is our view, therefore, that medical ethics must strive to propose policy decisions which respect as many values as possible. The test of a good policy is not so much how the policy preserves only one absolute moral principle but how the policy is congruent with the principles and obligations derived from the philosophical foundations of the physician-patient relationship.

What does this view mean for the normative status of the principles and axioms proposed? How can one move from the position of relative ranking of goods to proposing a professional code of medical morality, as we will do in the next chapter? The answer to this question leads to the second corollary.

From the previous discussion, it should be clear that the normative force of the axioms, which are rooted in the relative aim or value of health, depends upon the primacy of health as a value, as judged by both physician and patient. Thus, "Do no harm" is not considered a deontological principle unless both physician and patient rank health as primary, a situation which sometimes, but not always, holds true. On the other hand, we do not mean "Do no harm" as a simple counsel of prudence. As we shall show in the next chapter, such an interpretation will be viewed as a professional rule of ethics which itself can be developed from the axiom. Nonharm is more than a counsel of prudence because it describes a moral principle of a relative enterprise–that is, the enterprise of medicine judged as beneficial.[23]

In other words, our interpretation of the axioms attempts to draw a fine line between the position of Hare–that there are universal prescriptive norms in medical ethics–and the position of Morgenbesser–that there may not be special moral principles for medicine.[24] We have argued that there are special moral principles for medicine but that these are not, per se, universal prescriptive norms.

This point is worth pursuing for a moment, for the notion that one can draw upon an application of general moral principles to medicine only by first filtering them through more specific axioms or rules is not widely accepted by those writing in medical ethics. Most philosophers tend to apply a favorite philosophical theory from the past, a theory such as Utilitarianism (Hare), Deontologism (Ramsey), or Natural Law Theory (McCormick).[25] Attempts to make these theories lead to practical policy, such as the famous disagreement between Ramsey and McCormick on research on children, result in valuable insights about the presuppositions of medicine and culture. But no practical moral policy, as called for by Arthur Dyck, for example, ensues.[26] The reason is threefold.

First, applications of general principles neglect the specific moral rules of medicine, doubted by Morgenbesser but herein developed. Hence the application lacks adherents in medicine itself, where the practices are carried out for the good of patients.[27]

Second, applications of general principles must methodologically proceed through what John Ladd calls secondary principles (namely, rules, practices, moral notions) in order to bring about a relation between abstractions and concrete decision making.[28] Although Ladd does not stress this point, the secondary principles ought to be those arising from the value of healing for greatest applicability.

Finally, and most tellingly, without the limited axioms such as those we have developed, or at least a set of moral principles of medical practice, as superbly developed in the Belmont Report of the National Commission for the Protection of Human Subjects,[29] those who simply apply standard moral theory to medicine require policy makers to adhere to one or another mutually exclusive moral theory. But these theories are not universally accepted, a point which led MacIntyre to despair of any role for philosophy in medicine.[30] Lack of acceptance could lead, very naturally, to lack of compliance with policies suggested in this abstract approach to moral decision making.

Instead a moralist recognizing the limited nature of the axioms proposed can both develop arguments for them from standard moral theory and develop policy proposals from them, as we shall do in the chapters to follow. In other words, the limited axioms can be supported by different moral theories as well as interpreted in different decision-making contexts. They are sufficiently content-free to be capable of a wide range of interpretations while simultaneously being of sufficient moral force to guide in the process of making ethical decisions. Mill's observation, quoted by Ladd, can serve as an excellent summary of our theme: "Without such middle principles [axioms] a universal principle, either in science or in morals, serves for little but a thesaurus of common places for the discussion of questions, instead of a means of deciding them."[31]

It should be clear, therefore, that the limited axioms are relative to the concrete situations of medicine and culture, but absolute guides to decision making when certain conditions are met:

1. That *health as value* is ranked as primary among foundational goods.

2. That health is understood as a living condition of a human body.

3. That health is not totally identified with any particular scientific conception of well-being.

When these conditions are met, as they frequently are in clinical medicine, the axioms derived from the principles acquire a normative function. That is, neglect of the norms in the practice of medicine is a neglect of the nature of medicine itself. When the norms are adopted or professed by health care professionals, as we shall show in the chapters to follow, the norms acquire a prescriptive force.

In effect, then, norms describe a theory of the good which is at the moral center of medicine and prescribe action when this theory of the good is professed in dedication to healing.

9

A Philosophical Reconstruction of Medical Morality

Introduction

The central issue in medical morality today is whether or not there is some justifiable philosophical foundation for a set of obligations which bind all who profess medicine–or better still, all who profess to heal. Does such a foundation exist which is anterior to, and independent of, the position the physician takes on specific medical moral dilemmas?[1]

The question is urgent and significant for several reasons. First is the obvious wide divergency of opinions about the resolution of the moral dilemmas of medical progress: abortion, prolongation of life, recombinant DNA research, behavioral manipulation, and all the other issues that make up the content of contemporary biomedical ethical debate. Antithetical and logically incommensurable positions on these questions divide physicians and patients and expose serious conflicts of value systems and conceptions of the good.

Then there is the gradual erosion of the traditional sources of medical morality in the Western world. Fewer physicians accept a religious foundation for professional ethics,[2] and even fewer could claim to be faithful to all the injunctions of the Hippocratic oath.

This chapter is based upon an article by Dr. Pellegrino, "Toward a Reconstruction of Medical Morality: The Primacy of the Act of Profession and the Fact of Illness," Vol. 4, No. 1, *Journal of Medicine and Philosophy* (March 1979), 32–56.

Indeed, almost every one of its injunctions is violated in good conscience by some physicians: abortions are done; surgery is practiced; the patient is exposed to dangerous drugs; confidentiality is violated in the interest of public safety; the sexual mores and the Pythagorean vision of the "pure" life enjoined by the ancient oath are both far removed from the life-styles of many contemporary physicians.

In addition, codes of professional ethics–the recent proposed revisions of the AMA code are a good example–are becoming less committed morally and more legalistic in spirit. They seem designed more to protect against litigation than as voluntary statements of recognized obligations. To be sure, new codes have appeared to protect patients against the dangers of human experimentation, but little has been added to address the far more subtle but more common moral dangers in everyday clinical decisions.

All codes to date have been devised by the profession, for the profession, and without the participation of patients or society. They promulgate the profession's view of what is owed and "noble." These codes are all unilaterally derived and can hardly be considered contracts or covenants, as some would have them.

Lastly, and this defect pervades even the most ancient codes, the principles guiding physician behavior have rarely been justified on philosophical grounds. The sources of medical morality have been located invariably in existing philosophical or theological systems applied to medicine. Professional ethics has yet to be formally and systematically derived from a theory of medical acts.

The result is that two alteratives seem open at present. One is to abandon the possibility of a common set of moral principles which binds all physicians and return to the simpler, less demanding ethics of a craft. The other is to attempt a more philosophical reconstruction of professional ethics, one derived from the nature of medicine and medical acts, and specific to them. In earlier chapters, we developed a concept of the nature of medicine and its relationship to ethics. This chapter uses these concepts to develop the theoretical basis for the morality of the professional acts of professed healers.

While the physician will be used as the example, it must be understood that we believe these principles are intrinsic to, and binding upon, all who profess to heal, all who are included under the rubric of "health professionals"–nurses, pharmacists, dentists, allied health workers, psychologists, social workers, optometrists, podiatrists. We are seeking a common basis for the ethics of professional behavior and, hopefully, for a common code of moral conduct in the patient-healer relationship.

The foundations of medical morality derived herein are consistent with a wide variety of value systems, insofar as specific moral questions are concerned. These foundations are in fact minimal and irreducible prior requirements for the moral conduct of the human interaction specific to healing activity. They can be intensified, expanded, or illuminated by the additional obligations of theologically based value systems or of secular humanism. They are the common ground for a reconstruction of professional ethics in post-Hippocratic terms and are therefore more congruent with the state of contemporary society, medicine, and the health professions.

The argument advances in three stages: First, the philosophical sources of medical morality are examined and found wanting; a philosophy of the physician-patient (patient-healer) relationship is proposed; and the obligations which flow from the nature of this relationship are adumbrated.

The Sources of Professional Ethics

Although rarely stated explicitly, all codes of professional ethics reflect certain assumptions about the *nature of medicine,* the *nature of the relationship with the patient,* and *the nature of the good man who happens to be a physician.* The codes usually combine elements of these three sources of medical morality inextricably, and we tease them apart at some risk. Yet, we must do so to comprehend the anatomy of any system of medical morality. Only a few examples can be considered.

The Physician as Good Man

We can start with the idea of the physician as good man as a source of professional ethics. The central feature of this source of ethics is the promulgation of a variety of philosophies of life and of the good in the behavior of the physician. This is essentially the source of the oldest and most influential medical code in the West–the Hippocratic oath. As Edelstein has so cogently argued, the oath is an almost pure transcription into medicine of Pythagorean ethics–asceticism enjoining a life of purity.[3] The injunctions against abortion, euthanasia (poisons), and surgery, the strict sexual mores, and the keeping of confidences–all are peculiarly Pythagorean precepts. They were not shared by the majority of physicians in Greek times. The non-Pythagoreans violated the tenets of the oath. The same applies to the Pythagorean idea of the father-son relationship of student and teacher, urged in the covenant portion of the oath.

When we turn to the other books of the Hippocratic corpus, we encounter a profusion of philosophies, most of them applied in post-Hippocratic times by a variety of authors. These books reflect various combinations of the philosophies of Plato and Aristotle, Stoicism, Epicureanism, Sophism, and Skepticism. Physicians turned to the physiological and cosmological theories of these philosophies to elaborate their theories of medicine and therapeutics (the Methodists, Empiricists, and Dogmatists). They also imbibed the ethics of these philosophies in their definition of what the good physician should be. For example, each of the deontological treatises have somewhat different ethical emphases: *The Physician* is Aristotelian, emphasizing justice and fairness; *Precepts* is Epicurean, stressing gentleness and kindness; *Decorum* is Stoic highlighting duty; and the *Law* is Democritean. These philosophies of the good man were intermingled, as we shall see shortly, with a variety of notions of the physician-patient relationship. They were succeeded in the following centuries by an even stronger infusion of the ethics of the middle and late Stoa as exemplified by Scribonius Largus, Libanius, and Sarapion in the first and second centuries A.D. They spoke, for the first time, of love of mankind, of *humanitas,* compassion, and *misericordia,* mercy.[4]

It was in the early Middle Ages that the ethics of the Hippocratic oath were first universalized. The concept of the physician as a religious man–Christian, Moslem, or Jew–required him to serve the sick as brothers under the fatherhood of God. The oath was cleansed of its pagan references and found its sources refurbished by the humanism of the great religions. This is the wellspring for much of medical ethics in nineteenth-century America.[5] A good example of this transformation is the book on medical ethics published in 1849 by Worthington Hooker, who says bluntly, "How important he [the physician] should be right upon the great moral questions which agitate the community and that his morality should be strictly that of the bible."[6]

Many physicians today, perhaps the majority, still see the religious humanism and the modulations it impressed upon the Hippocratic oath as prime sources of professional ethics. The oath still retains an unparalleled viability. Yet, in our increasingly secular society, ever greater numbers of patients and physicians reject any religious source of professional morality.

The Nature of Medicine

The second source to which we now turn is the nature of medicine itself, and the ways in which obligations of physicians derive from what the physician is conceived to be. In early Greek times, as reflected in many of the Hippocratic books, medicine is seen primarily as a *tekné,* a craft (such as carpentry, for example). A craftsman has certain obligations to his craft: to preserve it against fakes, to practice it competently, to teach it, and to advance its knowledge and skill. This idea of a *tekné* is developed in both Plato and Aristotle as any pursuit of a special skill and as an understanding of why things are done a certain way. It is important to the personal reputation of the craftsman, his craft, and his practice that he practice with a certain kindliness, *philanthropia.* But this was not the love of mankind we find in the Christian ethics or even the Stoic ethic of Cicero, Panaetius, or Scribonius Largus. It was a practical matter essential to successful healing and a good reputation in practice.

Medicine was not referred to as a "profession" until the first century A.D., when Scribonius Largus, a physician in the time of Claudius, wrote his treatise *On Remedies.*[7] Here, medicine is classified as a profession, a vocation, in which the nature of medicine, which is to heal, raises certain expectations on the part of the patient and imposes certain obligations on the physician. Following the middle Stoa of Panaetius, Scribonius averred that we must play the role required by our profession–one which we choose voluntarily. Commiseration and humaneness are the doctor's unique professional virtues, as truth is for the judge. Each profession has its own ethics, according to Panaetius, whose book *On Duties* Cicero paraphrased in his *De Officiis*.[8]

This is a very different concept from the earlier notion of the physician as craftsman; it is more demanding and implies a certain nobility of dedication. This idea of a profession as a special calling is reflected later in Galen's *De Placitis* and in the eighteenth-century code of Thomas Percival, as well as in the AMA code of 1848 and its subsequent revisions.

The later and the modern view of a profession was, however, not as philosophically sound as that of Scribonius. It tended to promulgate the image of a special calling with certain prerogatives of authority and paternalism–combining technical and moral authority. The view of medicine as a gentlemanly profession, as Percival insisted, required that the physician be courteous, kind yet firm, interested yet objective, taking his patient's concerns into account and acting in his behalf. His comportment must be proper; he should inspire confidence.[9] These are the very same qualities prescribed in the Hippocratic corpus. What we inherit from the nineteenth century is the concept of medicine as a gentlemen's profession–the word "profession" now conveying the idea of privilege rather than certain specific obligations of the kind Scribonius emphasized.

Since the seventeenth century, there has been a growing supposition that medicine is really a science, more akin to chemistry and physics than to the arts or crafts. Beginning with Descartes, his disciple La Mettrie (in *L'homme Machine*), and then Claude Bernard, the concept of a quantifiable, experimental, and mechanistic reductionistic enterprise was introduced and developed. The modern positivistic and reductionistic bias of medicine, and the believers in medicine as high technology, are their linear descendants. The unprecedented successes of the scientific method in medicine are strong arguments in favor of their presuppositions. The ethics which emerges from this conception of medicine places its greatest emphasis on competence, scientific certitude, and the advancement of knowledge and clinical experiment.[10] It tends to depreciate caring and in its most severe form would assign the nonscientific aspects of care to others–not to physicians.

Finally, one more example will suffice–that of medicine as a commodity. The egalitarian spirit of modern democracy finds the privileged status of medicine as a profession with unique obligations unappealing. Instead the idea is growing that medicine is not at all unique; that health is a commodity that should be dealt with like other commodities; and that the basis of the physician-patient relationship should be a contract for services. The ethics of medicine should therefore be based on the legal ethics of the contractual arrangement. Such a view detracts from the notion of a profession as something unique in Scribonius' sense or even in Percival's. In the contractual model, courtesy and respect for the dignity of the patient would be closer to the practical kindliness exhibited by the physician-craftsman of Greek times rather than the loftier concept of special obligations contained in either the Stoic or religious concepts of profession. A contractual model for the physician-patient relationship requires courtesy and consideration as a practical matter. They are essential to a constructive negotiation of the terms of the contract and their satisfactory fulfillment. They do not require "love" or "humanity" as Scribonius argued, but only amicable relationships, as in buying any other commodity.[11]

The Patient-Physician Relationship

The third source of professional ethics is the patient-physician relationship. This central phenomenon of medicine has, until recently, received little formal philosophical attention. Pedro Lain-Entralgo has attempted a formulation largely in terms of the concept of brotherly love, drawing heavily on his own reading of the Hippocratic texts.[12] His view of the Greek physician's *philanthropia,* as we have already suggested, is at variance with Ludwig Edelstein's. Edelstein makes a distinction between the kindliness of the Greek physician-craftsman and the *humanitas* of the later Stoic or the religiously inspired physicians.

Though no formal philosophy of the patient-physician relationship was simultaneously developed, it is implicit in every professional code or ethical system. It is usually drawn from, and determined by, what we consider the physician as a good man to be and what we consider the nature of medicine to be. These prior philosophical considerations express themselves in the behavior of physicians and patients. The historically dominant notion of that relationship is the one derived from the Hippocratic authors. This notion of ethics can serve as an example of the third source of professional ethics, and deserves some detailed attention.

Historical Sketch: Professional Ethics

The Hippocratic Ethic

A fairly consistent image of how the Hippocratic physician regarded his relationship with the patient can be extracted from the Hippocratic corpus, especially the deontological books. That relationship was centered in the physician. It was a creation *of* the profession and meant *for* the profession. The physician, at first a craftsman and later a more elite personage, had great concern for his corporate and personal reputation.[13] The physician's moral behavior was as much a practical matter of economic success as it was a moral matter. By virtue of his greater knowledge and skill, the physician was presumed to act as a benevolent authority in both technical and moral matters. He took upon himself the cares of the patient, decided what was best and whom he would treat. He was expected to be competent, freely to seek consultation, and to set reasonable fees with some regard for the patient's ability to pay. He was not to harm the patient and was to safeguard confidence. Edelstein has shown that the more austerely moral proscriptions of the oath—those against abortion, surgery, giving of poisons, and the injunction to lead a pure life—were Pythagorean precepts, not by any means uniformly held by all Greek physicians. Something of the same pluralism we experience today must have characterized Greek medical morality.

The ethical books are notable for their silence on a number of moral questions involving the physician-patient transaction which are of intense interest today. There is little mention of the patient's part in the relationship except to urge that he not impose upon the doctor impossible or dangerous treatments which might fail and thus harm the doctor's reputation. "The Art has three factors, the disease, the patient, and the physician. The physician is the servant of the art. The patient must cooperate with the physician in combating the disease."[14]

But the cooperation required of the patient is that of the child or servant following the order of the master. Thus, "If the physician is to help, his relationship to the patient must be that of the person in command to one who obeys."[15]

There is even a sense of the patient as antagonist: "Keep a watch on the faults of the patients, which often make them lie about the taking of things prescribed."[16] For this reason, too, the physician is urged to visit frequently, or leave one of his pupils, never a layman, in charge. This assures that failures in treatment will not be held against the physician's reputation. We see here again the recurrent concern about reputation which seems to have obsessed the Hippocratic physician.

Edelstein attributes this partly to the fact that the early Greek physician was a craftsman, and his ethic was that of a good craftsman: doing the job well and distinguishing himself in the public eye from the charlatan or quack. According to Edelstein, this craftsman's ethic was the foundation for the humanism of the Greek physician, "Where there is love of man, there is love of the Attic precepts."[17] This was not a love of mankind in the sense of the religious or secular humanism of today. Rather, it bespoke a friendliness and kindliness essential to gaining the confidence of the patient, which helped to heal him and to convince him of the physician's capability.

In none of this is the patient seen as a partner in the decision but, rather, as someone to be protected against the anxiety of too much knowledge. The physician knows what is best: "Perform all this calmly and adroitly, concealing most things from the patient while you are attending him." "Sometimes reprove sharply and emphatically and sometimes comfort with solicitude and attention, revealing nothing of the patient's future or present condition. For many patients through this cause have taken a turn for the worse."[18] The physician clearly is expected to decide *for* the patient. "Patients in fact put themselves into the hands of their physician."[19]

If he did not participate in the physician's decisions, the Greek patient was nonetheless expected to decide who was a good physician. The book *Affection* is devoted to instructing the layman so that he can make some of these judgments himself. In the book *On Joints,* the physician is urged to publish his cases and admit when his treatments are bad.[20] These injunctions seem at odds with the recommendations in other books of the Hippocratic corpus. They illustrate an interesting feature of the whole corpus in its therapeutic as well as its moral contents. The Hippocratic books often seem to be commentaries on each other, giving contrary opinions on key topics or elaborating and refining them.

There is very little in the corpus to indicate an obligation to obtain the patient's consent as we would understand consent today. Nor is there any hint of the existence of conflicts of obligations and opinions between patient and physician or what to do about them. The Hippocratic physician's relationship with the patient is one of benign, authoritarian paternalism, and to some degree, the patient enters it at his own risk. It is left to him to know how to tell the good physician from the charlatan.

The Hippocratic books are moral in the sense that they espouse a set of strongly held beliefs about what is right and wrong in the physician's conduct. They are not really ethical in any formal sense of the term; that is, they do not give a systematic justification of philosophical principles for the relationships and obligations they enjoin. The moral precepts themselves are not problematic but simply stated as true. What genuine ethics there is–in the sense of justification of beliefs–is only implicit. No dialectic or analysis of contrary opinions is offered–except possibly between books, but not within them.

There is in the corpus, therefore, no explicit formal theory of the physician-patient relationship. A range of philosophies are adapted in a very pragmatic way to meet the requirements of medical practice. This was especially true in the Hellenistic period when theories of medicine and philosophies formed the basis of the physician's personal behavior as well.

The physician's "moral virtuosity" to which Edelstein refers was displayed on an instrument of his own choosing.[21] He vested himself with moral as well as technical authority–a serious confusion of his obligations which persists today.

The physician's obligations to his patient, as portrayed in the Hippocratic corpus, were not drawn from a philosophical consideration of the nature of medicine, or of his relationship with the patient. Even in those philosophies with a strong moral component, the idea of obligations of the physician toward the humanity of the patient is very inadequately developed. Indeed, the full force of these obligations to the patient as a human being was not felt until the oath and the deontological books were adopted by the Jewish, Christian, and Islamic religions. Then the obligation to act humanely and with compassion was justified because the patient was a fellow human, a brother, created by the same God who loves all men. Only when the major religions gave their benediction to the oath did it become the universal normative guide of physicians–a status it had not achieved in the pagan world.

Philosophical Basis

The first discernible attempt to provide a philosophical basis for the physician's moral obligations to his patient is found in Scribonius Largus, who lived at the time of the Emperor Claudius. Medicine, he says, incurs the obligation to sympathy, humaneness, and a true love of mankind because it is inherent in the nature of the profession, the vocation or calling, of the doctor. Edelstein traces Largus' view back to its origins in Cicero's *De Officiis* and in the second century Stoic philosopher Panaetius.[22] Panaetius held that we must be faithful to the role we have assumed in life. The physician has assumed a role that demands compassion and humaneness. These are the physician's professional virtues, though they are not, of course, exclusive with him. The same sentiments are expressed by Sarapion in the second century A.D. and by Libanius. The latter's speech to young physicians represents the pagan epitome of the obligations and empathy a physician owes his patients.[23]

These noble sentiments of Libanius derive from some of the loftier elements of the Stoic philosophy. They present a theory of the physician-patient relationship based on the duty of the physician to be benevolent, kind, and loving, for that is the role he has voluntarily assumed. We are not told whether that kindliness and love of humanity extend to treating the patient as an independent person with an identity of his own, which can be smothered even by a loving but authoritarian physician. In fact, evidence would indicate that the "loving kindness" is that of a father and not the respectful solicitude of one adult for another.

The image of the good physician and the content of his morality in the Hippocratic corpus underwent some transformations in ancient times, from a craftsman's ethic of work done well to the Stoic's ethic of duty and obligation to mankind and humanity. This is a truly remarkable moral image, considering the inhumanity of so many other sectors of ancient life. It was refined by infusion not only with religious values, as evidenced in the Christianized Hippocratic oaths of early centuries, but also with the "Fifty Admonitions to Physicians" of Isaac Israeli and the code of Ishaq Ibn Ali al-Ruhawi–both of the ninth century.[24]

Many scholars have traced the unbroken line of medical moral tradition from Hippocrates' books through their later religious associations to the codes of the present time. The codes of Thomas Percival in eighteenth-century England, the first and subsequent revisions of the AMA code, the codes of the World Medical Association (Geneva), and the Nuremburg and Helsinki codes all share the same provenance.

What is most significant in all these codes is the ethos–not a formally developed ethic–of the patient-physician relationship which we inherit. That ethos, which is still the dominant influence on how physicians see themselves, is that of the benign, authoritarian, dedicated, and competent craftsman who acts in the interest of his patient out of motives as practical as a good reputation and as lofty as love of mankind. The transaction is, with minor exceptions however, unilateral. It centers in what the physician does for the patient, who is in the main a passive recipient, one who cannot penetrate the mysteries of what is happening to him, and whose illness would be adversely affected if he knew the truth about his condition. There is no sense of accountability to the patient, only to the physician's own conscience; no opportunity for valid consent; no sense of responsibilities to society or to other health professions; no sense of the corporate obligation of the profession for quality of care, accessibility, and the like; and no sense of the obligation of the patient, as a member of the human race, a class instance as we have called it, to participate in medical work which may benefit only future generations.

The concept of the relationship with the patient inherited from ancient times rests on a set of strongly held beliefs, but it is not, strictly speaking, an ethical relationship. That is, the moral beliefs are rarely problematic, nor are they systematically derived, their logic examined, or their philosophical foundations demonstrated. In fact, one interpretation of the ancient medical ethos would forbid this kind of open examination. The physician was a member of a secret society, if we are to accept Jones' interpretation of the closing sentences of the treatises on *Law* and *Decorum*.[25] In this view, his morality was therefore his own and protected from the eyes of the uninitiated.

Contemporary Medical Morality

The image of medical morality each physician carries with him today is a highly personalized compound of these multiple historical sources. There may be considerable logical incompatibility among the individual formulations and interpretations of what a physician thinks medicine is, what the good man as physician should be, and what is the appropriate patient-physician relationship. Some physicians are impressed by economic forces; others want medicine to be a science, an art, or an hieratic enterprise. Some are highly pragmatic and would adapt to forces as they are, emphasizing the need for political defenses–unionization, strikes, and so on; some yearn for a return to the oath which, for them, takes on a quasi-scriptural significance.

Lacking a formalized theory of medicine or a philosophically derived notion of the relationship with patients, our society finds it more and more difficult to codify the principles of moral behavior for the good physician. Witness the serial transformations in the professional code of the AMA from 1848, when it was introduced, to the latest suggestions for revision in 1978. The first document was much lengthier, more specific, and strongly shaped by Percival's concept of the physician as gentleman. The 1978 revisions are the slimmest yet, consisting of ten brief paragraphs, pragmatically stated and increasingly wary of terms which might suggest some personal or humane commitment of a higher order than we might expect in a contractural relationship. The result is a cautious, legalistic, noncommitting document.

As with all previous codes, the latest revision is created *by* the profession and *for* the profession. Yet the preamble states that the code is to aid the physician in relationships with "patients, colleagues, members of allied health professions and the public." If there was consultation with any of these other groups, it is not mentioned explicitly. The unilateral spirit common to all medical codes dominates this latest version as well.[26]

The proposed revision, like its predecessor, contains elements essential to good professional conduct. Nonetheless, it perpetuates the unilateral and authoritarian determination of a physician's obligations. Like the ethos of the Hippocratic corpus, the current AMA decalogue makes no reference to the patient's consent, to the possibility of conflicting values, to the mutual obligations of patient and physician, to the mutual moral obligations of the members of the health care team, or to the physician's obligations when practicing in the hospital.

These omissions are serious when we consider the magnitude and direction of the external pressure which now intrudes from all sides on the physician's relationship with the patient. There is, for example, no acknowledgment of some of the major concerns expressed in the various patients' Bill of Rights, no recognition of the pluralism of today's value systems, no acknowledgment of any specific social responsibility or of the conflicts in accountability to society and to individual patients. Most of the major sociopolitical forces transforming medicine–the bureaucratization of medical care, the rise of consumerism, the demands of third-party payers, and the growing volume of government regulatory and legislative incursions–are simply not addressed.

The medical profession seems to have carried an honorable but dated philosophy of the physician-patient, physician-society relationship into a world which seriously questions almost every tenet of that ancient model. Patients today are educated; some live in democratic societies; they already have the legal as well as the moral right to decide how to dispose of their bodies; many want to define health in their own terms, or at least to decide for themselves what is worthwhile.

These revised AMA principles seem unmindful of the natural death acts, or of the swelling demand for partnership in the social decisions about resource allocation, the uses of technology, and the types of services to be provided. They also ignore the signals coming from the self-care movement, alternate medical systems, and the increasing popularity of quasi-mystical therapeutic models.

Moreover, all qualitative phraseology alluding to service, or suggesting a special obligation to compassion such as Scribonius Largus might urge, is eliminated. One senses a legalistic constraint, no doubt in response to the ambience of malpractice and litigation. This spirit is disappointing, nonetheless, in a profession with the noble traditions of medicine. It is one thing to answer questions in court succinctly and to be mindful of the fact that overstatement too often provides material for a new line of embarrassing questions. It is another thing to take a legalistic stance in setting forth what should be the moral goals for a profession so deeply enmeshed in human concerns, as medicine must of necessity be.

The trend of the suggested emendations in the latest AMA code seems to take us back to the ethics of the physician as craftsman-businessman, a pragmatic ethic more a protection of reputation than an assumption of special obligations. The overtones of individualism and autonomy in the physician-patient relationship are also very obvious.

To its credit, the code does not try to give specific answers to or prescriptions for the many vexing medical-moral issues of the day, such as abortion, euthanasia, behavior control, experimentation, and organ transplantation. In this sense, it does qualify as a set of principles directed to the physician-patient relationship. But these principles are not derived from an explicit, formally derived philosophy of the physician-patient relationship. They are therefore subject to the unpredictable vacillations of political, social, and legal events. It is the force of these events which seems to be shaping the evolution of the AMA code and its more recent emendations.

The philosophical deficiencies of codes of professional ethics—as we have outlined them thus far—raise the central question of this chapter: Is a philosophical basis derivable for professional ethics, one which arises out of the nature of the relationship of doctors with patients, and which could serve to reconstruct future codes more suitable to a democratic, educated, morally pluralistic society?

A Philosophical Basis for the Physician-Patient Relationship

The remainder of this chapter attempts to establish a philosophical foundation for professional ethics on three phenomena specific to medicine: the *fact of illness,* the *act of profession,* and the *act of medicine.* The interrelationships of these three phenomena are sufficiently unique to medicine to constitute a specific and special kind of human relationship which ought to be conducted in certain specific ways to be morally defensible. In developing these points, we will draw on the conclusions of Chapters Five through Eight–specifically, that the fact of illness involves one in a bodily condition vis-à-vis others and the world; that clinical judgment is aimed at providing good decisions for patients; that within the physician-patient relationship, discretionary space is needed because of the individualized nature of the transaction; and finally, that the normative aspects of medical ethics flow from the values inherent in the relative aim of medicine as healing. We will draw especially on the axiom of vulnerability.

The Fact of Illness

Medicine and physicians exist because humans become ill. Illness is a subjective state, one in which a human being detects some change, acute or chronic, in his mode of existence based on anxiety about the functions of body or mind.

As we have already indicated, illness may or may not be associated with demonstrable pathology. It is, rather, the perception of an altered state of existence, one in which the patient interprets some symptom or sign as an indication that he is no longer "healthy" according to his own definition of that fluid and multi-interpretable word.

A person who arrives at the conclusion that he is "ill" becomes a patient–one who bears some disability, some deficiency or concern, one who is no longer "whole," one who perceives special limits on his accustomed activity.

The person who becomes a patient suffers what is essentially an ontological assault. In our usual state, we see ourselves identified with our bodies, facing the world and acting on it in essential unity. In illness the body is interposed between us and reality; it impedes our choices and actions and is no longer fully responsive. The body stands opposite to the self. Instead of serving us, we must serve it. It intrudes on our existence rather than enhancing and enriching it. We can no longer use it for transbodily purposes.

With this assualt on the ontological unity of body and self, illness erodes the image we have fashioned of ourselves over the years. That image harmonizes our deficiencies and our strong points; we carefully and laboriously protect and refurbish it; we delicately balance it against the external exigencies of human life. Illness forces a reappraisal, poses a threat to the old image and the need to fashion a new image, opening up all the old anxieties and imposing new ones–often including the threat of death or drastic alterations in life-style.

This ontological assault of illness is aggravated by the loss of certain specific freedoms which we identify as peculiarly human. The patient is no longer free to make rational choices among alternatives. He lacks the knowledge and the skills necessary to effect a cure or to gain relief from pain and suffering. In many illnesses, the patient is not even free to reject medicine, as in severe trauma or other overwhelming, acute emergencies. Voluntarily or not, the patient is forced to place himself under the power of another person, the health professional, who has the knowledge and the skills which can heal–but also harm. This involuntary need grounds the axiom of vulnerability from which follows the obligations of the physician.[27]

When a person becomes ill, he is therefore in an exceptionally vulnerable state, one which severely compromises his customary human freedoms to use his body for transbodily purposes, to make his own decisions, to act for himself, and to accept or reject the services of another. The state of being ill is therefore one of wounded humanity, of a person compromised in his fundamental capacity to deal with his vulnerability.

How unique is the state of illness? Is it not a common condition in many other human situations? After all, the prisoner is deprived of his freedom and civic rights; the poor and the socially outcast are constrained even in the most mundane matters of life; none of us is totally free; we must all conform to some set of social conventions. But in none of these situations is our capacity to deal with our vulnerability so impaired as in illness. We feel, usually, that we can cope with almost all of the other states of vulnerability if we have our health. After all, we perceive health as a means toward freedom and other primary values. We ask only to be released from prison, given a job or money, and if we are healthy, we can rebuild our humanity and the integrity of our person. In illness, none of these things will help. Our essential existential mechanisms for coping with all other exigencies have been compromised, and more essential than that, we face the threat of loss of life itself, or we are suddenly asked to live a life not worth living.

There is a special dimension of anguish in illness. That is why healing cannot be classified as a commodity, or as a service on a par with going to a mechanic to have one's car fixed, to a lawyer for repair of one's legal fences, or even to a teacher for repair of one's defects in knowledge. The teacher-student, lawyer-client, and serviceman-customer relationships have some of the elements of the physician-patient relationship in that there is also an inequality of knowledge and skill, and one person seeks assistance from another who professes to provide it. What is different is the unique ontological assault of illness on the body-self unity, and the primacy of the freedom to deal with all other life situations which illness removes. Without denying the possible analogy with, let us say, the lawyer-client relationship, it would be difficult to argue that the degree of injury to our humanity and the kind of injury we suffer in litigation are identical in their existential consequences to being ill.

The Act of Profession

In the presence of a patient in the peculiar state of vulnerable humanity which is illness, the health professional makes a "profession." He "declares aloud" that he has special knowledge and skills, that he can heal, or help, and that he will do so in the patient's interest, not his own. That is what entering a profession means—not simply becoming a member of a defined group with a common education, standards of performance, and a common ethic. These are all accidental to the central act of profession, which is an active, conscious declaration, voluntarily entered into, and signifying willingness to assume the obligations necessary to make the declaration authentic.

Health professionals make this act of profession publicly when they accept a degree at graduation, when they take the oath of their profession, and most importantly, every time they present themselves to a patient in need who seeks their assistance in healing. They make the act of profession implicitly, but nonetheless undeniably. The expectation is thus induced in the ill person that the declaration will be true and authentic, that the professional knowledge and skill are there, and that the professional concern for the patient's interest will be truly exercised.

Medicine is, of course, not alone in making an act of profession which invites specific expectations of performance. Lawyers, teachers, and ministers similarly declare a special competence and its use in the interests of those who seek their aid. Their clients also lack something they need and are, like the patient, vulnerable to varying degrees. The ethics of each profession rests on the authenticity of its claim–the physician's claim to restore health, the lawyer's to seek justice, the teacher's to redress ignorance, and the minister's to teach the way of salvation.

The act of profession is a promise made to another person in need and therefore existentially vulnerable. The relationship between the professional and those he serves is characterized by an inequality in which the professional holds the balance of power. All the usual ethical obligations of making and keeping promises apply, but with a difference: The inequality of power imposes special obligations on the person who professes. The professional-client relationship is not simply a contract between equals in which each party can negotiate in his own interest, since one party is not free to avoid negotiating. Medicine, law, teaching, and the ministry do not supply products in the usual legal and commercial sense.

Each profession fulfills the promise inherent in its act of profession by a specific action which identifies that profession. This central act is the vehicle of authenticity and the bridge which joins the need of the one seeking help with the promise of the one professing to help. We can examine that central act only for medicine, though analogous analyses are applicable to the other professions.

The Central Act of Medicine

A patient in need who consults a physician wants to know what *is* wrong, what *can* be done about it, and what *should* be done. These three questions, and the subsets of questions which contribute to answering them, taken together, constitute the anatomy of clinical judgment previously developed. The final question–What should be done?–is the major focus of the patient's attention and the end toward which the whole process must be directed. It eventuates in a recommended action. While all the other questions leading to it can be reopened, the recommended action is, as an event, irretrievable. The end of medicine, formally considered, is therefore a right and good healing action taken in the interest of a particular patient. All the science and art of the physician converge on the choice: among the many things that *can* be done, that which *should* be done for this person in this particular situation of life. It is a choice of what is *right* in the sense of what conforms scientifically, logically, and technically to the patient's needs, and a choice of what is *good,* what is worthwhile for this patient. The recommended action intermingles technical and moral dimensions which may not always be immediately reconcilable.

This culmination in a right and good healing action is what constitutes medicine *qua* medicine. Diagnosis and therapeutics, singly and together, are propaedeutic only. The physician acts as a physician only when he particularizes the conclusions about what is wrong and what can be done in a decision about what *ought* to be, *must* be, *may* be, or *should not* be done for this patient, here and now. In making this claim, we do not wish to belittle the necessity for scientific research and application. Bear in mind our discussion of the role of theory in the epistemology of medicine in the first section of Chapter Four.

The patient expects the end of medicine to be an action which is right and good for him. This is the promise he perceives in the *act* of profession, collectively from organized medicine and singularly from his personal physician or physicians. It is what he expects also from medical and health organizations–the team, the hospital, or the agency.

The medical act combines technical and moral decision making in a way which makes it a moral enterprise of a special kind. Each medical decision involves the complicated interplay of several value sets–those of the physician, of the patient, and of society. In a pluralistic society, these value sets may differ sharply from each other. The possibilities of conflict in the conception of the good between physician and patient are many. A very special problem in medical decision making is how to resolve these conflicts in a morally defensible way.

Value conflicts occur in a relationship of inequality inherent in the vulnerability of the patient, as outlined above. The assault of illness on the usual freedoms of the human being presents an immediate and present danger that the patient's values might be violated or that the physician may confuse technical with moral authority. The patient's moral agency is at risk, and a special obligation of the act of profession is to protect that moral agency while treating the patient.

By virtue of his act of profession, the physician raises specific expectations and thus voluntarily assumes certain specific obligations. It is these obligations, as well as those of the patient to the physician, which we shall examine next.

Obligations Arising from the Special Nature of the Patient-Physician Relationship

The obligations which arise from the construal of the patient-physician relationship outlined here form the philosophical basis for a professional ethic–one which would obtain regardless of the position the physician might take on any of the specific moral dilemmas of medicine. A cursory examination of these obligations can illustrate the primacy of the *acts* of profession and medicine taken in the face of the *fact* of illness.

Let it be clear that no new moral principles need be elaborated. The well-adopted moral principles of truth telling and promise keeping, as well as the principles of nonharm and vulnerability, will suffice, but modulated by those special existential circumstances which define the relationship of one needing to be healed confronting one professing to heal. The same principle would apply analogously to the lawyer-client, teacher-student, and minister-subject relationships, each modified by the specific expectations generated by the act of profession each makes when confronting a patient or client who is seeking assistance.

To begin with, the act of medical profession is inauthentic and a lie unless it fulfills the expectation of technical competence. If the special knowledge upon which the act of profession is based is wanting, then the whole relationship begins with a lie. The decision may even fortuitously turn out to be the right and good one for the patient, but if it does, it is based on chance, not knowledge. The patient has been deceived into believing that the advice he received is the fruit of the physician's competence. The far greater likelihood is that the incompetent physician will not make the right or good decision. Then he becomes worse than a quack. The latter at least follows a system which makes no claim to being scientific, while the incompetent physician shrouds his ignorance in a mantle of science.

The moral obligation to be competent is lifelong and a matter of daily concern. It begins with a sound medical education and house staff training and goes on to a dedication to continuing education, a willingness to subject his decisions to peer review, an openness to criticism by his colleagues, a willingness to confess ignorance or error to the patient, and a concentrated and sustained effort to deepen his clinical craftsmanship. Competence, then, is a moral imperative and a clear statement of that fact together with its fullest implications; it should be an essential element in any professional code. Competence is explicitly required by the first four principles of the latest revision of the AMA code. It is equated therein with "scientific" medicine. Such a formulation is correctly applicable to the technical steps involved in diagnosis, prognosis, and therapeutics. It also includes the art and skill needed to perform the recommended procedures safely and with a minimum of discomfort.

But as our dissection (Chapter Six) of the complex anatomy of clinical judgments reveals, competence is a necessary but not a sufficient condition of a moral medical transaction and an authentic profession. Competence must itself be shaped by the end of the medical act–a right and good healing action for a particular patient.

Competence must be employed in the best interest of the patient, and wherever possible that interest must conform to the patient's values and sense of what it is to be healthy.[28]

Technically correct conclusions may not necessarily be in the patient's best interest when that interest is defined in the patient's terms–e.g., abortion for a Catholic, transfusion for a Jehovah's witness, prolonging life in someone prepared to die, or letting another die who wants to live what may seem to the physician an unsatisfying life. A scientifically correct medical conclusion, its "oughtness," can range from "must," "should," "may," or "need not" to "must not," depending upon the interacting moral agencies of patient and physician.

The physician has a special moral obligation to assure and facilitate the patient's moral agency, especially in light of the patient's special vulnerability. To assure a fully participatory moral agency, the physician must repair to the extent possible the wounded humanity and state of inequality of the sick person. He does so only in part by curing, or containing, illness or relieving pain and anxiety. These must be complemented by disclosure of the information necessary for valid choice and genuine consent[29] and by guarding against manipulation of choice and consent to accommodate to the physician's personal or social philosophy of the good life.

A first requirement, therefore, is to remedy the patient's information deficit as completely as possible. Information must be clear and understandable and in the patient's language. The patient must know the nature of his illness, its prognosis, the alternative modes of treatment, their probable effectiveness, cost, discomfort, side effects, and the quality of life they may yield. Disclosure must include degrees of ignorance as well as knowledge and the physician's own limitations.

The physician who is conscious of the special nature of his act of profession will not easily excuse himself from the obligation of disclosure on grounds that the patient cannot understand or will be harmed by the information. There is little if any evidence that such knowledge is deleterious, Hippocratic warnings to the contrary. Indeed, in those rare instances in which the matter has been studied, informed patients show a lower anxiety and complication rate than the uninformed.[30]

Reducing the inequality in information between patient and physician is essential in obtaining a morally valid consent, which is the vehicle for expression of the patient's moral agency. More is required than the minimal conditions of a legally valid consent, which is, after all, a guarantee against the grosser violations of the patient's right to decide. A morally valid consent moves closer to the realization of both senses of the word "con-sent," to *feel* and to *know* something *together*. Patient and physician therefore must both feel they *know* and understand the available facts, and both must *feel* they are truly part of the decision-making process.

When the patient cannot participate in the decision, the physician must deal with the patient's surrogate–the family, guardian, or court. The obligations to respect the patient's value system are the same. When dealing with surrogates, however, an additional obligation is imposed, and that is to be sure that they do in fact have the patient's interests at heart. In the case of the unconscious patient or the child, the physician must assure himself that the surrogate, parent or family, does not unconsciously wish the patient's demise.

This state of feeling and knowing together places the actual locus of decision making somewhere between physician and patient, and not really with one or the other. As in any relationship between humans, medical or otherwise, obtaining consent requires persuasion, a mutual accommodation of wills. It is extremely difficult to set limits on the degree to which manipulation of consent is morally permissible. It is important for this chapter only to indicate that the physician must be alert to those subtle choices of words, nuances of emphasis, or body language which tip the patient's consent in the direction of what the physician feels is good. It is unrealistic to expect even the most ethically sensitive physician not to wish that the patient would make certain choices. In certain cases, some degree of persuasion may even be ethically obligatory.

No set of rules can encompass all the subtle complexities of even the most ordinary relationship between two persons, much less the special dimensions peculiar to the medical transaction, in which one person in special need seeks the assistance of another who professes to help. What the preceding paragraphs underscore, however, is the weight of the obligations upon the physician. It is he who professes, in the face of the fact of illness, to act on behalf of the best interests of another person he presumes to help. The morality of clinical judgment goes well beyond the merely technical and scientific probity of the craft.

There are times when the physician can and should exert moral agency for the patient and make the value choice on his behalf. One instance would be when the patient or family requests him to do so even after the physician has attempted to provide the necessary information and has taken all pains to be clear and unequivocal about the choices. Some patients and families are either emotionally or educationally ill equipped to deal with such difficult decisions. They may ask the physician to decide. The physician then has a mandate to assume moral agency, and it would be a failure of the authenticity of his act of profession not to say what should be done. The same applies when the situation is of such an urgent nature that to consult the patient or even his family would be impossible or would delay emergency treatment. In the operating and emergency rooms, or the intensive care and coronary care units, the obligations we have stressed must be drastically modified because the patient's interest itself overrides even these fundamental requirements of medical morality. The retrospective examination of how, for what reasons, and according to what value sets the decisions were made is an essential antidote to the overzealous assumption of moral authority even in emergency situations.

Here, too, a caveat is in order. For the physician to say simply that he would treat the patient as he would treat himself or a member of his family is morally unsound. This misinterpretation of the golden rule would only reopen the possibility of overriding the patient's wishes. The golden rule in medical decisions is to be observed rather differently: *We should so act that we accord the patient the same opportunity to express or actualize his own view of what he considers worthwhile as we would desire for ourselves.*[31] This latter interpretation of the golden rule is fully consistent with the view of authenticity of the act of profession we have developed.

What obligations of this type require is a combination of conscious advertence to the meanings of the three elements–the fact of illness, the act of profession, and the act of medicine–with compassion. We do not think this has to involve the *iatrikê philia,* the love of which Pedro Lain-Entralgo speaks as the fundamental link in his superb phenomenological study of the physician-patient relationship. It does require the capacity to "feel with" the patient something of the existential situation he is experiencing in the condition of illness, whether it is somatic or physical in origin. Not to feel something of the patient's anguish and anxiety before the ontological assault of illness is to rely only on a rational adumbration of the obligations which inhere in the act of profession. But even this is superior to the more traditional conception of the physician as benevolent agent of both technical and moral decision making who decides what is best for the patient.

Many aspects of the physician's obligations which could be derived from the philosophy of the medical transaction proposed here have not been touched upon. Those chosen are meant to be illustrative, not comprehensive. We have not discussed, for example, how to resolve conflicts in values between physician and patient, between the physician's social and patient responsibilities, the obligations of the profession as a corporate whole, or the applicability of these principles when the physician functions in a collectivity as a member of a team or an institution.

Also, on this view, there is a set of obligations which would bind the patient so that we can begin to develop an ethics of the good patient. If the physician construes his act of profession as a special promise given under special conditions, and if the patient understands it that way, then the patient incurs certain obligations as well. He must be truthful in the information he gives the physician; he must avoid manipulating the physician in consent; he must follow faithfully the recommendations mutually agreed upon; he must educate himself sufficiently to comprehend the facts disclosed to him and take the trouble to be sure he does understand; and he must not consult another physician without informing his medical attendant unless he suspects dishonesty or malpractice. Further, he is partially obligated, by the fact that he is a member of the human race, to participate in reasonable experiments which are either aimed at healing his disease (therapeutic) or at discovering possible cures of this disease for others (nontherapeutic), provided the other rules for professional behavior are followed. We say "partially obligated" because the vulnerability of the patient excuses him from any absolute obligation. The principle of autonomy and the principle of partial obligation enunciated above represent almost a classic example of the possible clash between two goods. On the one hand, the person who is ill is clearly given the opportunity and the freedom to attend to his needs for healing, a value which takes precedence over any altruism to be demanded of him. However, the ill person is also a member of the human race and has obligations to help foster the understanding of the disease so that either he or others might benefit. It is our view that the class-instance axiom, derived from the ontology of the body in the doctor-patient relationship, should receive more weight in discussions of human research and the future of medicine than it has to date in the literature.

The patient, in short, in the relationship we have described, owes the physician the same respect for his values and cannot demand that the physician violate them even when the patient might benefit. The patient cannot ask his physician to practice deception with insurance companies and government agencies. In sum, even though the vulnerability imposed by illness makes the patient more vulnerable, the tyranny of the patient is as wrong as the tyranny of the physician.[32]

This construal of the patient-physician relationship calls therefore for mutual respect and compassion, even though it involves one person who is less free and more vulnerable. That is why the relationship cannot be regarded as a contract or even a covenant. It is not an agreement between two parties more or less equal, more or less free, who can negotiate terms for the delivery of some service or commodity. Medical care is not a commodity one may choose as freely as one chooses automobiles or television sets.

What we propose is a mutually binding set of obligations, predicated upon a special kind of human interaction and deriving its morality from the empirical realities in the relationship which specify it among human relationships. These specifications could be the basis for a philosophically justifiable statement of principles—a code—common to all physicians, indeed to all healers. If their implications are expanded, we can even hope for a more general code applicable to all the health professions, at least in part, since all health professionals make an act of profession in the sense we have defined it here.

The post-Hippocratic reconstruction of professional ethics is therefore possible. We need not return to the ethics of the good craftsman, as in our Greek beginnings. We can instead extend and build upon the idea of Scribonius Largus and Panaetius that there is an ethics specific to each profession, based on the nature of that profession, and philosophically justifiable.

Conclusion

Looked at historically, our line of reasoning has taken us away from the dominant sources of medical morality–that is, the Hippocratic corpus and especially the oath, away from both the craft and the privileged status ethic. Our inclination has been, rather, to the extension and elaboration of the idea of profession as it was advanced by Scribonius Largus and Panaetius and the middle Stoics. We have suggested a derivation of medical ethics from the specific relationship of three phenomena of the medical transaction rather than applying philosophical conceptions drawn outside of medicine to medicine. In contradistinction to Scribonius Largus, we have not made *humanitas* the specific end of medicine, nor, as with Lain-Entralgo, the *iatrikê philia,* but rather a right and good healing action for a particular patient. This is what the physician professes, what the patient expects, and what must be offered in the presence of the state of wounded humanity we call illness. This is the foundation of professional ethics, the source of medical morality, and the leitmotiv of a more satisfactory professional code of how the physician should act *qua* physician. It is necessarily antecedent to whatever position may be taken in specific moral dilemmas. Indeed, sensitively attended to, it assures the morality of the personal transaction even when there is a difference between physician and patient or physician and physician about particular medical moral problems.

A summary of the obligations for a medical professional code of ethics might be schematized as follows:

1. *Technical competence.*
2. *Insuring moral agency of patient.*
    - *Information*
    - *Consent*
    - *Proxy consent*

3. *Respect for the individualized nature of the transaction.*

A corresponding set of patient obligations can be summarized as follows:

1. *Trust in competence.*
2. *Respect for the moral agency of the physician.*
3. *Truth telling about the illness.*
4. *Caution in asking more of medicine than it can provide.*
5. *Partial obligation to participate in medical research.*

With these considerations in mind, we will turn to some moral problems of contemporary medical practice that are rarely addressed.

III

Applications to Moral Agency: Social Ethics

10

The Social Ethics of Primary Care

Introduction

In primary care, as in all other forms of care, the moral and ethical issues are situated in a complex matrix of reciprocal obligations which simultaneously bind professionals, patients, and society. Some of these obligations are common to all forms of care, while others are modified in different ways specific to each form of care.

This chapter examines only one of the questions in this complicated matrix: Is the human need for primary care of such a nature that it implies some obligation on the part of the health professions and society to make it universally accessible? Is there a moral center to primary care, or is it morally neutral? If there is an obligation of society with respect to primary care, is it absolute or relative? If relative, under what specific conditions is the obligation binding?

By delimiting the question thus, we do not demean the importance of many other ethical issues in primary care. It is justified by reason of space limitation, but especially by the urgency of the

This chapter has been expanded and revised from an article by Dr. Pellegrino, "The Social Ethics of Primary Care: The Relationship Between a Human Need and an Obligation of Society," *Mount Sinai Journal of Medicine,* Vol. 45, No. 5 (September–October 1978), 593–601.

questions and the political, legal, and economic implications of the answer we give to it.

We argue that the need for primary care is a universal human need; that it imposes a claim on society and the professions; and that the claim is relative, not absolute, but nonetheless a strong one in a democratic, affluent, technologically capable society like ours.

This proposition will be developed in four steps. The first describes the moral center of the medical enterprise; the second locates the moral center of primary care; the third defines in what sense it might be considered a right or an obligation; and the fourth outlines the potential conflict between such an obligation and others already binding on health professions and society.

The Moral Center of the Medical Enterprise

That medicine as medicine is at heart a moral enterprise is clear from its central aim: a right and good healing decision taken in the interest of an individual patient or society in need (cf. Chapters Six and Seven). This moral quality has been acknowledged in the professional codes of Eastern and Western medicine for two millennia.[1] Ever since, physicians have felt bound to normative moral guidelines which transcended mere self-interest.[2]

What has not been so clear until very recently—and what puzzles many physicians today—is that medicine must also be an *ethical* enterprise. That is, the physician's actions must have some rational justification beyond simple conformity to one or another ancient or modern professional code, however admirable. It is now essential that ethics as a formal discipline be recognized to be as integral to the practice of responsible medicine as the basic and clinical sciences.

Medicine is intrinsically a moral activity because all its many functions converge upon one end: making a decision for a particular person who presents himself in need, as a *patient,* someone bearing distress or disease. Everything the physician does, all his skill and knowledge, must focus on a choice of which of the many possible actions should be taken for this patient. What is the right decision, the one which is good for this patient—not patients in general, not what is good for the physician, for the science of medicine, or even for society as a whole. This is a summary of our argument in Chapter Six.

The moment we introduce the words "right" with respect to an action, and "good" with respect to an end, we introduce morality—any system of strongly held beliefs and values against which behavior is judged. Behavior in accord with such values is considered to be moral; behavior contrary to them is immoral. Every aggregation of humans united for some common end—a society, an institution, or a profession—has some set of values it considers prescriptive and inviolate. Some of these beliefs are trivial and confined to arbitrary matters of choice or taste. Others are held as right for all men because they somehow reflect what it means to be human and to enter into relationships with other humans.

The Hippocratic oath and corpus, and its successors and analogues, codify the moral behavior for physicians. They perceive implicitly that values enter into medical decisions, and that the self-interest of the physician and the demands of his art are to be shaped by the nature of the special human relationship of healer and person seeking to be healed. They define guidelines for moral or approved decisions and actions in that relationship.

Medicine is therefore a moral enterprise in two senses: first, in that its central and most characteristic function focuses on a right decision for a patient; and second, in that it explicitly codifies the values which should guide the good physician's decisions. But these considerations do not automatically make medicine an ethical enterprise, even though these codes are often called "codes of ethics," and a physician who follows them is considered an "ethical" physician. To be "ethical" is not synonymous with following a code of moral principles.

Ethics comes into existence, properly speaking, when morality itself becomes problematic, when the validity of beliefs about what is right and good comes into question, or when a conflict between opposing moral systems or obligations must be resolved. Morality takes its values and beliefs for granted as presuppositions that apply to all men. Ethics emerged as a formal discipline when the Sophists and Socrates first began to question Greek presuppositions about the right and the good in political and social life. Among them, morality for the first time became explicitly problematic, and the history of ethics since then has been an attempt to examine the presuppositions about what is right and good and what *should* be normative for human actions.

Ethics, then, is a formal intellectual discipline, a branch of philosophy that systematically examines the rectitude of human actions. Classical ethics was normative in that it attempted to arrive at generalizable principles of right conduct together with their rational justifications. Modern ethics has concentrated on the meanings, usages, and logic of moral terms and statements, attempting more to clarify moral discourse than to make general rules about conduct. It is thus meta-ethical in its bias. Both activities, the normative and the meta-ethical, are, however, subject to disciplined thought which examines moral principles and statements for cogency, applicability, consistency, and the validity of the assumptions from which they derive.

If medicine is to become an ethical enterprise in the sense in which ethics has just been defined, then it must subject its traditional and current morality to systematic and critical examination. It must not only recognize the central role of values in the decisions it takes but must be prepared to justify the values it chooses as the basis for those decisions. Ethics, then, must become an integral element in the education and practice of the contemporary physician. Indeed, it has become indispensable if the profession is to fulfill its social responsibilities today and in the foreseeable future.

The Indispensability of Ethics for Modern Medicine

While most physicians recognize the essentially moral nature of their enterprise, many are confused by, and even resist, its conversion to an ethical task. Why, they ask, is a commonsense interpretation of the Hippocratic oath and its recent modifications no longer adequate?[3] While acknowledging the importance of the newer moral problems created by medical progress, it seems to them that all we require is amplification of traditional professional codes. What can ethicists, lawyers, and philosophers, inexperienced in the intricacies of clinical medicine, add except obfuscation?[4]

Moreover, many physicians hold to the common view that morals and values are not matters to be settled by rational discourse. A physician's values are learned "at his mother's knee" or in church.

Medical school is "too late" to try to teach what is right and good. Moral values, whether we hold them to be relative or absolute, cannot be settled by rational discourse, and anyway, we must follow our consciences, not theorizing ethicists.

These attitudes are by no means confined to physicians, but they are heightened by the positivist bias of modern medical education. Ethical discourse, and even more specifically, normative ethics are among those intellectual ventures that cannot be resolved by empirical or experimental method. They seem futile exercises, doomed to end in frustration at best and unnecessary enmities at worst. Medical students would better expend their energies in understanding disease mechanisms and solving practical problems.

These disinclinations of many physicians to ethical discourse are unfortunately reinforced by the openly critical, oversimplified, and adversarial attitudes of some ethicists. Those who take the trouble to teach and function at the bedside emerge with a deepened respect for the complexities of the physician's moral choices. But ethicists without these insights have generated an unfortunate backlash which hinders precisely the critical engagement of the moral issues in clinical decisions contemporary medicine needs.

Many physicians, like other educated people, may hold that morals are created by social attitudes. What is right and good is therefore determined and defined differently in different societies. It is useless, they hold, to argue about generalizable principles of right conduct. The same can be said by those who equate the good with whatever makes you feel comfortable. Any attempt at a rational consideration of such a relativistic subject as morals is certain to lead only to clashes of irreconcilable opinions in which no one is convinced. The inadequacy of this position is shown by the following.

First, simple reliance on professional moral codes is inadequate to cope with the complex obligations imposed on the modern physician. Professional codes are of necessity couched in general terms, terms often vaguely defined and open to serious differences of interpretation in their application to specific cases. Commendable as they may be, codes may also contravene each other or create conflicts of obligation not resolvable in the codes themselves. The older codes, moreover, were developed without the challenges to values posed by recent technological advances. For this reason, we described principles of current medical morality in Chapter Nine.

These limitations are illustrated by such examples as the differing nuances in the provisions assuring confidentiality in the Hippocratic oath, the International Codes, and the codes of the American or British Medical Associations. Or we can cite the absence of any recognition of social obligations in the Hippocratic oath, their variable mention in the American revisions, and their overriding importance in the Soviet physicians' code. One of us has elsewhere pointed out the silence of the Hippocratic ethic on a variety of problems of urgent importance to modern medicine.[5]

Beyond these difficulties is another even more fundamentally important for our times: Professional codes, ancient and modern, have customarily been drawn up by the profession. While benevolent in intention, these codes enjoin the physician to do what he deems best for the patient. But no mention is made of the patient's participation in that determination. The physician is assumed to be the patient's moral agent, and no notice is taken of the possibility of a conflict between the physician's and patient's value systems. Recognition of this weakness led to our proposal for patient obligations as well.

Such a paternalistic construal of the physician-patient relationship is increasingly untenable and even immoral. For many urgent reasons, patients now wish to exercise their own moral agency.[6] They are better educated and can understand the alternatives in medical decisions better than ever before, and legal opinions in democratic societies assure the individual of the right to accept or deny treatment. Moreover, the capabilities of modern medicine now extend to preventing, prolonging, or discontinuing life at will, modifying generation, genetics, and behavior—offering possibilities of intrusion into man's most personal and intimate existence. Even in the more mundane medical encounters, striking the balance of efficacy against harm, expense and discomfort requires the most careful assessment of what is worthwhile or valuable to the patient.

If moral paternalism were ever justified, even in simpler times, it had to be on the basis of some commonly shared set of values. But if there is a moral characteristic of our times, it is pluralism—not just between societies, which has always been the case, but within societies and between individuals even in the same family. Each physician represents only one set of the divergent views we hold today about the value of life, health, or happiness.

In almost every medical encounter these days, there is the possibility of conflict between the intersecting values of physician and patient. Each may differ about what is right and most in the patient's interests, even when there is relative certitude about the clinical facts. Neither the physician's nor the patient's moral beliefs can justly be given automatic precedence. The older codified morality of the profession no longer suffices to resolve these dilemmas.

The physician's beliefs are particularly susceptible to critical examination because illness makes the patient so vulnerable. The physician possesses the advantage of knowledge and power in the relationship. The physician thus has the greater responsibility for assuring that the moral center of his acts as physician–choosing what is good for another human being–is morally managed. Ethics can provide the tools for recognition of the ethical issues, the values which underlie our opinions about them, and the conditions for a just and moral management of the whole decision-making process.

None of this contravenes the heavy emphasis placed by so eminent a clinician as Richard Clarke Cabot on the moral imperative of competence in differential diagnosis, and relating the pathophysiological disturbances to the needs of a specific patient. Chester Burns, in a recent study, asserts that Cabot's emphasis on the importance of clinico-pathological correlations constituted an abnegation of traditional professional ethics.[7] This seems a rather extreme view and a little out of focus. It certainly does not vitiate the assertion that ethics is as intrinsic to the physician's clinical functions as the basic sciences and the clinical methodologies.

As we indicated, accuracy of clinical diagnosis and skill in differential diagnosis in the Cabot tradition are still essential to clinical decision making. These skills are moral imperatives as well. But they are anterior to, and not synonymous with, the moral center of medicine, which is located at a precise point: recommending what *should* and *ought* to be done. No matter how accurate the diagnosis and how appropriate the therapy, most clinical situations involve choices which patient and physician may regard as being of different worth.

Clinical competence is necessary to moral decision making but not sufficient for it. It is obviously essential to diagnose disseminated cancer of the breast accurately, but this does not dictate whether treatment should be instituted and if so, what kind. It is indispensable to the decision to discontinue life support measures in a patient with irreversible brain damage that the diagnosis and prognosis be as precise as possible. It is one thing to discuss the need for blood for a Jehovah's witness or abortion for a Catholic, but another to expect patients to take the treatment or to manipulate their consent.

Clinical competence is in no way compromised by a knowledge of ethics. Ethics is enhanced only when the clinical issues it examines are defined as verifiably, as accurately, and in as much detail as possible.

Some Philosophical Questions at the Foundations of Ethics

We have thus far emphasized the practical utility and importance of ethics for medicine. But the three major domains of medical ethics–the biomedical, professional, and social–rest upon certain philosophical foundations. These form our opinions on each of the specific medical-moral issues of our day. The ethical examination of medicine uncovers the importance of the philosophical foundations of all ethical discourse. Ultimately the vast differences in these foundations must be recognized.

One very serious problem concerns the possibility of constructing a universally acceptable professional moral code in the pluralistic moral climate of our times, as we have discussed in Chapter Nine. Remember that the Hippocratic oath, which so many have taken as typical of the moral values of the Greek physician, has been demonstrated as quite nonrepresentative. Ludwig Edelstein showed that the oath represented Pythagorean views and that many of its precepts were foreign to the Greek ethos. Many of the proscriptions in the oath–such as those against abortion, euthanasia, and surgery–were violated by Greek physicians who held to philosophies other than the Pythagorean.[8]

When the Hippocratic oath was Christianized during the Middle Ages, it may have, paradoxically, been more representative of the dominant value system than it was in Greek times. Christianity and even Judaism were more influential in European culture than was Pythagoreanism in Greece, and they shared common views on the sanctity of life and the meaning of illness.[9]

Today, the problem of a universally acceptable professional code is vastly complicated for want of any generally held ethical theory. The influence of Judeo-Christian moral values is no longer prevalent, as it once was in Western society. Can ethical relativists and objectivists, utilitarians and consequentialists and Kantian deontologists or natural law adherents find common ethical ground? We need only look at the divergent views each takes on the most common moral dilemmas of clinical medicine to appreciate how far we are from any code acceptable to all.

Must we abandon the effort in consequence, and with it the idea of a morally united profession so long based on the Hippocratic oath and corpus? What will be the impact of that abandonment on a profession already so seriously divided that physicians can hardly communicate? It seems to medicine's severest critics that the common bond is not a common moral commitment but a defense of social and economic privilege against public and government intrusion.

Is the answer, as some suppose, to be found in an eclectic amalgamation of opposing ethical theories, adding a little Kantian deontology to Bentham and Mills' utilitarianism, and spicing both with natural law? The different philosophical construals of what is right and good are logically and metaphysically incommensurable. Indeed, the more possibilities technology offers us to modify human existence, the sharper these differences become. New technology always poses the question of purpose, which in turn uncovers fundamental divergencies among the philosophical foundations of ethics.

We think the best possibility to reconstruct a common professional code lies in the development of a common philosophy of the physician-patient relationship. Some common understanding is achievable in what that relationship means and the obligations it implies for both physician and patient. These obligations could become the commonly accepted guide for all physicians–indeed, for all health workers. This is the hope of such commendable efforts at constructing a sound moral basis for the physician-patient encounter as Robert Veatch's contractual[10] and Paul Ramsey's covenant theories.[11]

We proposed to found professional medical ethics in the *fact* of illness and the *act* of *profession.* The *fact* of illness wounds the humanity of the person who is ill and deprives him of some of the freedoms most fundamental to being human–freedom to move about as one wishes, freedom to make one's own decisions, freedom from the power of others, and freedom to construct one's own self-image. In illness, pain, disability, and disease rob us of these freedoms and create an essential inequality between patient and physician. Hence, the preponderance of obligations rests with the healer who voluntarily declares himself at the disposal of the person in need. That voluntary declaration raises certain expectations, not only that the disease will be cured but that the damage to the patient's humanity, the vulnerability of being ill, will not be ignored in the curing. This is the force of the axiom of vulnerability developed in Chapter Eight.

A new relationship must evolve between patient and physician to recognize that the clinical decision–the heart of medicine–the choice of what is to be done, cannot be the exclusive privilege of one or the other. That decision must arise somehow, in the ground between someone in need, a patient, and someone, the healer, who professes to alleviate that need. Manifestly, in this view the long-held notion of the benign but authoritarian or paternalistic physician deciding what is best for his patient needs drastic revision. A more adult relationship based on a mutual respect for each other's value systems is required. This involves full disclosure of what is to be done and an assessment of alternatives of what is worthwhile in the patient's estimation. Such an adult relationship also calls for a frank appraisal of the degree of congruence, or lack of it, in patient and physician value systems. Each party must be able to know when he reaches a point at which compromise would violate conscience.

The objection is often raised that asking the patient to participate in clinical decisions may be psychologically or even physically damaging. Illness induces a state of dependence in many patients, and some patients seek, rather than reject, the physician's paternalism.

There is no doubt that patients vary in their desire for disclosure and for the fullness of consent to what the doctor recommends. But an increasing number of patients emphatically reject the dependent role. Moreover, all the weight of legal opinion has been progressively in favor of full disclosure and patient participation. This is also evidenced in the patients' Bills of Rights now appearing in significant numbers.

It is one thing for the physician to assume that he has authority to decide what is good for a patient on his own, and quite another to assume this responsibility if the patient or family ask him to do so because they feel incapable of understanding or choosing the alternatives. It is certainly not improper for the physician to respond to such a request. But under these circumstances, he is responding to a mandate given to him by the patient or family; he is not automatically assuming that mandate. This is a distinction which traditional medical moral codes have not made clearly, or at all.

The philosophical groundwork for a morally acceptable physician-patient relationship is further complicated today because physicians rarely function in isolation, and explicitly or implicitly are members of a team in which other health professionals–nurses, pharmacists, allied health workers–share in the care of most patients. This matter will be addressed in the next chapter.

All of this is vexatious indeed for medicine, which considers itself the senior profession, and for the others that are striving for their own professional identity. Despite these realities, the health professions will only lose further moral credibility if they permit professional prerogatives to override the need for a more sensitive statement of their common moral obligation as professed healers. A common code for the health professions must emerge.

These questions at the foundations of ethics bring us closer to even more fundamental problems that we can only mention. What we think is right and good depends, after all, on what we think man is, what his existence is for, what medicine is, and what its role is in human existence. The metaphysics of medicine and of man are the wellsprings from which flow our theories of ethics as well as the criteria we use to judge the rectitude of human acts.

Having developed further the moral center of the medical profession, we now turn to the specific manner in which the vulnerability axiom affects primary care.

The Moral Center of Primary Care

Wherein lies the source of a specific claim, right, or obligation with respect to primary care? To answer this question, we need some operational definition of primary care. The admirable one recently advanced by a committee of the Institute of Medicine can, in part, serve this function. This definition is more a descriptive essay than a strict definition, but it should help to counter the laxity and multiplicity of existing definitions and make discussions and research studies more comparable.[12]

Nonetheless, even this admirable statement requires some modification and expansion for our purposes. It sets forth the necessary conditions for optimal primary care very well, but not the sufficient conditions. It lacks precision in distinguishing primary care, especially its first-contact component, from other forms of care which share with it the same characteristics. If we are to find something specifically moral in primary care, we must locate this distinction more clearly.

The IOM definition enumerates five characteristics of true primary care: accessibility, comprehensiveness, coordination, continuity, accountability. They constitute primary care regardless of the specialty of the provider. The committee avers further that primary care must be rendered by a team, and that it can be taught only in settings which exemplify these standards.

These characteristics are certainly qualifications necessary to optimal primary care, but they also qualify optimal care in any branch of medicine, no matter how narrow. If every physician adhered to them, all medical care would assuredly be improved. But the major deficiency which has generated so much of the public interest in accessibility to primary care would not necessarily be remedied. That interest centers on the mundane but ubiquitous human need for access to first-contact care, readily, efficiently, considerately, and competently ministered wherever one lives or is visiting in this country.

First-contact care is, of course, not the whole of primary care, as the IOM definition makes clear. It is, however, that part of the primary care spectrum which, unfortunately, can be most easily neglected, even if physicians follow the IOM prescription within their own particular specialties. Even the so-called primary care specialties sidestep it all too eagerly in favor of what they consider more sophisticated models of care. Each specialty circumscribes primary care with its own restrictions: general internists emphasize personal care for adults; pediatricians for children; gynecologists for women. To care for the family, they must form a troika. Family medicine comes closest, but it too is showing a tendency to retreat from high-volume first-contact care to the more sedate forms of low-volume care for families.

Quality first-contact care cannot result from the fortuitous convergence of the partial efforts of the several specialties–even the primary care specialties. What is needed is unequivocal dedication to a system of care, geographically and temporally accessible at all times, and designed to respond to felt needs for medical assistance. Need must be interpreted, at least at the time of contact, broadly enough to embrace what the patient, not the physician, perceives as a need.

Those who presume to provide this kind of care must be willing to meet the patient on his own terms, by his definition of an emergency, and to provide medical assistance. "Assistance" means several things in first-contact care–specific treatment for curable disorders, to be sure. But the bulk of what is required is the capacity, humanely and competently, to respond to the human need for help with ills, most of which are self-limited or irremediable by specific treatment, but calling for counseling, symptomatic relief, reassurance, or education. Throughout, there must also be assurance that the simple will be separated from the serious and referred expeditiously to the appropriate level of care; and that the patient will be assisted in threading his way through the seemingly perverse and insuperable obstacles of referrals, institutions, and procedures which obstruct the patient's progress to attention.

From the public point of view, what is wanted is the personal security of medical advice and assistance nearby, vested in some identifiable place and some person with whom and to whom the anxiety of a medical event can be shared, transferred, or discussed. The universality, and the intensely human quality, of this need is obvious even in seemingly trivial matters to anyone who has ever played a role in first-contact care or who has experienced the fact of illness. Even the critics of too much medical care, and those who make policy decisions–the economists, legislators, planners, and physicians–rapidly become advocates when they or their families find themselves in need in the circumstance of illness.

This is not to gainsay the value and necessity of the more comprehensive components of primary care, the preventive and educational aspects, and the continuity lauded by the IOM definition. But the moral center of primary care, that segment which generates a moral claim and leads inevitably in our kind of society to discussions of rights and obligations, is first-contact care. This is the moral fulcrum on which all rights and obligations in health care ultimately must balance. It is the highest priority entry point for all of us as persons; without it, further assessments of rights cannot proceed.

Primary Care as a Moral Issue

Moral obligations arise whenever some right exists–that is, whenever one person holds a strong claim on another or on society. Obligations can also arise as the result of some act or declaration by a person or by society which generates an expectation or promise that something will be done or given.

The philosophy of rights is a complex subject, and we cannot engage it here. Suffice to say that the concept of rights is a fairly recent one, deriving from John Locke and the seventeenth-century concern for protection against absolutist government. We have since come to regard some rights as absolute or well nigh absolute, such as the rights to life, liberty, justice, freedom of expression, and self-determination. This is because we regard these rights as intrinsic to being fully human, and because they are fundamental to many other more relative rights. They are restricted only under the most stringent conditions, usually only when their exercise by one segment of society limits the exercise of similar or other rights by others. Moreover, though we are all possessed of these rights, we need not exercise them always, else social intercourse would be well nigh impossible.

Other rights are more clearly relative, since they obtain only when certain conditions give them substance and reality. If, for example, a government declares that education will be provided for all, or that a vaccine will be distributed free, then all citizens would have an equal claim. This claim is relative, not absolute, because it would be meaningless if there were no teachers or no vaccines. The right in these cases might, by common consent, be set aside to achieve some other human good: food, jobs, or housing.

In what sense may primary care be considered a right in our society and in our times? This is a limited question, but it is prior to the larger one of a right or guaranty to health care, or to the even more expansive right to health itself. The complexities and conflicts of values in all these questions are not to be minimized, and they present formidable obstacles, especially in a time of economic constraint.[13] They are, despite this, unavoidable in any attempt at designing a socially just health care system. The possibility of a right to primary health care and to the first-contact component is a good point of engagement for all the larger issues as well.

The remainder of this chapter argues that primary care is a relative right in our times and our society and that it takes on substance because of the expectations and promises such a society implies.

All rights of any substance are based on some common fact specific to human existence. A right or claim to access to primary care could be based on the universality of human illness and the need all humans share for assistance in healing and being healed. Few events are more distressing and more threatening to our humanity than a medical event. When illness occurs, it immediately pushes aside most other considerations; other needs become subservient to the need to be restored to the freedom of movement, decision making, and independence we associate with health and the fullness of being human. In illness our bodies, or our symptoms, become the center of concern, and the source of anxiety about what will happen to us, and what we should do next.

To relieve that anxiety, to transfer it, and to know what is happening is to begin the process of healing or adaptation essential to the reconstruction of the individual's existence. The precise degree of any person's need, the extent to which disability and discomfort can be tolerated or integrated into living, are highly individual matters. But every person, at some time or other, will be in the state of illness and will have some need for first-contact primary care.

There are things more important than health, though not many. The claim to primary care is therefore relative and not absolute, like the right to life, liberty, freedom of expression, or justice. Yet these anterior absolute rights cannot fully be exercised when a person is ill. An argument could be made that health, while its definition is highly personal, is a prior condition to the full exercise of most of our basic human rights. In previous chapters, we have cited this view as it occurred in history.

Though a relative right, primary care becomes something of a moral imperative in our times and in our society. We claim to be a civilized society, one which, among other things, is sensitive to the fullest expression of each person's humanity. We also claim to be a democratic society, one which promises equity of access to at least the minimum of things essential to a humane existence. That we do not deliver fully on the expectations we generate, either in housing, jobs, nutrition, or health care, does not excuse us from the obligations we incur by virtue of our declarations. As a society we profess to be civilized, democratic, and humane; this is enough to raise reasonable expectations, and is constantly a promise and an obligation we must fulfill if at all possible.

These expectations are further enhanced by the enormous expenditures of both public and private funds for health care services and institutions, as well as the education of health professionals. The health professions justify public support by declaring that they act in the public interest. So do the bureaucrats, the insurers, and even the proprietary institutions–though they admit to doing so for a profit. The whole health care establishment implies that it is offering a human good. These declarations engender the expectation that the consumers' notions of the basic needs pertinent to that good will be given high priority. Judging from public and legislative concerns, first-contact care is high on that priority list, even if it is not with the providers.

These social expectations are much intensified by the peculiar place health occupies in our culture. Our technological society promises ultimate control of all the distressing elements in human existence. It no longer accepts the will of God or violations of a taboo as adequate explanations for illness. Illness loses its meaning, and together with its unpredictability creates a special anxiety known only to modern man. In no other age was medicine capable of suggesting the possibility of physical immortality, as it does for so many people today. Moreover, as affluence increases, the tolerance for even minimal discomfort decreases. Medicine has become the means not only for control of the more dire prospects in illness but the guarantor of a life free of even the more trivial discomforts.

This overdependence on medicine can have dire economic consequences, as we are being steadily warned. We are exhorted to remember that health has no greater value than many other good things in life and that there must be a limit to the amount we spend on what some observers see as a cult of health. But before our cultural anxieties can be reduced to more rational proportions, their present reality must be confronted–and we must be as wary of undervaluing as overvaluing health and medical care.

Much depends upon whether we view medicine as useful only when it offers radical cure, or whether we see it, in addition, as a more widely useful mechanism for caring, coping with, and containing those ills for which there is no radical cure. Granted its notable failings in caring, medicine can and does, in large part, provide human assistance in the existential distress of illness. This assistance is of variable worth to different people, but we must not therefore conclude that its social utility for many others is inconsequential even in economic terms. Primary care, especially its first-contact component, is particularly pertinent in this respect.

The crucial question, then, in the social ethics of primary care is not whether it is an absolute human right. Rather, we must ask ourselves whether in a professedly democratic, affluent society with an abundance of available medical resources, we can allow so fundamental and universal a human need to go unfulfilled. Primary care, within the explicit framework of the here and now of our society, can be considered a relative human right, and a very real and pressing one. In other cultures and other times, it might very well not be regarded as such.

Looked at in this way, primary care has more of the quality of an obligation incurred by all of us by our mutual declaration of the kind of society we profess to be than a strict legal right in the Lockean sense. Locke's view of right has an adversarial and coercive quality that could negate much of what the public seeks from its health care system. An ethic of obligations voluntarily assumed, even if implicitly, seems preferable to a legalistically framed assertion of an absolute right.

Implications of Primary Care as a Social Obligation: Potential Conflicts

To accept primary care as a relative right or obligation owed to citizens of a society such as ours has obvious far-reaching implications. We face the same knotty dilemmas posed by regarding health care *in toto* as a civil right. The social, economic, fiscal, political, and ethical implications of guaranteeing health care have been widely examined in recent publications.[14] These essays are mentioned to indicate that the few ethical dilemmas we select in the remaining pages must be placed in a much larger context. These complexities can be illustrated by two sectors of conflict in making primary care even a relative right: the conflict with other forms of care, and with other obligations imposed on providers.

Some difficult questions arise immediately if we take the view that primary care is even a relative right. Is it ethically justifiable to give it a higher priority than other needed forms of care? Primary care does not exist in isolation. To assure access to it will lead ineluctably to assuring access to all forms of care. Is it not more socially defensible to divert resources to prevention than to meeting primary care needs, so many of which do not require dramatic treatment? Alternatively, should not our resources go into the more complex technologies, or into research? If the argument for primary care as a human need is valid, does it not apply with equal force to other forms of care?

A similar set of questions may be asked about the relationship of primary care to other human needs outside the realm of health. Are we not overinfatuated with health and medicine? Are not housing and nutrition, jobs and personal security, just as essential–indeed, more essential to a satisfactory human existence?[15] More to the point, are the deficiencies in these matters not more deleterious to health than the absence of primary care? Or will easy access not mean more abuse, inefficiency, and overuse of medical services?

Another set of conflicts becomes obvious when we examine the impact on providers–health professionals and institutions. Perhaps the most significant factor limiting the access and availability of primary care services is the maldistribution by geography or specialty of health personnel, particularly physicians. The social and living conditions in poor, remote, underpopulated areas or crowded city precincts force physicians and other health workers to concentrate in the suburbs. They now exercise another right our society guarantees: the right to live and practice where and how one pleases. Current efforts to ameliorate maldistribution have centered on incentives to induce recent graduates to serve voluntarily for some period in underserved areas. These measures seem unlikely to assure equity of access anywhere approaching that required to fulfill an obligation of society with respect to primary care.

Some have suggested that the time has come when the obligation to provide equity of access to primary care should override the obligation of society to allow freedom of professional self-determination by requiring all recent graduates to spend a period of service in an underserved area. This is seen as a way to offset the privilege of a medical education made possible only by partial public subsidization. Lacking this, should government itself provide the needed service wherever it is deficient?

The trend in the last two decades toward the ever more detailed regulation of medical practice and education is also just as slowly making primary care a civil right, de facto if not de jure. It has been unofficially proclaimed as such in political rhetoric and clearly enunciated as a major goal of PL 93–641.[16] But coercion of health professionals, and the inevitable adversarial spirit it induces, might well be self-defeating. Health care by coercion is almost certain to be less satisfying to both patient and physician than an obligation voluntarily assumed by an ethically sensitive profession.

After all, the health professions do make a "pro-fession"–a declaration and a claim that all their acts are ultimately performed in the public interest. As we suggested in the previous chapter, do not these "professions" create expectations and impose a responsibility to make them authentic? Is there a corporate responsibility which binds the whole profession? Are not all members of the health professions to some extent culpable if the aggregate of their efforts neglects a fundamental need?

These are legitimate ethical questions and the substance for a debate just beginning to become public. Ordering the priorities among conflicting obligations is a crucial enterprise of ethical discourse. Resolution of moral dilemmas turns finally on what we consider to be good for individuals and for society. That resolution is seriously hampered by our collective inability as yet to define the acceptable conditions of social justice. Without such principles, it is not possible to choose rationally among competing claims.

By examining carefully the case for primary health care as a relative right, we may be able to clarify our stance on the somewhat more fundamental questions of ends and purposes for the health care system. In any case, those who examine or raise ethical questions have an obligation to offer some tentative way of resolving obligations in conflict with each other. With the intention of advancing the discussion, and avoiding apodictic pronouncements as carefully as possible, we offer the following as a reasonable order of priorities.

Primary health care, and specifically its first-contact component, seems the minimal health care claim a citizen may make on a society of our kind. It takes precedence over other forms of care because of its universality and its intensely human dimensions, and because it is the critical point of first entry into the entire system of health care. It is fundamentally a form of personal security, and one of the benefits which ought to follow on the formation of society. Following this would be access to treatments which can effect a radical cure or prevent occurrence of a disease entirely. Next would come the care and containment of established serious diseases for which no radical cure is available; then the more expensive, highly complex procedures of dubious or unproven benefit; and last, treatment for disorders with minimal disability, which, though distressing, are not incapacitating and need only symptomatic treatment or self-care.

A nation must determine how far down this list it will go, given its resources and the expectations its form of society engenders. Whether health is preferred to other human services will depend largely on how far down the list of health priorities one wants to go. Since sanitation, housing, nutrition, and environmental safety contribute to health, they might well take precedence over health care items lowest on the list. In fact, they might take precedence over primary care as well.

No matter what priority a society assigns to health among other human services, it quickly goes to the top for any individual when he becomes ill. Society cannot refuse help to a person who is suffering. The promises of prevention, the welfare of future generations, the value of better housing, or jobs cannot substitute for the here-and-now view of the sick. There is an inescapable immediacy about the call for help of a sick person that overshadows all other more remote social needs, no matter how important. Until first-contact primary care is secure for all, the options are really limited.

Economists point out, quite correctly, that polls often show that Americans place health low on their priority lists. But they do not tell us what the priorities are for those who are already sick. The transition from health, in which we exercise the fullness of our humanity, to illness, in which that humanity is compromised, is so profound that the priorities of the healthy are meaningless for the ill. There is considerable warrant, therefore, if not on grounds of economics, at least on grounds of the realities of human existence, to place medical and health care ahead of many of the other competing good things an advanced society can provide.

It should be noted, finally, that in this analysis no new moral or ethical principles have been introduced, except for the axiom of vulnerability. The case for primary care as an obligation of society is derived from the special vulnerability and the universal fact of illness. This vulnerability generates a need which takes on the substance of a relative right because of the promises inherent in our social and political structures.

We have, in a sense, all made a set of mutual promises to guarantee to each other a certain kind of society, one which is sensitive to and secures those things closest to our needs as humans. We would break our communal promise, tell a communal lie, and live an inauthentic social life if we neglected to exert every effort to assure the minimum security of access to primary care whenever it is neded. We need resort, therefore, only to the commonly accepted principles of promise keeping, truth telling, and fairness which govern any morally sound relationship between persons and between society and persons.

11

Social Ethics of Institutions

A reflection on aspects of institutional ethics, a field which has not yet occupied the professional ethicist to any significant degree, is essential to address the moral agency of hospitals and health care teams.[1] This reflection is mandated by the rise of health care services in institutions and the increasing utilization of team health care skills within these institutions. The thesis we develop is that hospitals and teams must become conscious, explicit, and responsive moral agents in the future. To a certain extent, the argument in this chapter builds on the reflections of the previous chapter, in which we articulated the professional and social concern for realizing obligations to other human beings. Institutions and teams that profess such help must make their commitment known.

The subject of "institutional ethics," as we call the category of problems herein discussed, has significance beyond hospitals. Our country is entering its third century in a state of moral disquietude. There is widespread confusion about moral values. We suffer from an obsession with means and a fear of ends and purposes. Institutions are particularly suspect. Most of them–whether we look at business, education, government, or the church–seem to have be-

Parts of this chapter are based on excerpts from E. D. Pellegrino, "The Ethics of Team Care: Some Notes on the Morality of Decision-Making," published from proceedings of the American Cancer Society's Second National Conference on Cancer Nursing, May 9, 1977, copyright The American Cancer Society.

come disengaged from their human purposes, for economic, political, and fiscal considerations and self-interest are too often their dominant justifying principles. Rarely do our government or institutional leaders speak convincingly, as the founders of our country did, of the moral purposes of their enterprise. The inescapable challenge for all our institutions in the next century, the one upon which the revitalization of our national life depends, is to recapture the sense of a moral purpose transcending self-interest and self-preservation. Because of the urgent and intensely human milieu within which it operates, the hospital must be among the first to attend to its institutional moral obligations. It can, in fact, be the paradigm which others might emulate.

Furthermore, medical and professional ethics have concentrated largely on the relationships of individual physicians to individual patients. There is, as yet, no fully developed ethical theory to define the obligations of a group of individuals (the team) making decisions which affect the well-being of another person, the patient.[2] What special kinds of moral questions are implicit in the action of a collectivity?

The issues are by no means limited to the care of special patients. Nor are they peculiar to any one of the health professions. They are problems inherent in any circumstance in which a group of health professionals make their collective knowledge and skills available to patients or families, especially within institutions.

In order to pose the questions and our responses properly, we must discuss (1) institutional and collective ethics; (2) the nature of the relationship between a hospital and a patient in today's system of health care; (3) the obligations derived from that relationship; (4) the nature of team actions; (5) the complexities of collective morality; and (6) the unanswered questions and practical implications of obligations to patients.

Institutional and Collective Ethics

It is essential to again clarify our understanding of ethics, institutional ethics, and the collective ethical issues we are to address. Along the way, we will rule out certain features which we do not subsume under the rubric of institutional ethical obligation. Further, the special problems posed by team care require some preliminary understanding of common terms, such as "social ethics," and the team itself.

Many health professionals still believe that ethics is either an intuitionist collection of unsupportable hunches and beliefs or a collection of assertions that have no ultimate justification. It should be clear at this point that we do not hold either of these opinions. We have offered a normative medical ethics (with the cautions expressed at the close of Chapter Eight) which is based upon the ontological nature of medicine itself. Hence it should come as no surprise that we consider ethics to be a branch of philosophy, practical philosophy, which rationally and systematically examines the rightness or wrongness of human action. It is normative in that it seeks generalizable rules of good behavior and the reasons on which they are based. It also examines the meanings and logic of ethical language. Ethics therefore is concerned with principles of conduct, with the nature of ethical knowledge, and with the nature of the good.

We may consider the moral quality of actions affecting either individuals or groups. Usually it is the former–the behavior of individuals–which receives major attention in ethical discourse. But increasingly, social ethics, which deals with the moral quality of actions taken by groups of individuals, or affecting groups, is coming under closer analysis.

Institutional Ethics

Institutional ethics consists of the general normative principles which define the way institutions should act with respect to their obligations. It is a branch of social ethics in that it pertains to men when they act as members of a group rather than as individuals. The problems of institutional morality, those which emerge from the actions of organized groups, are more complex than those of individual ethics.

Institutional ethics is not the sum total of the ethical beliefs of the people who make up the institution–the individual physicians, nurses, administrators, and board members. Each has his own set of values and beliefs, and in a pluralistic society must be permitted to express them as an individual.[3] In contrast, institutional ethics consists of a definable set of obligations which transcends these individual beliefs.[4] For example, individual physicians differ in their views on abortion and euthanasia, direct and indirect. What an institution must decide is whether or not it sanctions absolute or limited pluralism or whether, on this or that issue, it will take some specific stance to which it feels morally obligated above others. Institutions, as we shall see below, will be called upon increasingly to make their moral choices more explicit than has been customary.

Nor is institutional ethics to be equated with meeting only the legal requirements for accountability. Many obligations which derive from the nature of the hospital's mission in society are now being transferred to the realm of law. This is a forceful commentary on the tardiness of hospitals in sensing what should be ethical obligations. We refer to the sharpening of the definitions of legal and fiscal accountability of boards and administrators for quality of care, protection of the rights of consent, managerial efficiency, equity in provision of services, and assuring rights of due process. Most of these obligations would have, and should have, been derived from a conscious reflection on the moral obligations implicit in what hospitals are all about. Their translation in legislation, together with a plea for a variety of Bills of Rights by patients, are signs of the ethical lassitude of our institutions.[5]

But if these rights and obligations are now being expressed in law, is this not sufficient? A brief look at the differences between law and ethics will make the distinction clearer. Law and ethics may often coincide, but they are not necessarily and always the same. In fact, as recent history shows, they may often be antipathetic. Law is in many ways the coarse adjustment of society to assure that certain obligations are fulfilled. It has been undeniably a positive force in enhancing human rights and freedom in our country. But as our lagging progress in civil rights, or our Vietnam interlude illustrate, there is too often a disjunction between what is legal and what is moral.

Law, for example, can guarantee the validity of consent or minimum standards of quality by requiring hospitals to follow certain procedures, that they be recorded, and that penalties be imposed for violations. But law, by its nature, seeks standardized and bureaucratized, often impersonalized solutions. What is transferred to law is by definition taken out of the realm of the voluntary recognition of moral responsibility. Something subtle and exquisite is lost. Law cannot guarantee the quality of the human transactions even though it may protect the rights of the parties to the transaction.

If pressed, we would lay the source of increasing legal solutions to moral problems at the door of ineffective and sometimes nonexistent training in moral reasoning. This is especially the case in our schools. Consequently, dialogue and clarification of values have become lost arts among many today. Appeals are made instead to suits and taking those with whom we disagree to court. Such an approach is not only unhealthy, it tends to circumscribe too narrowly the range of personal relationships which should accrue even in health care.

Ethics, in contrast to law, is the fine adjustment of men for the voluntary assumption of obligations because they are demanded by the very nature of certain relationships between humans.[6] Ethics sets a higher ideal than law, simply because it is not guaranteeable. An ethically sensitive institution would take the full dimension of the medical encounter into account–all those things which flow from the existential condition of humanity in the state of illness.

Law and ethics can reinforce each other, as do the coarse and fine adjustments of the microscope. Law assures that patients' rights are guaranteed against those who do not act from ethical motives; ethics guarantees that the institutional conscience will transcend law and attend to obligations, whether guaranteed by law or not. It also guarantees that law is applied humanely, always in the spirit of serving personal needs rather than justifying itself. Government therefore must never be the sanction for ethics but only a recourse when human frailty obfuscates moral sensibilities. Law seems an indispensable condition of human life, but it cannot be a totally sufficient one for an institution consciously attending to its moral obligations.

Neither should ethics be confused with etiquette–the niceties of conduct between institutions and professionals which protect their mutual self-interests. Even in the so-called ethical treatises of the Hippocratic corpus, these domains are confused. Intermingled with a few true ethical principles are many more precepts as to the physician's mien, conduct, and comportment with patients and families and courtesies he should affort his fellow physicians. In our times, such things as the proscription against advertising, or unseemly publicity, or the rules of enlightened self-interest which govern the inevitable but subtle competition between institutions or professionals are in the "etiquette" category. There may be fragments of moral issues here, but they are not mandatory obligations whose violation undermines professional authenticity.

Finally, institutional ethics does not imply a single rigid set of principles, uniformly practiced by all hospitals. This is manifestly impossible in a society with such a wide range of values as ours. Indeed, our moral pluralism may itself require some declaration by the institution of its values, if the patient's own values are to be fully protected.

Some commonly applicable principles will undoubtedly emerge, so that the final declaration of institutional morality will be an admixture of shared and unshared beliefs. What is important is that the points we emphasize here be adverted to consciously by those in whom corporate responsibility is vested. We now summarize those points before moving to the next step in these reflections.

Ethics is a legitimate branch of practical philosophy which systematically examines and rationally justifies claims about how we should live as individuals and members of society. Institutional ethics seeks out these principles as they apply the moral obligations of institutions to the segment of mankind they profess to serve. There are several things institutional ethics is *not:* It is not the same as accountability to law; nor is it the simple addition of the ethical beliefs of those who work in the institution; nor is it professional etiquette or some unexamined set of norms which should be imposed upon all hospitals.

Collective Ethics

The ethics of the health care team focuses on the moral agency of a group of health workers whose collective decisions and actions are undertaken in the interests of a patient. The term, therefore, can apply to a moral agent as well as the individual health professional. "Collective ethics" comprises the principles which should guide this special kind of moral agency, locating and defining the obligations of the team members to each other as well as the patient.

The central question in any theory of collective action is the extent to which such actions differ from individual moral acts. Analysis of these differences is not as yet well developed, but a critical question is whether or not we should regard collective acts as distributive or nondistributive. In a distributive interpretation, collective decisions or actions are the arithmetic sum of the decisions of individual team members, and responsibility is allocated only to the individuals and not to the other members of the group. In this atomistic view, the only moral agents are individuals, and no such thing as a contract or a moral relationship with the team or the institution as a collectivity is possible. In a nondistributive interpretation, the decisions taken by a collectivity are not reducible solely to individual decisions; the group itself is deemed to act as a moral agent. Obligations to patients are incurred by virtue of the fact of being a member of the group, and the moral decision of an individual is never a totally isolated event. The patient, in effect, enters a contractual or fiduciary relationship with the group as a group.[7]

Resolution of this fundamental question is of more than theoretical interest. The precise allocation of moral responsibility, as well as legal accountability and liability, all depend upon the answer.[8] There is a great concern in our institutionalized society about how to fix responsibility and from whom to demand accounting when things go wrong. The necessity for collective activity within institutions and bureaucracies is not an acceptable moral shield for the individuals who make the decisions within a group.

The Hospital's Profession and the Patient's Need

We must first examine the genesis of the moral obligations of the hospital as an institution to the patient. It is useful to begin with what we call the hospital's "profession."[9] By this, we mean that a hospital, by the very fact of its existence in a community, makes a declaration; that is, it professes to concentrate and make available those resources which a person can call upon when he is ill. Implicit in that profession is the promise to assist the sick person to regain what he has lost—his health—at least to the maximum degree possible. Thus the profession of the hospital is analogous to the profession of individual health care providers and rests on the second ethical axiom developed in Chapter Eight.

As a community, voluntary, nonprofit hospital, the hospital makes a second declaration—namely, that it is available to all, that it will not profit from the patient's need, and that its self-interests are subservient to those of the community.

The hospital usually makes its resources available through the medium of the physician and the team of health care providers. But they too make a public declaration that they possess skills to be put at the service of those who are ill. In doing so, they incur all the moral obligations traditionally delineated in professional codes of ethics: They must be competent, act in the patient's interest, never do deliberate harm, protect confidentiality, and treat the patient honestly, considerately, and personally. These obligations bind the providers within the hospital as they do in their offices.

In using the hospital, however, the provider takes advantage of a community resource which he has not personally given. The community places this resource in the trust of a board of directors who act as surrogates for the community. The provider's moral obligations to the patient are no longer his sole concern. They now occur within an institutional framework which modulates the relationships with the patient in two ways. First, the provider's decisions directly or indirectly affect others. Second, he shares his responsibilities with the institution through its board, which must carry out the obligations it incurs by virtue of its own declaration.

In fact, today an increasing number of patients now enter the same relationships with a hospital which formerly was obtained solely with physicians. The patient with no personal physician, or whose physician is unavailable, or who has an emergency, expects the hospital to assume the same obligations for his care a physician would. When the hospital assigns a physician, technician, or nurses, it carries out its moral obligations through them but it is not absolved of responsibility for the way they are fulfilled. When the physicians are full-time employees of the hospital, the corporate obligation of the hospital is even more direct.

An even more fundamental and demanding source of the hospital's moral obligations arises from the special vulnerability of the person who is ill. The fact of illness is an insult to those aspects of existence most integral to being human. As we argued in Chapter Eight, illness deprives the patient of his distinctly human freedoms—to act, to make his own decisions, to be independent of the power of others. The integrity of the patient's self-image as a human is shattered, or at the very least, threatened.

This state of vulnerability and injured humanity of the patient is one of grave inequality. All the power rests with those who have made the declaration that they will assist—the physician and the hospital. Even the most highly educated, powerful, or wealthy patient becomes a petitioner. Healing cannot be humane unless it does everything possible to restore these impaired freedoms, in a sense restoring the patient's humanity along with relieving his pain or disability or curing his disease.

It is clear from the foregoing that hospitals as well as physicians incur serious moral obligations, both by the special nature of illness and the profession they voluntarily make to heal and assist. The central moral obligation is to make that profession fully authentic by fulfilling the expectations implicit in a relationship of such great inequality as exists between the helper and the one to be helped. A little closer look at the nature of the obligations themselves is now in order, and can be derived from their sources in a humane profession.

The Nature of Institutional Obligations

We have space to illustrate only a few of the specific obligations which flow from the special relationship we have described between patients and those who profess to heal them. Some have been touched upon already.

First, it seems clear that the institutionalization of so many aspects of medicine places the hospital increasingly in a moral relationship with the patient not too different from the doctor's. This means a great deal more than simply providing the setting in which medicine can be practiced safely and competently as well as assuring its managerial efficiency and fiscal integrity, though these too are obligations. What is called for is a sharing of the same range of ethical responsibilities which have traditionally been implicit in the relationships between physician and patient. The board of trustees must feel moral as well as legal responsibility for the actions of the professional and nonprofessional workers within its walls. This responsibility, even in presumably professional matters, cannot be delegated. Institutional morality, by necessity, must concern itself with every facet of the corporate life of that institution.

The result is an overlap and sharing of moral obligations in which the professional and the institution check and balance each other more intimately than is now customary. In this view, we would have to take some exception to Charles Fried's recent analysis of the partitioning of responsibilities between physicians and hospital authorities.[10] Fried assigns the hospital directors the bureaucratic decisions–those affecting efficiency, equity, and allocation of resources, excusing them from responsibility for the personal dimensions of care given. These latter he assigns wholly to the physician, excusing him from concern with allocational decisions and suggesting that he must work within the framework of efficiency/equity decisions made by administrators or government.

Fried's division of responsibilities is reasonable so far as primary operational emphases are concerned. But these domains must not be compartmentalized; they are always in dynamic equilibrium with each other. On the theses we suggest here, physicians and hospital directors are morally bound to see that their areas of primary responsibility do, in fact, interact. Each must fulfill the ethical obligation for the whole of what patients have a right to expect.

This mutuality of moral obligation becomes even more impelling when we turn to remediation of the injured humanity of the patient which illness entails. Both physician and hospital must reduce the inequalities in the relationship as well as the situation allows. The patient must be provided the knowledge necessary to participate rationally in the decisions which affect him. He must know what is wrong, what can be done, what the chances are for success, the dangers of treatment, and the alternative procedures. The physician and the hospital share this obligation to enable the patient to make as free and rational a choice as possible.

The obligation goes well beyond the mere legal requirement for valid consent. It demands consent of the highest quality and fullest sense of self-determination by the patient. The right to refuse specific treatment must be protected as well, while still caring for the patient. The physician, the patient, and the hospital share obligations to each other, but because of the patient's vulnerability, his needs are foremost.

This particular obligation assumes exquisite significance when the decision itself involves a moral question–a situation increasingly more pertinent as the capabilities of medicine expand the ways human life can be altered, shortened, or extended by technological means. The questions in this realm are already matters of widespread public debate–abortion, continuing or discontinuing life support measures, treatment or nontreatment of terminal or seemingly hopeless patients, participation in experimentation, and the like. The choices involve an intersection of the patient's values and those of the physician and the institution. Respect for the patient and humane treatment demand that these values be respected and that the patient be given the opportunity to act as his own moral agent if he wishes.

The problem of paternalism in health care is addressed most seriously when the patient's illness deprives him of the ability to speak about his values. Especially in tertiary care settings, we have observed that the values of the patient in decisions decline and the values of the institution or health care team rush to fill that vacuum. Establishment of a moral policy is seriously needed in these cases, such as when to "pull the plug," in order to avoid the legal problems that ensue (e.g., the Karen Quinlan case). But we stress again that legal reasons in themselves are insufficient for the establishment of such a moral policy.

There are clear indications that more and more patients will wish to be their own moral agents and not delegate this agency to physicians, as in the past. We live in a democratic society in which there is no uniformity of opinion on most medico-moral issues and no recognized authority to settle differences in ethical beliefs. There is also a growing tendency to distrust experts and institutions. The traditional moral authority of the physician has already been substantially eroded. The rise in hospital review boards, some devoted to ethics, highlights the radical change taking place in how moral decisions are made by and in institutions.

Under these circumstances, the moral responsibility of hospitals, like that of physicians, must be to make its values clear so that the patient can make his own choice among institutions and physicians. We can foresee a time, not too far distant, when hospitals will have to declare their positions on the major medico-moral questions for the patient's guidance. Catholic hospitals have customarily done so on certain specific procedures in the past. There is room for considerable variation in ethical practices among hospitals. A democratic society should offer each patient the possibility of being cared for in institutions which declare the same moral values he holds. This right can be actualized only if boards of trustees are willing to state clearly the ethical principles to which they subscribe in more specific terms than is now the case.

The immediacy of this issue is underscored in the recent excellent study by Diana Crane of the decisions physicians actually make in the care of the critically ill.[11] She shows considerable disparity between the official medical position, which holds that treatment is continued until the patient is physiologically dead, and the actual practice, wherein treatment is discontinued in those patients for whom the possibility of meaningful social interactions is nonexistent. Patients and their families should know of this disparity. Hospitals have an obligation to see that clear guidelines on terminating support measures are developed and monitored. Here again, we see the dynamics of interaction on a moral issue between the physician and the institution.

Katz and Capron have carefully studied the decision-making process in catastrophic illness. They outline the professional and institutional interactions necessary to assure that decisions are made rationally, equitably, and responsively.[12] Hospitals have the moral responsibility to provide these safeguards before they become matters of law.

What we suggest is that most of the decisions taken in a hospital are decisions in which technological and value choices are intermingled. Our society has developed a deep concern, not without foundation, that in deferring to the expert in technical matters, it has lost control of the values and purposes of that technology. We need ways in which to control technology democratically, as Arthur Kantrowitz has suggested. He called for the separation of the technical from the value components in the uses of technology, the delegation of decisions on mixed decisions to designated judges who are not themselves scientific advocates, and finally, wider publication of the deliberations and decisions of judges and advocates.[13]

Some parallel system is needed in hospitals and in society to distinguish between the professional medical advocacy for the introduction and use of high technology and the social values of its employment. Institutional morality, if it is to be exercised fully, must grapple with such sensitive and even dangerous issues. Institutions are not immune to irrationality, the abuse of power, or the usurpation of morals, as our own recent sad history amply illustrates.

If there is a single message in this section, it is this: An analysis of the obligations which emerge from the role of professionals and hospitals indicates the need for a new balance between them as moral agents. Neither institutional nor individual professional ethics is sufficient by itself to safeguard the humanity of patients. Heretofore, professional ethics has been the dominant and even the sole influence. We are now entering a new era in which a three-way interaction between the moral agencies of physicians, hospitals, and patients is necessary. This interaction is further complicated by the role of teams in providing care, a point to which we now turn.

The Nature of Team Actions

A team is a transitory social system comprising a group of two or more individuals held together by a common purpose. The team comes into existence because of the special function it is intended to carry out; its composition, leadership, structure, and the duration of its existence are all determined by the end it serves.

The health care team is any aggregate of health workers–professional or otherwise–directed to meeting certain specified needs of a patient, a family, or a community.

There is obviously no such thing as *the* health care team, but rather a whole array of teams. The composition of the operating room team, the primary care team, the rehabilitation team, and the dialysis team are all different since their functions are different. The major roles within teams may shift from one health professional to another. In the operating room the surgeon is clearly the captain. In primary care the family physician, the physician's assistant, or the nurse practitioner may, at different times or under different circumstances, take charge. In chronic care, the physician may be in command during the assessment period and the nurse during major portions of the patient's course. The same is true of the coronary care team. The nurse is really the captain in the first moments when the arrythmia occurs and during the initiation of its emergency treatment.

What is common to all teams is the fact of collective action. Decisions about what should be done, who should do it, how it should be evaluated and how communicated to the patient, the development of a detailed treatment plan and the decision about when to change it are all taken by a group of specialists *acting together.* The opinion of any single member of the group is invariably modified by the dynamics of the group. Only rarely can a team member identify a complex decision as solely his own. Some modification of individual positions inevitably occurs by the simple fact that the decision is made collectively. Each team member is enhanced, and also to a certain extent restrained, by being a member of the team. The allocation of responsibilities and the locus of final accountability for the final decisions belong in some real sense to each team member, and in another sense to the entire team.

It is essential to team action that some compromise be made. Yet each team member must also carry out his assignment reliably and competently. In carrying out a particular task–whether it is as general as a nursing plan or as technical as ligation of a bleeding artery–nurse and surgeon are each responsible for personal skills and competence. But the team also shares in this responsibility since it must assure that these actions are well carried out by team members to whom they are assigned and whether a particular person should have been chosen–or rather, entrusted–with the task of carrying it out.

Responsibility for team actions is, therefore, in reality both distributive and nondistributive. Thus, the usual moral obligations of a professional to his patient care are complicated by the superimposition of the moral agency of the team as a team. We do not as yet have a code of ethics common to the health professions which defines the new responsibilities which derive from taking decisions and actions interprofessionally, though our proposed principles of medical morality do support developing such a code. Each profession now establishes its own code of ethics. While it may define relationships between its own members, it says nothing of the way these professionals ought to act when they become part of the larger entity of the team, acting in unison with members of other professions.

Some such commonly accepted statement of moral principles is required today, for a variety of obvious reasons flowing from the progress of medicine and its institutionalization. First is the impossibility of any one profession embracing all the knowledge and techniques required in the care of any complicated illness. Then, to an extent unknown in the previous history of medicine, individual patients depend for their care upon institutions as much as they do on individual physicians. Consider the cancer patient. He may be admitted by a personal physician, but in a short while he becomes the subject of numerous consultations. Surgeons, chemotherapists, radiation therapists, psychiatrists, social workers, and nurses all have something to contribute to his care. These individuals are often institutionally assigned and employed. The patient does not really choose each one of them; even his physician is dependent upon whom the institution designates to carry out many of these functions. In effect, the patient enters a relationship with the institution which is not unlike that with his own physician. The institution has an obligation to provide competent, responsive, and personal care and to fulfill that obligation by virtue of the competence of those it employs and the degree to which it monitors their competence, as we discussed in the previous section.

The complexities of modern medical care and its institutionalization compel the institution and the team to become moral agents as well as the individual health practitioner. We would hold that the responsibilities of the health care team are both distributive and nondistributive. One of the delicate and difficult unresolved questions before us, then, is how to decide which of these principles applies in a particular action, and with respect to a particular member of the team.

This intermingling of distributive and nondistributive responsibilities complicates the moral and ethical behavior of every member of the health care team. A brief look at some of the implications of the collective actions implicit in team care will illustrate the nature of these ethical complexities.

Some Complexities of Collective Morality

We may assume that the health professional acting as a team member is subject to the usual moral obligations of any practitioner, as developed in Chapters Eight and Nine. The real complexities are introduced by the possibility and unavoidability of a distributive interpretation of team ethics. While these dilemmas will appear obvious, it is useful to outline a few specifically.

One such dilemma is the extent to which each team member is bound to monitor, correct, and reveal the incompetence of fellow team members. Team interaction affords a more intimate experience of a colleague's competence than isolated practice. The outcome, as well as the patient's responses to what each member does, is evidence to the entire team, inasmuch as each is charged with some part of the therapeutic plan. Each is simultaneously exposed to and dependent upon his fellows; each is compromised by any incompetence in his fellows. The ethical force of this point stems from the axiom to do no harm.

In the rare situation when there is evident or imminent danger for the patient, direct intervention to prevent the incompetent act is called for. More usually, however, the problem is a more subtle one, and therefore more difficult. When lapses of competence are habitual; where they pose some danger of unusual discomfort for the patient; where there is failure to use optimal measures–each of these circumstances will raise the question of corporate culpability, legal as well as moral.

In the presence of such lapses, what constitutes ethical group behavior? Who has the responsibility for monitoring individual and team competence? To whom are lapses reported–the erring colleague, the team, the captain, or the institution? The matter is especially delicate when one profession is critical of another, particularly if one–the physician's, for example–has traditionally seen itself as being in charge.

Does corporate responsibility extend beyond the more obvious breaches of good judgment and skill to include breaches in the moral obligations to patients–the right to valid consent, confidentiality, and humane, nonhumiliating treatment? To what extent is one obliged to carry out the orders of the team captain when they violate the team member's own value system? The physician, for example, may order the discontinuance of life support measures, while the nurse or other health professional may have serious doubts about its propriety, yet they may be expected to carry out his orders as team members.

The special vulnerability existentially inherent in being a patient renders violations of values and consent especially reprehensible. It is easy for health professionals to take advantage unconsciously of this vulnerability and thus to manipulate the patient's choice of alternatives. This would violate our second axiom about the vulnerability of those in need. On the other hand, a certain amount of persuasion may be ethical and, indeed, mandatory in the patient's best interests. Team members share the responsibility to see that each member, and the team as a whole, always steers carefully between the extremes of subtle manipulation and indifference.

In a collective decision, how can the values of individual team members be preserved against opposing values of the majority? When does the need for response to authority or to team decisions in the patient's interest override individual preferences? When must individual scruples be asserted? To what extent can a task be assigned without discussion or choice of alternatives?

Granting that each team member shares in the distributive nature of the moral obligations of team action, the danger of excessive moral scrupulousness must be avoided. Such moral rigidity could stifle decisions and paralyze any team action. There are some very delicate decisions to be made: When is an imputation of incompetence merely a difference in philosophy of patient care and when does it make an appreciable difference in outcome for the patient? How do we keep the team from endless bickering? It is manifestly impossible, and positively disruptive of patient care, to expose the patient to every difference of opinion among team members. Where and what are the limits of reasonable and responsible collective action in this regard?

These few questions and problems merely illustrate moral difficulties in team actions as yet, not very consciously addressed by ethicists. Some may think it better not to uncover still another area of professional activities to ethical scrutiny. "Let these matters be settled among the professions," they will say. Others will insist that the physician has final legal authority, and thus final moral authority; his decision, therefore, must be final. Even if the moral insensitivity in these positions were ignored, there are strong reasons dictating the opposite. The current climate of public concern for forestalling any usurpation of individual rights to participation in decisions which affect them would suffice to make further explicit discussions mandatory.

But the mandate for a more careful scrutiny of the ethical problems in team actions is founded on a more solid basis than political or legal considerations. It derives from the "profession" the team makes as a team. It professes, declares publicly, that it will put its combined knowledge and skill at the service of the patient. In this sense, it parallels the profession of the institution. The patient is therefore entitled to the expectation that the individuals and the group who make the decisions will observe the same ethical safeguards he expects from the individual health practitioner and from the hospital. The group is bound by the profession they make, just as the individual professional is bound by his. The group becomes, in this sense, a moral agent, subject, as a group, to certain principles of right action.

Unanswered Questions and Practical Implications

Many practical questions remain to be addressed. How does the hospital balance its moral obligations to individuals who work for it and with it, and its obligations to those it serves as well as to the community as a whole? How are obligations defined and deployed among professionals, nonprofessionals, and administrators? What mechanisms can be designed to implement the hospital's moral agency? What is the best way to allocate moral responsibility in team care? The team is, after all, a transitory social mini-system operating within the hospital. It illustrates in microcosm the difficulties of the ethics of group actions.

How are conflicts of values and principles among individuals in the institution resolved? To what extent and to what degree of specificity should the institution declare the values it subscribes to? How are the legal and ethical values of everyday decisions reconciled with each other? Law may lag behind ethics in some instances. Can an institution take a stance which society has not yet sanctioned in law?

These and related questions constitute the domain of institutional ethics. They will be subjected to deeper and more critical analysis in the years ahead. The field of ethics, as it applies to humans acting in concert, is in need of a sound theoretical base before practical steps can be rationally justified. But the issues are sufficiently urgent to require tentative actions even before a substantial body of theory can be elaborated. Hospital administrators and trustees are already engaging some of these issues. Some collaboration between ethical theorists and health care practitioners is essential if the principles developed in this special domain of social ethics are to be practicable as well as theoretically sound. We have suggested that some practical steps can be taken on the basis of the axioms and norms already developed.

Even while these fundamental explorations are being conducted, there is immediate need for a more open discussion of the issues of institutional morality among physicians, other health workers, and trustees. These are delicate issues of the kind generally eschewed in our society. The adherents of the intuitionist or skeptical views of ethics will protest the utility of such discussions. Others will shy away from the personal and sometimes emotional tone of ethical discourse. Some authorities even feel that the "tragic decisions" we must make in hospitals should not be the subject of public debate.

In our view, there is no alternative to a more concrete development of the issues in institutional morality at this time in our history. Everywhere, there is a rebirth of interest in questions of value and purpose. If this scrutiny is happening in professional medical ethics, can we realistically postpone consideration of the new relationships between institutional, professional, and personal ethics?

Moreover, as Renee Fox has pointed out, the new interest in ethical issues in medicine is simply an expression of a deeper concern in America with the values, meanings, and purposes of life and institutions in general.[14] The assumption of a more explicit role of moral agency by hospitals is entirely consistent with this trend. In fact, the hospital is a natural place to raise these questions because of the special sensitivity of its mission in society–one which is inextricably bound up with the most human of needs.

Rather than shying away from the undeniable challenges of moral agencies, hospitals can show the way toward a clearer conception of institutional morality. The nation must rebuild that sense of moral purpose in the probity of human enterprises without which much of human activity becomes meaningless. Our nation will regain a sense of its worth only if its institutions exhibit the courage to pursue higher ideals than can be accomplished in a lifetime. People are less disappointed with high ideals sincerely enunciated and imperfectly attained than with their abnegation out of cynical or practical motives.

In the matter of team health care, we need a more explicit statement of acceptance of collective responsibility by team members for the decisions, actions, and recommendations they make as a team. This may be implicit now with some team members, but it is certainly not for others. The public and the patient have the right to some such declaration which is at least morally binding. Such a declaration might appear appropriately in the moral codes of the separate professions, or in a common code. Such a declaration would lead inevitably to a greater openness in team decision making; laying out of alternatives; providing greater opportunity for expression of dissenting opinion: sharing of authority; and diminishing the gap, at least in moral authority, between different professions and between professions and patient.

All this means that regular mechanisms must be established to monitor incompetence, to deal with it openly and as a group, and to permit rehabilitation or reassignment of offending members when necessary. No profession should be immune from this openness and mutuality of surveillance of competence. The process must always be conditioned by the need to seek an optimal outcome for the patient. The preferences of professionals for their favorite modes of management and even their definition of what is good for the patient must take second place.

The captain or team leader must therefore more explicitly share his authority, whenever possible, to allow team members to dissent, and even to withdraw honorably, from a particular procedure or decision they find reprehensible. Tasks must be accepted as well as assigned; the physician's legal authority does not equate with moral authority. What is more, not only the team captain but also the administration and governing board participate and share in the moral agency exerted by any team of health professionals operating in their institution. The extent of this responsibility and how it is to be implemented have rarely been discussed.

If the locus of responsibility is thus to be pinpointed, there is a corollary obligation to disclose the facts about who is responsible for what procedures and decisions. The patient is entitled to hold the team as a whole responsible for an untoward event if it is avoidable by a skilled practitioner. Presumably, redress for damage done could legally be demanded from the group for an injurious collective decision. Each team member is compelled to take seriously the moral and physical effects of collective decisions to which he assents, and which are carried out in the name of the whole team. This mode of decision making is, of course, common in selecting among several alternative treatment plans available, e.g., for a cancer patient.

To justify these and other moral practical steps, there is need for a more careful explication of the theory of collective morality, a subject of increasing importance in every walk of our highly institutionalized lives. Pending such a formulation, professional ethical codes might take more specific cognizance of their ethical obligations, the duties they incur in collective activity with other health professionals.

Ideally, a code of collective morality should be arrived at collectively. The major health professions should elaborate a set of commonly held principles or guidelines which will recognize the special nature of their obligations to patients when they act as a team. We have offered three axioms which might form the groundwork of such a task.

Collective decisions are the order of the day in every aspect of contemporary life. The principles which emerge from a closer scrutiny of the distributive and nondistributive obligations of health professionals will be pertinent for legislatures, public commissions, institutional administrators, and governing boards. A morally sophisticated society will not be satisfied with the vagueness, and diffuseness of responsibility which now obtain in most collective actions and decisions. We must look as rigorously at the ethical dimensions of collective action as we are already looking at those of the individual professional.

As demonstrated already in the realm of personal and individual professional ethics, a failure voluntarily to undertake moral obligations inevitably generates legal alternatives. Granting the utility of law in a democratic society, it cannot fully replace the more sensitive–and more humane–modulations of human relationships which inhere in an ethic of obligations based on the needs of patients, as afflicted human beings.

Strange as it may seem to team members accustomed to treating all decisions as medical, the very nature of team care and the moral force of medicine we have described in previous chapters require team members to discuss norms, axioms, and an axiology of human life in order to be most effective. The same moral force of the vulnerability of a person in need of help requires hospitals to engage in the justification of moral beliefs they publicly profess.

12

Medical Morality and Medical Economics: The Conflict of Canons

"Cost containment" and the economic considerations that have inspired it are fast becoming an ideology. That is, they are being uncritically accepted as self-justifying arguments for a wide variety of policies and actions in health and medical care. Indeed, in the minds of some, they are identical with what is right and good for the health of society.

The phrase "cost containment" now seasons the exhortations of health planners, economists, legislators, and physicians. Friends and foes of the present system use these words to cajole, threaten, warn, or promise. Can anything so well intentioned and so shrouded in the aura of "good" economics be anything but enthusiastically supported?

After all, we are told, most of the world's ills are economic, and they cry out for economic solution. There is sufficient truth in that claim to give the whole notion of good economics a quasi-moral tone, making it a determinant of ends as well as a deviser of means to ends otherwise defined. The canons of economics then are assuming a normative quality which may obscure some very fundamental moral questions which should include but also transcend economics.

This chapter is adapted from an article by Edmund Pellegrino, "Medical Morality and Medical Economics: The Conflict of Canons," in *Hospital Progress* (August 1978), 50–55, copyright The Catholic Health Association of the United States.

Indeed, the more the economics of cost containment takes on a moral tone, the more it comes into conflict with the canons of an older morality–the traditional morality of medicine expounded in these pages. Before we accept the measures being proposed, and without derogating the importance of economic considerations, it is essential to examine the points at which economic and moral canons may conflict.

The purpose of this final chapter is threefold: to examine the canons of good economics in health, to describe the canons of good medicine, and finally, looking at the potential conflicts, to indicate modes of equilibration of the opposing tendencies.

The Canons of Medical Economics

The provision of health services has become a serious economic problem even in relatively affluent societies. The magnitude of health care expenditures and the importance of health in an advanced society more than justify careful examination of the way resources are used, allocated, paid for, and organized. On the whole, the widespread scrutiny of these questions by economists has been necessary and salubrious.

These economists' view of things, as succinctly stated by Victor Fuchs, is rooted in three observations: (1) resources are scarce relative to wants; (2) these resources have alternative uses; (3) people have different wants and assign different values to them. The economists' central problem is how to allocate resources optimally to meet human needs. If needs judged as good are values, as we have suggested, then medical economics must deal with health as a value.[1]

The difficulties inherent in implementing the goal of economics toward meeting human needs are significant. They are well epitomized in the current slogan, "Quality health care at a cost we can afford." This slogan has become a goal of national health policy. Words such as these have a superficial attractiveness that easily deludes us into thinking that we know what we mean when we utter them. But any debate on the issues of resource allocation amply illustrates how sharply divergent may be the construals of the key words in the slogan–"quality," "care," and "affordability." It is impossible to optimize three such concepts simultaneously, since there are mutual contradictions between them. Compromise is essential. The critical question becomes, Where, precisely, do we set the line of that compromise?

Economics as a discipline is competent to deal with the means and methods of allocating resources, but nothing in its methodology endows its practitioners with special expertise in determining what values should predominate in our society. Economic considerations undeniably shape goals and purposes. This is an inevitable consequence of any definition of matters such as cost, price, productivity, efficiency, and priorities. Economics, of necessity, limits the range of possible services and forces choices among them.

Sophisticated economic analyses are necessary to structure realistically our choices and allocations of resources. What they cannot do is assign "worthwhileness" or values of those choices as ends and goals of society. Such limitations are recognized by all but the more expansive economic theorists. Unfortunately, this is often not the case with those at the periphery of economics as a formal discipline–the regulators, legislators, policy makers, and consumers. In their frantic attempts to "do something" about rising costs, dubious quality, or excessive use of medical services, they can easily mistake good economics for a good health care system.

We know, for example, that the health care market violates many of the supposedly immutable laws which rule in other commodity markets. The usual forces which enable supply and demand to exert reciprocal restraint are absent or obtunded. There is a scarcity of providers; the entry of new providers is limited by licensure and credentialing by those already in the field; providers set the prices, dictate a large part of the need and demand, and are free to locate where they wish and provide what services they wish. The demand for health services is seemingly insatiable despite price and cost increments. These demands increase as a society becomes more affluent. There is an excess supply of some services in certain locations and a paucity in others. The cost of obtaining the information needed to choose among providers and services is high; increasing the input of resources does not have a linear relationship with improved health; the incremental value of research may be dubious or difficult to measure.

These violations of good economics are held responsible for most of the aberrances in the health care system: excessive demand; excessive utilization; provider dominance; uninhibited technological expansion; indiscriminate use of procedures with only marginal benefit; maldistribution of personnel and resources; duplication of resources and services; and a growing disjunction between expenditures and discernible improvements in the nation's health.[2]

Economic pathology understandably elicits rigorous prescriptions. These remedies take a variety of forms: control of price; a cap on total expenditures; rationing of services; limiting resource input; reducing inefficiency and duplication; reducing demand; reallocation of resources to more directly health-related activity; withholding expensive care from the hopelessly ill; substituting lower paid health workers for physicians; and utilization review and quality control.

All or some of these measures are being or will be tried in an attempt to gain control of the runaway health care market. These measures are subsumed under the cost containment rubric. There is little question that many of these measures should be tried, and many will be found necessary. There is, however, the real danger that measures primarily economic in their motivation will come increasingly into conflict with the more traditional morality of medicine and health care institutions. Before examining some of these conflicts, we will briefly review the traditional obligations of those who profess to care for the sick.

The Traditional Canon of Medical Morality

In this section, we do not intend to review codes of professional ethics. Rather, we wish simply to recall the expectations a patient customarily holds when he is ill, and when a physician professes to cure or care for him. The physician is understood to have special skills which he promises to use in the interests of the patient when that patient presents himself for care. The prime focus of the physician's intention, therefore, is the good of the patient who presents himself here and now–not some distant patient, not even the good of society or the greatest good for the greatest number. The physician, and by implication the health care institution, become agents of the patient's well-being at the moment of engagement. They are expected to cure and to care as well.

The patient ordinarily assumes that the physician is his agent and will take all measures which may benefit the patient. The physician is expected to do everything possible for the good of the patient. This may mean, in some instances, desisting from doing things as well as doing them. But the essential matter is the patient's expectation that the physician, and the hospital, will act in his behalf. This is, in fact, the moral center of medicine, the moment of clinical truth, that which makes medicine what it is. It is the point of convergence of the sciences and the arts of medicine. It is expressed in a decision to take this rather than that action for the good of *this* patient.

The patient does not expect the physician to be an instrument of social and economic policy–whether that policy is dictated by the physician's or society's value system. Clearly the physician operates within certain publicly established policies. He cannot be totally independent of them. But he also has the responsibility to resist those policies when they are detrimental to the welfare of his patient. The physician is obliged to make some effort to advocate this patient's welfare unless that welfare is immediately and urgently a danger to others (e.g., the patient with a contagious disease, the dangerous psychotic). Here the good of the patient may itself dictate the same action which is good for society as well.

The complexity of the issue of competence for mental patients is one example of the struggle to maintain a priority of moral principle in this regard. Resolution of the complexity is partially provided for by law, which stresses that the patient must be a clear and present danger to himself or others before being treated against his will. However, the issue of senility is less clear. At what point may an elderly person, usually regarded as "eccentric," be permitted to refuse life-saving therapy? What is the good of society in this case? It seems best that the physician, not society and the courts, determine with the patient what is the good to be pursued, based on the patient's values, especially those which span a lifetime. If the physician becomes an agent of society's values, to whom could such persons turn for help?

None of this implies that the physician should be socially irresponsible, that he must satisfy the patient's every whim, or that he should not participate in planning and decisions for optimal use of resources, their allocation, and their efficient application. The physician-patient relationship takes place in a societal framework, to be sure, and neither party can totally evade social responsibility. But when that responsibility is in conflict with what both conceive to be in the interest of his patient, that interest can be overridden only in the most exceptional circumstances.

This interpretation of medical morality creates the possibility of considerable conflict between the physician's obligations and economic measures that may be legislated to contain costs. How does the physician exercise his responsibility in a national policy of "quality care at a cost we can afford"? There is an inevitable conflict between quality and cost containment which refuses to go away, no matter how ardently we may wish to control medical care costs and for whatever good purposes.

A few examples will illustrate some ways in which economic justifications may conflict with moral justifications in decision making.

One much debated issue is that of the so-called CAT scanner (computerized axial tomography). Physicians have hailed this new and expensive technological advance as an indispensable tool, especially in neurological diagnosis. Economists, administrators, planners, and consumers, on the other hand, have seized upon it as an example of irresponsible cost escalation.[3] In the interests of cost containment, they have demanded demonstrations of cost effectiveness and called for a limitation on the number purchased, as well as centralization and sharing.

It is already very clear, if we confine ourselves to neurological uses for the moment, that the CAT scanner offers distinctive clinical advantages over other methods of neurological diagnosis of brain tumors, hemorrhage, infection, and trauma. It is a noninvasive, complication-free, ambulatory technique which in specific situations is at least as good as pneumoencephalography, angiography, and radionuclide scanning, and in some instances demonstrably better. In the case of acute trauma, it is especially useful in reducing craniotomies (reportedly 94 percent).

Much remains to be done to demonstrate the comparative effectiveness of the CAT scanner with other measures, the degree to which other tests will be replaced, significant changes in therapy made, the use or need for beds reduced, and cost effectiveness achieved. The question now is whether we can deprive any patient with a possible brain tumor, cerebral hemorrhage, and especially acute head trauma the benefit of this new device. At the moment, charges for CAT scanning are high and savings are difficult to demonstrate, if at all. In good conscience, can physicians and hospitals–or health regulators and planners, for that matter–withhold this modality, even if it is not cost effective? What is the value of a noninvasive versus an invasive procedure, one which gives a faster answer or more quickly assuages the anxiety of a patient and physician who fear a brain tumor?

More pointedly, can we insist on centralization and sharing of a procedure of such apparent use in acute head trauma? Head trauma does not distribute itself according to size of hospital or availability of CAT scanners. Moving patients with head trauma can be risky and life threatening; decision about craniotomy usually cannot be postponed safely.

A philosophy of cost containment comes into conflict with the good of the patient under these circumstances. Economic factors must somehow take second priority, and CAT scanning will have to be provided wherever there is a competent neurologist or neuroradiologist to interpret the results. The economic factors must of course be analyzed, and answers provided to cost-benefit questions, but the whole must eventually yield to the canons of medical morality, or at least be shaped by them.

Another kind of conflict between economics and medical morality is raised in the current interest in reallocating funds from curative to preventive medicine. Here the conflict is less dramatic and immediate, though more far-reaching than in the case of introducing an effective new technology. There is no question that the economic impact (disability, loss of productive days, cost of care) consequent on poor personal habits is enormous. If we could eliminate smoking, alcohol, poor driving, poor diets, sedentary living, and dangerous working environments, billions of dollars would be available for reallocation for other needed human services. Why not deviate limited funds from the care of those in whom there is marginal benefit from treatment, or who have incurable or minor disorders?

The question is a reasonable one, but again the seeming perverseness of human existence intrudes. What do we do when the funds allocated for curative medicine are exhausted? Those who are healthy may agree to a policy of prevention. When they become ill and are in immediate need, however, they are far less likely to think about the economic impact of care versus cure and prevention. What physician or hospital can turn away the sick in favor of the future social benefits of those who will not get sick?[4] Where do we draw the lines between effective and palliative treatments, or needed and unwarranted care? Is there a moral justification for not treating those who persist in smoking or drinking? What advanced society, let alone what health professional, could justify this kind of statistical morality?

Again, the traditional canons and expectations of medical morality demand help for those who are ill now and present themselves for care. No matter what large-scale policy decision may have been made, the medical professional cannot reject the person in need and remain faithful to the obligations he incurs in agreeing to treat. It is unlikely that society would wish to change its expectations of physicians so drastically as to make them instruments of economic policy rather than advocates for the patient.

The same considerations obtain in a variety of other measures being generated as part of our cost containment efforts. Let us suppose that we place a "cap" on all hospital construction, as has been proposed. On the surface, this seems very reasonable. We are all aware of excessive and unused beds in many locales. Limiting the number of new beds should encourage better use of existing beds and avoid unjustified utilization and duplication of facilities. There is much logic in this position. It is less in conflict with medical morality than perhaps some other measures.

But again, we must see what the moral implications might be. For example, when do existing beds become so obsolete that they are no longer suitable for caring for the sick? What is the proper use of a hospital bed? So often the crucial factor in recovery may be getting the patient out of his home or work environment for a medical condition that might be less effectively treated on an ambulatory basis–peptic ulcer, for example. What dollar value do we place on those extra days in the hospital for a young mother recovering from pneumonia or surgery? Or the days consumed by the elderly man medically ready for discharge but as yet unable to cope with daily life without completion of family arrangements? One answer is to send them both to a nursing or convalescent home, which is less expensive. Is this justifiable for three days? Are our resources so constrained that standardized rules about how many days treating a disease justifies should take precedence over the number of days treating a patient justifies?

Many more examples could be offered, from the problems created by the recently published HSA regulations, to the definition of what minimal services every citizen might be entitled to in an advanced society or under national health insurance, to just what it is society wants from its investment in health services. Every measure aimed at rationing scarce resources entails such dilemmas. That they exist, however, is no excuse for yielding to one extreme or another. Cost containment and "everything for every patient" are twin ideologies equally to be avoided. Neither is morally acceptable. In our world, we face the necessity to balance these opposing slogans as explicitly and as rationally as possible.

Equilibration of Morals and Economics

If there is an inherent tension between medical morals and medical economics, and if neither can be accepted as an unexamined ideology, how can the balance between them be managed? Obviously, no formula is at hand to set the balance point on any particular issue, even those we have used in illustration. Yet, there are some principles and some questions which need specific confrontation, and these can at least be outlined.

To begin with, the *primary* obligation of the physician to his patient does not excuse him totally from social and economic concerns. We have already noted those exceptions when the patient's good might be a threat to public safety. In those cases, the principle of the common good takes precedence over the nonharm and vulnerability principles of medical ethics. However, strict safeguards must be formulated to ensure that the patient is not deprived of the consent possible in his condition, so that the principle of the common good rests on its condition of possibility. The physician cannot take advantage of the vulnerability of the sick patient to advance his own, or even his nation's social and political philosophy. This is a first principle derived from the fact of illness, the act of profession, the principle of nonharm, and the ethical axiom of vulnerability developed in Chapter Eight. The historical dangers in ignoring this principle are too recent and too numerous to be recounted here. The appalling use of medical professionals for political purposes, even torture, are the consequences of ignoring this first principle.

The physician is also obliged, as an individual and as a member of a profession with a corporate responsibility to society, to take both economic and social concerns very seriously. Physicians therefore are obliged, as citizens and as expert citizens especially, to take an active part in decisions which determine health care policies and expenditures.[5] They have the obligation to define alternatives, to explicate the moral dilemmas of a policy, and to help frame modulations which will prevent any policy from overriding human concerns. They must conscientiously provide reliable data on efficacy, efficiency, and optimal utilization of resources. They must provide the technical input needed to make sound economic decisions.

As physicians participate in public decisions, they must not seek to protect medicine or their vested interests, or even to propound absolute dicta about what is good for all patients. They must appreciate that, as experts, they have considerable prerogatives in technical matters, but no special prerogative in the matter of values. Ultimately, the decision to take a particular social or economic position must turn on questions of value: what we think the good life may be; what is worthwhile and what not. On such questions, the physician is free to propound his personal values, but not as an *expert* on values. Failure to make this last distinction often weakens a physician's effectiveness in policy-making bodies.

Whatever may be his personal values, the physician has a choice, like any other citizen, to conform or oppose a public policy. But in dealing with the individual patient, his preferences must take second place. If they are so important to him that he must promulgate them in his treatment, then he must make that fact known beforehand so that the patient may reject him in favor of another physician. Under no circumstances can the physician use economic constraints to punish patients whose values he abhors.

These caveats notwithstanding, there is much a physician can do to be sensitive to economic factors, even in the care of individual patients. Here we prefer the idea of "cost consciousness" to "cost containment." The former attitude permits more flexibility than the latter, which announces its goal in advance of actual engagement with the patient. "Cost consciousness" can be consistent with good economics and good medicine as well. Some principles of cost consciousness might include the following: The first is to cultivate diagnostic "elegance"—that is, to order only those tests which answer a specific question and which lead to some decision. Much more critical attention to what is sufficient evidence for a diagnosis, or better, for taking a clinical action, is needed. "Shotgun" and "roulette" work-ups to cover all bases are expensive, nonconclusive, and even dangerous. Clinicians need to know when a test makes only a marginal contribution, when diagnostic certitude is possible, and when it is an illusion. They must understand something, too, of their own diagnostic and therapeutic style. The compulsive diagnostician keeps testing beyond the law of diminishing returns; the therapeutic enthusiast keeps trying medications beyond the limits of reason and safety; the action-oriented physician likes to "do things"; and the meditators do nothing judiciously. Each may produce excessive costs, which on critical examination are indefensible clinically as well as economically. Too many tests and procedures, too many drugs, too many consultations, and too many x-rays are the mark of disorderly clinical thinking, as well as cost insensitivity. In this sense, good economics is good medicine.

Even more fundamental is a mastery of the basic skills of history taking and physical diagnosis. Costly errors in diagnosis most often result from failure in these basics and not in the failure to order enough tests. Unfortunately, lawyers and courts are as ignorant of this fact as the poor clinician. Excessiveness in procedures, tests, and x-rays is defensive. This is yet another example of judging medicine by standardized criteria when the criteria themselves have not been rigorously justified.

The cost-sensitive clinician is just as rigorously critical in his use of the hospital, of other health personnel, and in choosing his consultants. His criterion is not his own convenience–unconsciously exercised usually–but what is good for the patient. He must avoid surgeons with relatively high morbidity rates (and they are discernible); he must convince the patient of the efficacy and desirability of ambulatory care when it is justified; he need not accede to his patient's every whim. That too is poor medicine, and economically unsound as well. Penicillin for a viral infection, a tonsillectomy on demand, or even a new drug when the patient demands it is an invitation to unnecessary expense and to a serious side effect.

To practice cost sensitivity requires, first of all, that the physician be expert in the basic tools of his own craft. Properly understood, these tools will make him discriminating enough to use only those means which are most effective in meeting the patient's needs and no others. He must, in short, practice an economy of means in his daily work. This is the precise point at which medical morality and medical economics can be equilibrated in the care of individual patients.

But this is not enough. There must also be some equilibration on the broader scale of social and public policy. Even the cost-sensitive clinician must function under policies and in institutions which can reinforce or frustrate his efforts in caring for individual patients. Certain fundamental questions upon which policies ultimately depend must be faced much more explicitly than they have been to date.

For example, some economists and physicians suggest that the American people do not place health very high on their list of priorities. This view is based on surveys mainly among healthy people. The priorities of those who are ill can be drastically different–as any clinician will attest who has attended even the most ardent cost-containing economist or health planner. Of course, we do need to know more accurately where the American people place medical care, to what extent they are willing to compromise their customary expectations of physicians and hospitals that "everything possible" will be done in their interest.

The compromises contained in many of the decisions now facing us have not been made clear enough to enable the public to make choices. Instead, planners and legislators respond frenetically to one crisis after another–cost escalation, variable quality of care, Medicare and Medicaid abuses, excessive demand for new technology, and needless prolongation of life in the incurable, to mention a few. Piecemeal legislation is promoted with catchy phraseology to answer each crisis, but rarely are the solutions embodied in one piece of legislation related to other needs and services. We hear constantly of limited resources, but only infrequently are we told what a shift in priorities means for those services we now demand.

The public debate on resource allocation, health policy, and legislation must be conducted in a more considered way. Alternatives must be more clearly delineated. For example, many planners speak of limiting health expenditures to 10 percent of the Gross National Product. What is the justification for this figure? Everyone speaks glibly of the "American people" and what they will or will not tolerate, or what they "want" in addition to health care. Granting they receive their "money's worth" and granting it is efficiently and honestly provided, the figure may be higher or lower.[6]

Nor do we really know what people want medicine for. Some argue that medicine should confine itself to high technology and only effective therapeutic measures. Others take the contrary view that medicine is really the instrument of total health and happiness. Still others emphasize the helping and caring functions as being of equal value with the specifically curative. Which of these alternatives we choose will profoundly alter our expenditures, the kind and number of health professionals we educate, the types of institutions we build, and the minimal benefits we will provide under national health insurance. This choice is more crucial than any adjustments and fine tuning we may make in efficiency, increased productivity, fee regulation, or expenditure ceilings within the system.

Ultimately we, as a nation, must decide what it is we expect in the way of health and medical care in an advanced democratic society. Is primary care a human need so basic that it is an obligation of a civilized society? If, as we have suggested, health is one of three or four fundamental human values, then it very well might be. Does such an obligation apply to other forms of care as well? Is it possible to be a free human being and to pursue other human ends if one is ill or in distress?[7] Is health, with security, food, housing, and civic liberty, among the first principles of civilized life?

These are questions of value, of what we as a society consider to be the things for which we will sacrifice. Would this sacrifice include providing the most humane care even for those whose social utility is marginal or questionable? An economically inspired morality would answer that question one way; a morality inspired by care and solicitude for others would give a different answer. How much of our amusements and diversions–the tremendous expenditures, the almost universally accepted forms of chemical coping, alcohol, coffee, tobacco–would we sacrifice for the security of medical care available and accessible to all?

We cannot presume to answer these questions for others. Our policy makers have assumed certain answers as the basis for their recommendations. How well do they reflect public opinion? The questions have, in our view, not been put directly, clearly, understandably, and so we do not have reliable answers. In the moment of illness, when the need for care is immediate and urgent, almost every person would put all these other things aside for considerate, compassionate, and competent care. Does illness have to be the only prerequisite of a compassionate human society?

These are moral questions, turning on what we as a society believe to be good for humans as individuals and as communities. In short, what kind of society do we want to be? In Chapter Eight, we suggested the critical need for establishing a new cultural teleology, an assignment of ends, so that our *tekné* may aim at a good human life. Before we accept cost containment as the new slogan that will lead us to a well-ordered and responsive health and medical care system, we must face these values critically and as a society. The cynics will immediately protest that society cannot partake of such a critical inquiry. The only reply we can make is that if it does not, it cannot remain democratic. So important a matter as health and its impact on all other human services can be intelligently and justly disposed only if we are clear about our ends and purposes. Such critical examination would establish a moral policy about health care.[8]

Undeniably the physician, all other health professionals, and health care institutions have a crucial role in the equilibration of economics and medical morality. Their efforts in individual and personal medical transactions must be reinforced by a context of moral policy decisions which also attempts to reach some equilibrium between the inherent tensions of the canons of morality and economics.

Epilogue

This book has, we believe, taken a first step toward a philosophy and ethics of medicine and healing. A more complete philosophy of medicine requires that we examine not only what medicine is but also what kinds of knowledge it generates; what logical tools it uses; what its social, political, and aesthetic dimensions might be; and how that philosophy relates to the more general issues of the good life, the good man, and the nature of man and the cosmos.

We have intentionally concentrated on one portion of the large spectrum of topics which make up the philosophy of medicine. We have chosen the nature and conduct of medicine as practice because we hold these to be the most distinctive traits of medicine as a human activity. It is these two facets that most justify a philosophy of medicine which is more than a branch of the philosophy of science or of biology.

In our Preface, we claimed that a philosophy of medicine could benefit both medicine and philosophy. Of the philosophical tenets we have proposed, the most helpful to medicine would be the description of medical activity, the moral nature of the medical act, the meaning of the act of profession and the fact of illness, and the principles and axioms of professional ethics (Chapters Eight and Nine).

Our description of medicine working in and through the body provides a telos for the whole medical enterprise. This telos becomes the definable goal against which the moral quality of a medical act of decision can be judged. The moral nature of medicine is rooted therefore in the goals of health and healing, both of which are biological values proper to the living human body. Thus the profession, as well as the discipline, of medicine is morally centered.

There are also tenets important for philosophy which medicine can reveal, such as the role of the body in epistemology and ontology and the normative basis for medical ethics. The richness and concreteness of medical knowledge about man are indispensable requisites for philosophical anthropology as well. Some of the views we have set forth in Chapter Five point toward the post-Cartesian analysis of human judgment and anthropology which has engaged philosophers as various as Marcel, Merleau-Ponty, Scheler, and Dewey. The fact that cures do occur forces philosophy to take a realistic rather than an idealistic stance toward philosophy in general and philosophy of medicine in particular.

We have posited a normative basis for the act of profession—a basis common to all health professionals. The ethic derived from our philosophy of the patient-physician interrelationship is prior to, and independent of, the particular position we may take on the common medical-moral issues of the day. This ethic is compatible with a variety of value systems because it emphasizes the moral quality of an interhuman relationship and not the particular choice which may come out of that relationship.

The philosophical framework we have suggested for the act of profession in medicine has possibilities for an analogous ethic of the other professions. Law, teaching, and the ministry, for example, also confront humans in some state of special need, and thus of vulnerability. Each professes to address some need; each does so by an act peculiar to its profession. Lawyers, teachers, and ministers are bound to their fellows by a commonly shared ethic arising from the nature of their acts of profession.

General philosophy is served, finally, by the attention the philosophy of medicine directs to the most ancient and fundamental questions. The physician, we aver, is obliged to facilitate the patient's moral agency, to take one example. But moral agency is contingent upon rationality, freedom, and information. How these are defined depends upon our prior conceptions of what constitutes the good life and the good man and what we mean by freedom and rationality. Is the good what the patient perceives as good? Or is it what the doctor or society think is good *for* the patient? Is the patient's autonomy defensible even when he chooses what is patently harmful? Or do we hold that the sick person is never free and that the doctor is obliged to take the burden of decision from him? These questions are not resolvable in the domain of a philosophy of medicine, but a philosophy of medicine cannot proceed without their clarification. Philosophy itself is thus challenged to a renewed engagement with some of its oldest and most perennial problems.

We will perhaps be chided for our apparent neglect of the noncurative, caring, and preventive aspects of medicine. We would include these under the obligations of the physician, and they therefore become part of the expectations generated by the act of profession. It is possible that prevention and health promotion may in the future not be included in the scope of medicine. This depends very much upon how far our society goes in the medicalization of daily life. This will also determine how many more of the issues of social ethics will need to be embraced in the normative schema we have proposed.

Finally, it is unlikely that even profound changes in the way medicine is practiced will alter the fundamental philosophy of medical activity we posit. Computers will surely enter the medical transaction increasingly, just as will institutionalization, bureaucratization, and regulation. Physicians may well undergo a bifurcation in functions, some becoming technician specialists in organ systems and techniques, others tending more to coordination and generalist functions.

But none of these transformations will alter the fundamental human phenomenon we see as specific to medicine—the placing of trust and expectation in some person or institution. The mechanization and impersonalization of medicine and physicians will only underscore the urgency of the personal interaction in which decisions and actions are taken by one or a group of humans in the interest of one in need.

We find congenial the position of American pragmatist philosophers that the true test of ideas rests in their applicability and not in the rigor and logic with which they are posed or with which they withstand debate and refinement. We therefore invite development of ideas and indeed their improvement. For we strongly believe that to be practiced responsibly and to become an integral element in our culture, medicine needs a more explicit theoretical foundation than it now enjoys.

Notes

PREFACE

1. "Preface," to Pedro Lain-Entralgo, *Mind and Body,* tr. A. M. Espinosa, Jr., (London: Harwill, 1955), p. vii.
2. Enthusiasm for the cure rate, however, should be tempered by the lack of a relationship between cost and outcome. "Longevity has changed little, and the major illnesses such as malignancy and cardiovascular disease remain unimpeded. Illnesses disproportionately affect the poor, major environmental and occupational causes of illnesses receive little attention and less action, and malpractice charges intensify. Clearly, there is a crisis in health care, both in its effect upon health and in its cost. Simultaneously, medical institutions characterize themselves as excellent" (H. R. Holman, "The 'Excellence' Deception in Medicine," *Hospital Practice,* April, 1976, 11).
3. Ibid., p. 18.
4. Cf. G. B. Risse, " 'Philosophical' Medicine in Nineteenth Century Germany: An Episode in the Relations Between Philosophy and Medicine," *The Journal of Medicine and Philosophy,* I:1 (March 1976), 72–92.
5. This is the well-developed thesis of S. Gorovitz and A. MacIntyre, "Toward a Theory of Medical Fallibility," *Journal Of Medicine and Philosophy,* I:1 (March 1976), 51–71.
6. For example, G. H. Stollerman writes: "There are growing within our academic midsts professional ethicists . . . who sometimes challenge our qualifications and our competence to make appropriate ethical decisions. While we can and should welcome any critics of our performance, our desire not to surrender these deci-

sions to other professional advocates of ethics stems from our conviction that those who are granted and who assume the responsibility for the physician-patient relationship should be most ready and best prepared to make such decisions." ("Consumerism and Clinical Investigation," *Journal of Laboratory and Clinical Medicine,* 87:2 [February 1976], 182–183). Garrison is particularly strident against unhelpful philosophy: "It is thus due to lack of funds and facilities for experimentation that we find continental Europeans turning to such comparatively sterile fields as . . . the maundering of 'medical philosophy' which, far from helping toward the 'logical clarification of thoughts,' seems as confusing and unrewarding as in the days of Hegel and Schelling." (F. Garrison, *History of Medicine* [Philadelphia and London: Saunders, 1960] 4th edition, p. 801).

7. The identical problem of medical ethics is sketched by A. Jonsen and A. Hellegers, who argue that medical ethics has traditionally rested on a theory of virtue and a theory of action. With the increased complexity of modern medicine, however, the authors suggest the need for a theory of the common good to underline many ethical issues (A. Jonsen and A. Hellegers, "Conceptual Foundations for an Ethics of Medical Care," in *Ethics of Health Care,* ed. L. R. Trancredi [Washington: National Academy of Sciences, 1974], pp. 3–20).
8. E. B. Strauss, "Preface," p. ix, says: "In my opinion until medicine and surgery in all their aspects come to form part of a true *anthropology* in the Thomistic sense, a Science of Man in health and disease, it is best as a first step to try to clarify our concepts of aetiology." (author's emphasis)

Prologue

1. James, W. *The Meaning of Truth, a Sequel to Pragmatism* (London: Longmans Green, 1909), pp. xi–xii.
2. Zaner, R. M. *The Way of Phenomenology* (New York: Pegasus, 1970), p. 220.

Chapter One

1. This is the view of E. Cantore, "Humanistic Significance of Science: Some Methodological Considerations," *Philosophy of Science,* Vol. 38, No. 3 (1971), 395–412.
2. *Bioethics: Bridge to the Future* (Englewood Cliffs, N.J.: Prentice-Hall, 1971).
3. C. Bernard, *Philosophie: Manuscrit Inedit* (Paris: Boivin, 1937), p. 35.
4. W. Jaeger, *Paideia: The Ideals of Greek Culture,* Vol. III (New

York: Oxford University Press, 1944), pp. 3–45; L. Versenyi, *Socratic Humanism* (New Haven: Yale University Press, 1963), pp. 33–35.

5. Plato, *Symposium,* 186, *The Dialogues of Plato,* Vol. I, B. Jowett tr. (New York: Random House, 1937), p. 313; S. Rosen, *Plato's Symposium* (New Haven: Yale University Press, 1969), pp. 90–119, 273–77.
6. Plato, op. cit., 211, p. 335.
7. Plato, *Phaedo,* 67, ibid., p. 450.
8. Cf. the debate between Isocrates (*Antidosis* 271) and the early Aristotle (*Protrepticus,* frag. 47) on the proper ends of a good human life.
9. Hippocrates, *Precepts,* I, p. 313.
10. Hippocrates, *Ancient Medicine,* XX, p. 53.
11. C. Bernard, quoted in "Philosophical Presuppositions of Present-Day Medicine," by Walther Riese, *Bulletin of the History of Medicine,* Vol. XXX (1956), 164.
12. S. Buchanan, *The Doctrine of Signatures, A Defense of Theory in Medicine* (London: Kegan Paul, Trench and Trubner, 1938), p. x.
13. *Timaeus,* 82D.
14. R. Descartes, *Correspondence,* II, edited with an Introduction by C. E. Adams and G. Milhaud (Paris: Felix Alcan, 1936–63 in 8 volumes), p. 32.
15. M. W. Wartofsky, "Roundtable Discussion," in H. T. Engelhardt, Jr., and S. F. Spicker, eds., *Evaluation and Explanation in the Biomedical Sciences, Philosophy and Medicine, Vol. I* (Dordrecht, Holland: D. Reidel, 1947), p. 228.
16. L. Edelstein, "Hippocrates of Cos," in *The Encyclopedia of Philosophy* (ed. in chief P. Edwards), Vol. III (New York: Macmillan, 1967).
17. W. Jaeger, Ibid.
18. Hippocrates, Corpus of works attributed to Hippocrates, Littre edit. "On Wellbeing," Hab. 5, IX, p. 232.
19. Aristotle, *De Sensu,* in *The Works of Aristotle,* J. I. Beare tr., W. E. Ross ed. (New York: Oxford University Press, 1931), Ch. I, p. 436a.
20. *Claudii Galeni,* C. Kuehn, ed. (Leipzig: Opera Omnia, 1820–1833), I, pp. 53–63, cited in John S. Kroffer, *Galen's Institutio Logica* (Baltimore: Johns Hopkins Press, 1964).
21. G. B. Risse, "The Quest for Certainty in Medicine: John Brown's System of Medicine in France," *Bulletin of the History of Medicine,* Vol. 45 (1971), 1–10; G. G. Risse, "Kant, Schelling and the Early Search for a Philosophical Science of Medicine in German," *Journal of the History of Medicine,* Vol. 27 (1972), 145–58; I. Galdston, "The Romantic Period in Medicine," *Bulletin of the New York Academy of Medicine,* Vol. 32, No. 5 (1956), 346–62.

22. E. McMullin, "Two Faces of Science," *Review of Metaphysics,* Vol. XXVII, No. 4 (1974), 655–76.
23. P. Edwards (ed. in ch.), *The Encyclopedia of Philosophy* (New York: Macmillan and the Free Press, 1972).
24. W. Szumowski, "La Philosophie de la médecine, son histoire, son essence, sa dénomination, et sa définition," *Archives internationales d'histoire des sciences,* Vol. 2, No. 9 (October 1949), 1097–1139.
25. A. de Waelhens, "The Ontological Encounter of Human Science and Philosophy," in *Begegnung: Rencontre: Encounter,* F. B. Sullivan, tr. (Utrecht: *Uitgeverij Het Spectrum,* 1957), pp. 492–507, reprinted in *Philosophy Today,* Vol 3 (Spring 1959), 52–64.
26. G. Marcel, "Incarnate Being as the Central Datum of Metaphysical Reflection," in *Creative Fidelity,* R. Rosthal, tr. (New York: Noonday Press, 1964), pp. 11–37.
27. M. Merleau-Ponty, *The Spatiality of the Lived Body and Motility,* C. Smith, tr., in S. Spicker, ed., *The Philosophy of the Body* (Chicago: Quadrangle Books, 1970), pp. 241–71.
28. S. Spicker, "The Lived Body as Catalytic Agent: Reaction at the Interface of Medicine and Philosophy," in Engelhardt and Spicker, eds., *Evaluation,* pp. 181–204.
29. E. Straus, *Phenomenological Psychology,* Selected Papers, tr. in part by E. Eng (New York: Basic Books, 1966).
30. E. Straus, M. Natanson, and H. Ey, *Psychiatry and Philosophy,* ed. M. Natanson (New York: Springer-Verlag, 1969).
31. M. Grene, "People and Other Animals," *Philosophia Naturalis,* XIV (1973), 25–38.
32. H. T. Engelhardt, Jr., "The Philosophy of Medicine: A New Endeavor," *Texas Reports on Biology and Medicine,* Vol. 31, No. 3 (Fall 1973), 443–52; H. T. Engelhardt, Jr., "The Concepts of Health and Disease," in Engelhardt, *Evaluation,* pp. 125–42.
33. F. J. J. Buytendijck, *Prolegomena to an Anthropological Physiology* (Pittsburgh: Duquesne University Press, 1974).
34. P. Lain-Entralgo, "The Health and Perfection of Man," *Diogenes,* No. 1 (Fall 1970), 1–19; P. Lain-Entralgo, *La Relación Médico-Enfermo* (Madrid: Revista de Occidente, 1974); P. Lain-Entralgo, *The Therapy of the Word in Classical Antiquity,* L. J. Rather and J. M. Sharp, tr. (New Haven: Yale University Press, 1970).
35. M. W. Wartofsky, "Organs, Organisms and Disease: Human Ontology and Medical Practice," in Engelhardt, *Evaluation,* pp. 67–83.
36. R. Zaner, "The Radical Reality of the Human Body," *Humanitas,* Vol. 2, No. 1 (1966), 73–87; R. Zaner, "Context and Reflexivity: The Geneaology of Self," in Engelhardt, *Evaluation,* pp. 154–74; R. Zaner, "The Unanchored Leaf: Humanities and the Discipline of Care," *Texas Reports on Biology and Medicine,* Vol. 32, No. 1 (Spring 1974), 1–18.

37. H. T. Engelhardt, Jr., and S. F. Spicker, eds., *Evaluation and Explanation in the Biomedical Sciences, Philosophy and Medicine, Vol. I* (Dordrecht, Holland: Reidel, 1974).
38. J. Shaffer, "Roundtable Discussion," in Engelhardt, *Evaluation,* pp. 215–22.
39. S. Toulmin, "Concepts of Function and Mechanism in Medicine and Medical Science" (Hommage á Claude Bernard), in Engelhardt, *Evaluation,* p. 54.
40. W. Szumowski, "La Philosophie," in Engelhardt, *Evaluation,* p. 1138.
41. E. Husserl, "Philosophy as Rigorous Science," in E. Husserl, ed. *Phenomenology and the Crisis of Philosophy* (New York: Harper & Row Torchbooks, 1965); M. Heidegger, *An Introduction to Metaphysics,* R. Manheim tr. (New York: Anchor-Doubleday, 1961); M. Merleau-Ponty, *In Praise of Philosophy* (Chicago: Northwestern University Press, 1963); J. Ortega y Gasset, *What Is Philosophy?* Mildred Adams tr. (New York: Norton, 1960).
42. Toulmin, ibid.
43. H. Jonas, "Technology and Responsibility," *Social Research,* Vol. 40 (1973), 31–54.
44. O. Temkin, "On the Interrelationship of the History and the Philosophy of Medicine," *Bulletin of the History of Medicine,* Vol. XXX, No. 3 (1956), 241–51.
45. W. Osler, *A Way of Life and Selected Writings* (New York: Dover, 1951).
46. K. D. Clouser, "Medical Ethics: Some Uses, Abuses and Limitations," *New England Journal of Medicine,* Vol. 293, No. 8 (1975), 384–87. Of course, philosophy does make judgments about medicine, for even to classify what is the case is to separate what appears important to us from what does not. This is an important judgment.
47. R. Straus, "The Nature and Status of Medical Sociology," *American Sociological Review,* Vol. 22 (1957), 203.
48. M. Heidegger, *What Is Called Thinking?,* F. D. Wieck and J. G. Gray, tr. (New York: Harper Torchbooks, 1963), p. 33.
49. H. Dreyfus, "The Critique of Artificial Reason," in Marjorie Grene, ed., *Interpretation of Life and Mind* (London: Routledge and Kegan Paul, 1974), pp. 99–116.
50. M. Buber, *Between Man and Man,* R. Smith, tr., (New York: Macmillan, 1972); E. Cassirer, *An Essay on Man* (New York: Bantam, 1970); M. Scheler, *Man's Place in Nature* (New York: Noonday Press, 1961).
51. G. S. Stent, "Limits to the Scientific Understanding of Man," *Science,* Vol. 187, No. 21 (1975), 1052–57.
52. S. Gorovitz, "Bioethics and Social Responsibility," *The Monist,* Vol. 60, No. 1 (1976), 3–15.

53. J. Bronowski, *Science and Human Value* (Baltimore: Penguin Books, 1964), pp. 63–64.
54. G. Holton, "Modern Science and the Intellectual Tradition," *Science,* 131 (1960), 1187–93.
55. H. Jonas, ibid.
56. D. K. Price, *The Scientific Estate* (Cambridge, Mass.: Harvard University Press, 1967), p. 105.
57. E. D. Pellegrino, "The Most Humane Science: Some Notes on Liberal Education in Medicine and the University," The Sixth Sanger Lecture, *Bulletin of the Medical College of Virginia,* Vol. 2, No. 4 (Summer 1970), 11–39.
58. Foucault, *The Birth of the Clinic: An Archaeology of Medical Perception* (New York: Random House, 1973).
59. A. MacIntyre, "Moral Philosophy and Medical Perplexity: Comments on 'How Virtues Become Vices,'" in Engelhardt, *Evaluation,* pp. 97–111.
60. M. W. Wartofsky, ibid.
61. "Human Values Teaching Programs for Health Professionals," Institute on Human values in Medicine (Philadelphia: Society for Health and Human Values, 1977).
62. C. Fried, *Medical Experimentation: Personal Integrity and Social Policy,* distributed by American Elsevier (Amsterdam: North-Holland, 1974).
63. Buchanan, ibid.

Chapter Two

1. S. Marcus, "The Demoralized Humanists," *Chronicle of Higher Education* (1975), 32.
2. Ibid.
3. C. J. Bontempo and S. J. Odell, eds., *The Owl of Minerva: Philosophers on Philosophy* (New York: McGraw-Hill, 1974).
4. D. Callahan, "Year of the Ethics Backlash," *Hastings Center Report,* Vol. V (1975), 18.
5. M. Merleau-Ponty, *In Praise of Philosophy,* John Wild and James M. Edie, tr. (Evanston, Ill.: Northwestern University Press, 1963), pp. 27–28, 51–54.
6. Ibid., "Philosophy Is an Architecture of Signs," p. 57.
7. Ibid., pp. 52–56.
8. M. Scheler, *Die Stellung des Menschen im Kosmos* (Darmstadt: Reichl, 1928), pp. 13ff, quoted in E. Cassirer, *An Essay on Man* (New York: Bantam, 1970), p. 24.
9. This binary nature of experience is noted by virtually every modern thinker cited. Merleau-Ponty observes, for example, that the "distinction between fact and essence rests on my ability to distinguish the fact that I am living through something and what it is" (*Phe-*

nomenology of Perception [London: Routledge and Kegan Paul, 1962], p. 54). James M. Edie, reflecting on Husserl's observations about this binary nature of experience, states that concrete universals, empirical necessities, and material a prioris always exist as part of factual concretizations–that is, as structures of experience; see W. Von Baeyer and R. M. Griffith, eds., "Phenomenology and Psychiatry: The Need for a 'Subjective Method' in the Scientific Study of Human Behavior," *Conditio Humana* (Berlin: Springer-Verlag, 1966), p. 68.

10. A. N. Whitehead, *Modes of Thought* (New York: Capricorn, 1958), pp. 1–27. Also see W. A. Christian, *An Interpretation of Whitehead's Metaphysics* (New Haven: Yale University Press, 1967), pp. 19ff.
11. S. Spicker, ed., *Organism, Medicine and Metaphysics,* Vol. 7 of *Philosophy and Medicine* (Dordrect, Holland/Boston: Reidel, 1978), p. xviii.
12. E. Husserl, *Krisis der Europäischen Wissenschaften* (Den Haag: M. Nijhoff, 1954), p. 130.
13. A. Gurwitsch, "Problems of the Life-World," in *Phenomenology and Social Reality,* ed., M. Natanson (The Hague: Nijhoff, 1970), pp. 36–37, argues that the lifeworld is an important concept in modern philosophy because it does set limits to theoretical constructs.
14. L. W. Beck, "German Philosophy," *Encyclopedia of Philosophy* (New York: Macmillan, 1967), III, pp. 301–302, argues that this was Kant's preoccupation.
15. M. Grene observes how Heidegger, Bergson, and Dewey all revolted against the simple world picture of Descartes and Newton by focusing on man as a maker in a social environment in her article "Martin Heidegger," *Encyclopedia of Philosophy,* III, p. 459.
16. R. M. Griffith, "Golden Coins and Golden Curls: Lived Aesthetics," in *Aisthesis and Aesthetics,* ed. W. W. Straus and R. M. Griffith (Pittsburgh: Duquesne University Press, 1970), p. 63.
17. Merleau-Ponty, *In Praise of Philosophy,* pp. 23, 40, 46.
18. M. Natanson and E. W. Straus with H. Ey, *Psychiatry and Philosophy* (New York: Springer-Verlag, 1969), p. viii.
19. C. Burns, "Diseases Versus Healths: Some Legacies in the Philosophies of Modern Medical Science," and A. MacIntyre, "How Virtues Become Vices: Values, Medicine and the Social Context," in *Evaluation and Explanation in the Biomedical Sciences,* ed. H. T. Engelhardt, Jr., and S. F. Spicker (Boston: Reidel, 1975), pp. 29–50, 97–112, respectively. MacIntyre continued this same theme in his later "Patients as Agents," and Burns explored the variety of sources of American Medical Ethics in his "American Medical Ethics: Some Historical Roots," in *Philosophical Medical Ethics:*

Its Nature and Significance, ed. H. T. Engelhardt, Jr., and S. Spicker (Boston: Reidel, 1977), pp. 197–212, and 21–26, respectively. Background on this point can also be found in C. R. Burns, ed., *Legacies in Law and Medicine* and *Legacies in Ethics and Medicine* (New York: Science History Publications, 1977), 2 vols.

20. (New York: Modern Library, 1955), p. 509.
21. Husserl, *Krisis,* p. 136. R. J. Baron, "Clinical Distance: Toward an Ontology of Illness," M.D. thesis, Yale University School of Medicine, 1978, notes that the study of disease in medicine is a study of paradigmatic sets (Kuhn) of ideal objectivities rather than the existential meaning of illness for the patient. Using Husserl, Baron argues that the prescientific lifeworld, a world of unmediated direct experience, forces medicine to direct attention to the problems of an ill person. Thus a dualism between experience with the patient and objectivity or distance from the patient is necessarily formed (pp. 68–72).
22 S. Buchanan observes that reflective reasoning is a power which goes along with ordinary direct knowledge. "Therefore not only do I think, I know that I am thinking as I think (*Embers of the World, Conversations with Scott Buchanan* [Santa Barbara: Center for the Study of Democratic Institutions, III, No. 2 of the Center's Occasional Papers], p. 30.) Because all the world consists of relationships, "human beings symbolize these relationships in their reasoning power, connecting in concepts what was interrelated in direct experience" (p. 200). Buchanan therefore considered the liberal arts as the power of handling symbols, as he articulates in his writing of the St. John's College Catalogue of 1937–1938 for a "Great Books" curriculum.
23. Ibid., p. 30.
24. L. Wittgenstein, *Philosophical Investigations,* 2d. ed. (New York: Macmillan, 1953).
25. Husserl, *Krisis.*
26. Merleau-Ponty, *Phenomenology of Perception.*
27. A. MacIntyre and S. Gorovitz, "Toward a Theory of Medical Fallibility," *Hastings Center Report,* Vol. V (1975), 13–23. W. Ong, "Foreword," in *Therapy of the Word,* by P. Lain-Entralgo (New Haven: Yale University Press, 1970), pp. xii–xiii, offers some comments on Aristotle's therapy of *Katharsis* which can serve as a corrective to the MacIntyre and Gorovitz relentless condemnation of Aristotle throughout their article on the grounds that Aristotle neglected individuality. Ong's remarks on *Katharsis* show that Aristotle was profoundly interested in individuality and the human condition, and that he must have been aware, as they are, that medicine treats a different class of individuals than science does.
28. J. Dewey, "Soul and Body," in S. Spicker, ed., *The Philosophy of the Body* (Chicago: Quadrangle Books, 1970), p. 119.

29. We caution the reader that the use of "forms" is meant more in an Aristotelian than in a Platonic sense.
30. H. Fabrega, Jr., "The Need for an Ethnomedical Science," *Science* 146 (1975), 969–75. C. Leslie, ed., *Asian Medical Systems: A Comparative Study* (Berkeley: University of California Press, 1976).
31. J. Locke, *An Essay Concerning Human Understanding,* 2d. ed., Book I, Chapter I, ed. by J. W. Yolton (London: J. M. Dent & Sons Ltd., 1961), I, p. 129.

CHAPTER THREE

1. This is the view of Dr. Eichna, for example, who pronounced it at an address made to the Association of Professors of Medicine in 1977. Dr. Eichna is a distinguished former chairman of medicine at New York Downstate Medical Center. His view is representative of many physicians today.
2. P. Lain-Entralgo, *La Medicina Hipocratica* (Madrid: Revista de Occidente, 1970), pp. 225–48, clearly sets out the subordination of diagnosis to prognosis in Hippocratic medicine. Judgments were made on the state of health of the individual to discern the balance between health and disease prior to any intervention. In fact, *diagignoskō* meant primarily to distinguish or discern.
3. P. Lain-Entralgo, *Doctor and Patient* (London: World University Library, 1969), traces a change in this anti-hubric attitude during the rise of the Christian era. By the additional notion of divine law, Christians were able to relativize the givens of nature, thus giving rise to the development of modern science in the Middle Ages and thereafter, and laying the groundwork for a more interventionist model of medicine.
4. Democritus, *Fragment* 37.
5. Here we use the term as Plato did, an *ars medica,* or *tekné iatrikê.* The term is derived from the Hippocratic corpus. Plato's notion of *tekné* more closely approximates a practice with knowledge than Aristotle's more refined sense of the word. In the next chapter, we will trace the development of the concept. For the moment, the term is used to mean a practice depending on experience. Knowledge of the theory alone, in Plato's view, could not suffice.
6. The *Charmides* is normally placed by scholars seventh among nine early works depicting the historical Socrates. Charmides was Plato's uncle.
7. Georgias, *Fragment* 23 (Plutarch *de gloria Athen.,* 5, 348c).
8. St. Thomas Aquinas, *In Boethii de Trinitate,* V, a. 1, obj. 5.
9. Avicenna, *Canon Medicinae* I, fen. 1, doctr 1, prologus (Venice, 1608, I, 6, a 33–40).

10. P. Lain-Entralgo, *La Historia Clinica* (Madrid: Consejo Superior de Investigaciones Cientificas, 1950), pp. 6–8.
11. E. Cassell, M.D., "Healing," *Hospital Physician,* Vol. 12 (1976), 28–29, offers a brief outline of an argument later appearing in his book on medicine as the art of healing. In the article he argues that medicine is inherently a moral profession because practitioners are committed to action in the service of a good, an argument with which we have no quibble. However, in support of this thesis, he also argues that were medicine completely technological, it would not be a moral discipline. Here we detect a confusion about why medicine is an art, as will become evident later in the text. This confusion leads one to Cassell's conclusion that physicians act as applied moral philosophers.

    Equally confusing is the proposal by A. MacIntyre and S. Gorovitz that medicine is a science of individuals–not just an applied science, but a science about an individual. Unless the authors mean classes of individuals, it is difficult to reconcile this view with any standard notion of science. See Gorovitz and MacIntyre, "Toward a Theory of Medical Fallibility," *Journal of Medicine and Philosophy,* Vol. 1 (1976), 51–71.
12. See E. Pellegrino, "The Most Humane Science," Sixth Sanger Lecture, Bulletin of the Medical College of Virginia, 2, No. 4 (1970), 11–39.
13. S. Buchanan, *Embers of the World* (Santa Barbara, Calif.: Center for the Study of Democratic Institutions; Vol. III, No. 2 of the Center Occasional Papers), p. 36, argues that the power of handling symbols rests in the liberal arts, and that all professions manipulate symbols. He would presumably class medicine as a liberal art.
14. See E. Pellegrino, "The Humanistic Base of Professional Ethics in Medicine," *New York State Journal of Medicine,* Vol. 77, No. 9 (1977), 1456–62.
15. See E. Pellegrino, "Interdisciplinary Education in the Health Professions: Assumptions, Definitions, and Some Notes on Teams," *Report of a Conference: Educating for the Health Team,* Chap. II (Washington, D.C.: National Academy of Sciences, Institute of Medicine, 1972), pp. 4–17.
16. Thus J.-C. Sournia, M.D., *Mythologies de la Médécine Modern* (Paris: Presses Universitaires de France, 1969), explores the language and considerable magical thinking present in modern medicine. His argument is that a search for causes of disease is rarely a step away from magical thinking and imprecise language (pp. 36–42). Some causal examples he cites are: "inflammation" (Middle Ages), "tumor" (nineteenth century), "rheumatism" (sixteenth-century France), "irritation" as a form of animism, a "cold" causing a temperature, "spontaneous nerve paralysis," "cancer," and

"lipid." He concludes that medicine, especially surgery, gets results from comparable cases, not from rigorous scientific experimentation and refined language (p. 40).

17. As quoted in the texts collected by W. A. Wallace, *Causality and Scientific Explanation* (Ann Arbor: University of Michigan Press, 1972), Vol. II, pp. 141–54.
18. P. Lain-Entralgo, *La Historia,* pp. 23, 489–90.
19. See, for example, the articles by Burns, Engelhardt, and Wartofsky in T. Engelhardt and S. Spicker, eds., *Evaluation and Explanation in the Biomedical Sciences* (Boston: Reidel, 1975).
20. Relationships are often thought of as things or functions. In fact, they are neither. They are abstractions appropriate to describing observed data. T. S. Szasz and M. Hollender use this viewpoint to examine "The Basic Models of the Doctor-Patient Relationship," *A.M.A. Archives of Internal Medicine,* Vol. 97 (1956), 585–92.
21. "Foreword," in E. R. Babbie, *Science and Morality in Medicine* (Berkeley, Calif.: University of California Press, 1970), p. ix.
22. Babbie, *Science and Morality in Medicine,* p. 12, states this case clearly: "Why are interpersonal relations so important in medicine? The patient-physician relation, like other social relationships, reflects the general values of human morality in a given society. Those values, in turn, are founded on basic ontological beliefs about man's nature and that of society. The character of the relations between physicians and their patients, then, ultimately supports or threatens the basic beliefs held in general society."
23. *Phaedrus,* 270b. P. Lain-Entralgo, *La Historia,* p. 8, calls the clinical interaction the elemental condition of medicine, and further notes that it involves a nosological and anthropological set of tacit assumptions.
24. *Lysis,* 218e–219d.
25. Aristotle called wholes which have qualitatively similar parts *ta homoiomere.* By contrast, a whole not having similar parts was *to anomoiomeres.* An example of the former would be gold; cut in half, it would still be gold. An example of the latter would be a dog; cut in half, it would cease to be a dog. Our concept of a unitary discipline is parallel to anhometic wholes: Parts of medicine are not medicine, but other disciplines. For this reason, we have also stated that medicine is a *derived* discipline.
26. J. Bergsma, *Somatopsychologie: op zoek naar psychosociale dimensies van de geneeskunde* (Lochem: de Tijdstroom, 1977), pp. 204–205, argues that the imbalance of the doctor-patient relationship is not due to knowledge but to the power stemming from the art of medicine as viewed by society. However, it seems difficult to deny the importance of scientific knowledge in creating this imbalance.
27. *de Beneficiis,* VI, 16.
28. Ramsey's argument in his *Patient as Person,* that this relationship

should be grounded in a religious conception of covenant, has a positive side in that it illustrates a more profound source of medical morality than adherence to codes. However, its negative side is that it explains something clear, the need for trust, by something more obscure to many Americans, a covenant.

29. See Plato, *Republic,* 406b.
30. P. Lain-Entralgo, *Mind and Body* (London: Harwill, 1955), p. xvii, quotes Kant as observing that "Each man has his particular way of being in good health." We cite this quote because of its obvious good sense. The motive of the physician must include the personal and subjective values of patients.
31. These motives also lead to three different parallel forms of pathological explanation: etiological (social usefulness), symptomatology (personal clinical sign), and entitative (objective, human condition). See P. Lain-Entralgo, *Mind and Body,* p. xviii.
32. As reported by Siebeck; cf. ibid, p. xv.
33. P. Medewar, "Scientific Method in Science and Medicine," *Perspectives in Biology and Medicine,* Vol. 18, No. 3 (Spring 1975), 346–47.
34. As quoted in F. Garrison, *History of Medicine* 4th ed. (Philadelphia and London: Saunders, 1950), p. 44.
35. For an historical development of medicine as a relationship, consult P. Lain-Entralgo, *Doctor and Patient,* op. cit.
36. *The Art of Worldly Wisdom,* tr. J. Jacobs (New York: Ungar, 1892), p. XIX.
37. Cf. W. J. Stein, "De-Animation: The Sense of Becoming Psychotic," in E. Straus and R. Griffith, *Aisthesis and Aesthetics* (Pittsburgh: Duquesne University Press, 1970), pp. 77–101.
38. G. Marcel, "The Existentialist Fulcrum," in R. Zaner and D. Ihde, eds., *Phenomenology and Existentialism* (New York: Putnam Capricorn, 1973), p. 214.
39. This activity represents the *Lebenswelt* of Husserl or the "world of the street" discussed by W. James. The "facts" of this world of consciousness are concrete and pervaded by value. For a developed discussion, cf. J. Wild, "Husserl's Life-World and the Lived Body," in E. Straus, ed., *Phenomenology: Pure and Applied* (Pittsburgh: Duquesne University Press, 1964), pp. 10–28.
40. K. E. Rothschuh, "Der Krankheitsbegriff," *Hippokrates,* Vol. 43 (1972), 3–17.
41. Cf. A. Neale, "An Analysis of Health," *The Kennedy Institute Quarterly Report,* Vol. 1, No. 1 (Autumn 1975), 1–9.
42. L. Thomas, *The Lives of a Cell* (New York: Viking, 1974). This view is expressed in a number of essays contained in the volume.
43. Thus L. Kass, "Regarding the End of Medicine and Pursuit of Health," *The Public Interest,* Vol. 40 (Summer 1975), 11–42, checks some false ends of medicine such as happiness, civic or

moral virtue, or the prolongation of life, by arguing that disease and health have an organic base.

44. E. Straus, *The Primary World of Senses: A Vindication of Sensory Experience* (New York: Free Press, 1963), p. 18.
45. For the distinction between sign and symptom, cf. M. Merleau-Ponty, *Signs* (Evanston: Northwestern University Press, 1964), pp. 39–83; *The Primacy of Perception* (Evanston: Northwestern University Press, 1964), p. 7.
46. R. Hudson, "The Concept of Disease," *Annals of Internal Medicine* (1966), Vol. 65, 595–601.
47. Cf. E. Cassell, "Disease as an 'It'," *Social Science and Medicine* Vol. 10 (1976), 143–46, develops his observation of patient-facility in this regard.
48. Cf. E. Pellegrino, "Medicine, Philosophy and Man's Infirmity," in *Conditio Humana,* ed. W. Von Baeyer and R. Griffith (Berlin: Springer-Verlag, 1966), 272–84.
49. Cf. P. Lain-Entralgo, *Mind and Body,* pp. 132–33.
50. As quoted in ibid., p. xv.
51. C. Reynolds, "Somatic Ethics: Joy and Adventure in the Embodied Moral Life," unpublished paper, argues that theology views God as a unitive power beyond us yet an Ideal Participant in our social reality.
52. Cf. P. Lain-Entralgo, *The Therapy of the Word* (New Haven: Yale University Press, 1970).
53. P. Lain-Entralgo argues that Freud reintroduced into medicine persuasive psychological action which heals, a feature of Greek medicine which used *epode* (charms or conjurations) to produce *sophrosyné,* a calmed, enlightened, and orderly person (Ibid). However, Socrates, Plato, and Aristotle saw medicine in a more scientific light and suggested that cure of the soul be left to philosophy. Because Western medicine followed this advice, verbal therapy has never been fully integrated in modern medicine–indeed, in psychiatry itself.
54. E. Straus, *Reason and Unreason in Psychological Medicine* (London: H. K. Levis, 1953), p. 10.

Chapter Four

1. F. Hartmann, "Ietros Philosophos Isotheos," *Niedersächische Artzeblatt* (Feb. 19, 1977), 52–56. Also see H. Gadamer, "Apologie der Heilkunst," in *Kleine Schriften* (Tübingen: Max Niemeyer Verlag, 1967), Vol. 1.
2. As quoted in O. Temkin, *The Double Face of Janus and Other Essays in the History of Medicine* (Baltimore: Johns Hopkins University Press, 1977), pp. 179–89.
3. In "Philosophy and Medicine: The Clinical Management of a Mixed Marriage," K. D. Clouser discusses topics of interest to

medicine and suggests that clinical concerns, mutually interesting to philosophers and physicians, constitute a "critica." It is analogous to this more general sense of the term that we employ. Cf. *Proceedings of the Institute on Human Values and Medicine* (Philadelphia: Society for Health and Human Values, 1972), pp. 47–80. Kant's own understanding of "critical" was a science of the limits of human knowledge, an analytic search of the powers of reason while simultaneously constructing a rational approach to the problem. Thus the *Critique of Pure Reason* examines the form of experience of thought without identity or matter. We use "critique," therefore, only in the sense of an examination of the form of medical experience or clinical interaction. Through analysis of the forms of interaction, the uniqueness of each is laid aside to discover what, if any, conditions of possibility remain.

4. Cf. J. Dewey, *Experience and Nature* (New York: Dover Books, 1963), pp. 396–403. It should be noted that Dewey's theory of criticism is relative to ends in view. Because we argue later that health is a perduring value of human beings, the result of our critique, we hold, is less relativistically conceived.
5. Cf. L. Edelstein, *Ancient Medicine,* ed. O. Temkin and C. L. Temkin (Baltimore: Johns Hopkins University Press, 1967), chaps. 1 and 2; Hippocrates, *The Book of Prognostics.*
6. *Charmides,* 156e-157b. *Sophrosynē* is often translated as "temperance."
7. Medicine is referred to as an art and a science. *Charmides,* 165c; 170c.
8. Ibid., 170–175.
9. *Timaeus,* 88a. Plato here says that professors of medicine frequently do not know anything about it.
10. P. Lain-Entralgo, *The Therapy of the Word in Classical Antiquity,* L. J. Rather and J. M. Sharp, tr. (New Haven: Yale University Press, 1970), pp. 120ff. Also see Plato's attack on medicine in his day in *Republic*/III, 405–406.
11. *Phaedrus,* 268–270b.
12. *Philebus,* 56 a–b.
13. *Laws,* IV, 720. It is interesting to note that medicine which neglects the whole person calls forth the same criticism today. Thus H. M. Graning, *RX: Education for the Patient* (Carbondale: Southern Illinois University, 1975), pp. 16–17, is critical of "Professionals [who] prefer to have patients behave as children. They want patients to be obedient . . . to do the things they are told without argument." In light of Plato's view that the medical event should be one of friendship, two features of dehumanizing interaction destroy the nature of medicine: custodianship rather than fellowship and the breakdown of trust. Of the former, O. Guttentag says: "clear differentiation between fellowship with someone and responsibility in the

sense of partnership on the one hand, and care of something and responsibility in the sense of an engineer's responsibility for optimal functioning of a machine on the other is especially difficult" ("Foreword," in Babbie, *Science and Morality in Medicine,* [Berkeley: University of California Press, 1970], p. xi.) On the breakdown of trust, M. Merleau-Ponty notes: "to obey with one's eyes closed is the beginning of panic; to choose against what one understands, the beginning of skepticism" (*In Praise of Philosophy* [Evanston: Northwestern University Press, 1963], p. 60). We regard Plato's observation about the poor practice of medicine an enduring truth about the structure of the medical event.

14. *Symposium,* 193 c.
15. *Lysis,* 217. It is difficult to say where medicine would be placed in Plato's famous passage in the *Republic* about degrees of knowledge (509d). *Doxa* is knowledge through images, while *epistemé* is knowledge of ideas. Is medicine a pure *noesis* of health? Or is it *pistis,* a state of imagination?
16. *Nichomachean Ethics,* VIII, 1155a. P. Lain-Entralgo, *Doctor and Patient* (London: World University Library, 1969), pp. 1–40.
17. *De Partibus Animalium,* I, 640 a.
18. *Metaphysics,* XII, 1070 a.
19. *De Partibus Animalium,* I, 639 a.
20. *Politics,* III, c. 11, 1282 a.
21. Ibid., III, c. 11, 1281 b.
22. *Posterior Analytics,* I, c. 2, 71 b.
23. Ibid., I, c. 13.
24. *Rhetoric,* I, c. 1, 1355 a.
25. Ibid., 1355 b.
26. Ibid., 1356 a. Aristotle's clue that rhetoric, of which medicine is an analogue, is also like ethical studies, is important.
27. Ibid., c. 5, 1361 b. Temkin reproduces the prologue of an Alexandrian commentary on Galen's *De Sectis* which highlights the role of medicine in healing the body by which all other goods come to man: "Bonum Aliquid divitiarum et vite nostre oportunum adinventa est ars medicine. Sanitatem enim operari et conservare promittit et exercere: per quam magna bonorum utilitas hominibus additur: per quam etas et tempus et omnis medicatio et disciplina procedit: et ipsius anime operationes" (O. Temkin, *The Double Face,* p. 181).
28. Ibid., II, cc 3–18, 1381 a–1391 b.
29. P. Lain-Entralgo, *Therapy of the Word,* pp. 123–24.
30. O. Temkin, "Studies on Late Alexandrian Medicine," in *The Double Face,* pp. 179–97. Aristotle's real opinion can be found in his *Nichomachean Ethics,* VII, 15.
31. See P. Lain-Entralgo, *Doctor and Patient,* pp. 55ff, for a sketch of this change. His thesis in *Mind and Body* (London: Harwill, 1955)

is that modern medicine inherits the naturalism of the Greeks and the personalism of the Semites. The former permitted the distinction between myth and nature, leading to the patient, rather than the gods, as therapeutic object. The latter permitted the distinction, through the development of Christian thought, between the moral realm and the physical.

32. *In Boethii De Trinitate,* Q5, a. 3; *Summa Theologiae,* I, 40, 3; *In III Meta,* lect. 7 n. 405.
33. *In II Meta.,* Lect. 5, n. 335; *In Boethii,* op. cit., Q5, a. 1, reply to 2 and 3.
34. *In I De Caelo Et Mundo,* lect. 3, n. 7; II, Lct. 17, n. 2; *Summa Theologiae* I, 32, I ad 2, Aquinas notes that the Ptolemaic system of astronomy "saves the appearances" but may not be true because they might be saved by some other system not yet devised. This observation later proved to be the case.
35. *In Boethii,* op. cit., Q5, a. 1, obj. 4 and 5.
36. Ibid., reply.
37. Ibid., ad 2. For Aquinas, bodily activities are not among the liberal arts.
38. *Canon Medicinae,* I fen 1, doctr. 1, prologues (Venice, 1608) I, 6, a 33–40.
39. *In Boethii,* Q5, a. 1, ad 4. Of course, this point of view does not address the Kantian critique of the relation of theory to practice, a point we will pursue in developing an ontology of the body.
40. Ibid., ad 5.
41. Ibid., a. 2. The entire article is devoted to the question of the individual in scientific knowledge.
42. Cf. M. Wartofsky, "The Mind's Eye and the Hand's Brain," in H. T. Engelhardt, Jr., and D. Callahan, eds., *Science, Ethics and Medicine* (Hastings-on-Hudson: The Hastings Center, 1976), pp. 167–94; "Organs, Organisms and Disease: Human Ontology and Medical Practice," in H. T. Englehardt, Jr., and S. Spicker, eds., *Evaluation and Explanation in the Biomedical Sciences* (Boston: Reidel, 1975), pp. 67–84; C. Whitbeck, "The Relevance of Philosophy of Medicine for the Philosophy of Science," *Proceedings of the Philosophy of Science Association* (Ann Arbor: Edwards, 1976), S. Suppe and P. Asquith, eds., pp. 123–135.
43. Cf. Whitbeck, op. cit., M. Grene, "Philosophy of Medicine: Prolegomena to a Philosophy of Science," Ibid., pp. 136–44. Whitbeck criticizes Aristotle for not basing theoretical knowledge on the practical, yet seems ignorant of Aristotle's insistence that science regard what is real insofar as it allows us to say determinate things about it. Nevertheless, her discussion of causation in medicine reflects the quasi-Aristotelian nature of the search for proximate causes specific to disease and to that disease alone. We agree that medical practice does not arise out of an application of theory, but that theory arises

out of clinical practice. E. Cassell, "Preliminary Explorations of Thinking in Medicine," *Ethics in Science and Medicine* Vol. 2 (1975), 1–12, argues that analytic, scientific thought is driving out valuational, synthetic thinking in medicine. The latter he holds to be characteristic of clinical medicine and value clarification. It is based on syntheses against which the object of thought is compared.

44. Whitbeck, op. cit., is one exception to this generalization, disagreeing with Engelhardt that the concept of disease involves a therapeutic imperative. Cf. H. T. Engelhardt, Jr., "The Concepts of Health and Disease," in Engelhardt and Spicker, eds., *Evaluation,* pp. 125–42.
45. Gorovitz and MacIntyre, "Toward a Theory of Medical Fallibility," *Journal of Medicine and Philosophy, I* (1976), 51–71. Jacob Bronowski, *The Ascent of Man* (Boston: Little, Brown, 1973), p. 13 notes that a change in the temper of science is taking place due to a shift from the physical to the life sciences in the past twenty years. This shift is accompanied by a scientific interest in individuality.
46. Cf. W. A. Wallace, *Causality and Scientific Explanation,* Vol. I (Ann Arbor: University of Michigan Press, 1972), pp. 117–59.
47. M. Wartofsky, "The Mind's Eye."
48. Wallace, *Causality,* pp. 184–93.
49. P. Lain-Entralgo, *Doctor and Patient,* pp. 105–108.
50. Cf. O. Temkin, "Zimmerman's Philosophy of the Physician," in *The Double Face,* pp. 239–45, esp. 240–44.
51. As quoted in J.-C. Sournia, *Mythologies de la Medicine Modern* (Paris: Presses Universitaires de France, 1969), p. 27.
52. Cf. the collection of relevant texts in Wallace, *Causality,* Vol. II, pp. 141–54.
53. M. Foucault, *The Birth of the Clinic: An Archeology of Medical Perception* (New York: Pantheon, 1973), pp. x–xiv.
54. Ibid., p. xv.
55. Wartofsky, "The Mind's Eye."
56. Sournia, *Mythologies,* p. 27.
57. S. Buchanan, *The Doctrine of Signatures* (New York: Harcourt, Brace, 1938), p. xii. The book was written under a grant to spend one year at Hopkins to develop a philosophy of medicine suitable for a socialized medicine program in the United States.
58. Ibid., pp. 200–201.
59. P. Lain-Entralgo, *La Historia Clinica* (Madrid: Consejo Superior de Investigaciones Cientificas, 1950), pp. 3–5.
60. P. Lain-Entralgo, *Mind and Body,* pp. xvii–xviii.
61. *La Historia Clinica,* pp. 11–16.
62. E. Gilson, *The Unity of Philosophical Experience* (New York: Scribner's, 1937), pp. 147–64.

Chapter Five

1. L. Mumford, *The Myth of the Machine, The Pentagon of Power* (New York: Harcourt, Brace, Jovanovich, 1979), p. 420, argues that "If we are to save technology itself from the aberrations of its present leaders and putative gods, we must in both our thinking and our action come back to the human center; for it is there that all significant transformations begin and terminate."
2. We have deliberately left out the category of medical ethics research, both because it would divert us from the purpose of this sketch and because it has become highly specialized. However, the concern for a normative base and the reconstruction of professional ethics occupy the second section of this book.
3. E. D. Pellegrino, *Humanism and the Physician* (Knoxville, Tenn.: University of Tennessee Press, 1979), p. 20.
4. E. D. Pellegrino, "Philosophy of Medicine: Problematic and Potential," *Journal of Medicine and Philosophy,* Vol. 1, No. 1 (1976), 5–31.
5. S. Levinson, "The Search for a Philosophy of Medicine," *The Pharos* (Winter 1979), 6.
6. M. Gelfand, *Philosophy and Ethics of Medicine* (London: Longmans, 1968).
7. G. Canguilhem, *On the Normal and the Pathological,* C. R. Fawcett, tr. (Dordrecht/Boston: Reidel, 1978), p. 143.
8. J. Cody, "The Arts Versus Angus Duer, M.D.," in D. Self, ed., *The Role of the Humanities in Medical Education* (Norfolk, Va.: Biomedical Ethics Program, 1978), pp. 45–61.
9. R. M. Zaner, "The Unanchored Leaf: Humanities and the Discipline of Care," *Texas Reports on Biology and Medicine,* Vol. 32, No. 1 (1974), 2.
10. V. S. Yanovsky, *Medicine, Science and Life* (New York: Paulist Press, 1978), p. 58.
11. Cf. J. Bergsma, *Somatopsychologie* (Lochem: De Tijdstroom, 1977), Chap. 1, which details current theory on the relation of the body to self-consciousness, self-image, and personality.
12. H. T. Engelhardt, Jr., "Introduction," in H. T. Engelhardt, Jr., and S. Spicker, eds., *Mental Health: Philosophical Perspectives* (Dordrecht/Boston: Reidel, 1978), p. VII.
13. Cf. S. Spicker's comments on Straus' critique of theories of consciousness, in "The Psychiatrist as Philosopher," ibid., p. 147.
14. Engelhardt, "Introduction," ibid., p. VII.
15. Kant, *Critique of Pure Reason,* tr. by Norman Kemp Smith (London: Macmillan, 1967), p. 359, A392.
16. S. Spicker, "Introduction," in S. Spicker and H. T. Engelhardt, Jr., eds., *Philosophical Dimensions of the Neuro-Medical Sciences* (Dordrecht/Boston: Reidel, 1976), p. 2.

17. Cf. H. T. Engelhardt, Jr., "Explanatory Models in Medicine: Facts, Theories and Values," *Texas Reports,* Vol. 32 (1974), 231; J. G. Scadding, "Diagnosis: The Physician and the Computer," *Lancet,* Vol. 2 (1967), 877–882.
18. A. Feinstein, *Clinical Judgment* (Baltimore: Williams and Wilkins, 1967), esp. Chap. 16.
19. K. D. Clouser and A. Zucker, "Medicine as Art: An Initial Exploration," *Texas Reports,* Vol. 32 (1974), 271: "The practitioner is more like a detective; he is using what he already knows in general to see what will happen in the *particular* case. Thus medicine's art would seem to operate in that interface where generalities (formulas, recipes, theories, laws) are either used or sought in the particular instance."
20. E. Cassell, "Moral Thought in Clinical Practice: Applying the Abstract to the Usual," in *Science, Ethics and Medicine,* pp. 147–60.
21. E. Cassell, "The Conflict Between the Desire to Know and the Need to Care for the Patient," in *Organism, Medicine and Metaphysics,* op. cit., pp. 57–72.
22. S. Spicker, "The Execution of Euthanasia: The Right of the Dying to a Re-Formed Health Care Context," ibid., pp. 73–96.
23. O. Guttentag, "Care of the Healthy and the Sick from the Attending Physician's Perspective: Envisioned and Actual," Ibid., pp. 41–56.
24. A. Lowe, "Prometheus Unbound? A New World in the Making," Ibid., pp. 1–12.
25. J. N. Findlay, "The Contemporary Relevance of Hegel," in *Hegel: A Collection of Essays,* ed. by A. MacIntyre (Notre Dame: University of Notre Dame Press, 1970), p. 11.
26. Yanovsky, *Medicine, Science and Life,* pp. 149–50.
27. P. Romanell, "Medicine as a New Key to Locke," *Texas Reports,* Vol. 32 (1974), 275–85.
28. "Explanatory Models in Medicine," pp. 225, 232.
29. M. Lipkin, *The Care of Patients* (New York: Oxford University Press, 1974), p. 35.
30. J. G. Bruhn, "The Diagnosis of Normality," *Texas Reports,* Vol. 32 (1974), 241–48. ". . . in assessing a patient's degree of normality the physician must weigh both the patient's current functioning against established clinical 'norms' and the patient's past functioning against that of the present" (p. 242).
31. Engelhardt, "Explanatory Models in Medicine," pp. 226, 235.
32. "It is diseases which have stimulated physiology; and it is not physiology but pathology and clinical practice which gave medicine its start. The reason is that a matter of fact well-being is not felt, for it is the simple awareness of living, and only its impediment provokes the force of resistance." (Kant, *Werke,* Akademie Ausgabe,

15^{2}, *Anthropologie,* p. 964, as quoted in Canguilhem, *On the Normal and the Pathological,* p. 141).

33. Ibid., p. 73.
34. H. Jonas has constructed what he calls an "ontological imperative"—namely, the duty of humanity to continue to exist. H. Jonas, "Technology and Responsibility: Reflection on the New Tasks of Ethics," *Social Research,* Vol. 40, No. 1 (1974), 35–36. Evidence from survivors of concentration camps indicates that, when all civilized behavior and the self constructed in that civilization were stripped away, the survivors experienced a simple but forceful urge just to survive. See T. des Pres, *The Survivor* (New York: Oxford University Press, 1976).
35. C. H. Waddington coined the phrase "biological wisdom" to indicate how the living organism "chooses" from a range of possible options for defense and repair. Thus a cellular "biogram" is postulated by students of biology because, as J. Z. Young notes, "living things act as they do because they are so organized as to take actions that prevent their dissolution into the surroundings." Cf. C. H. Waddington, *The Ethical Animal* (London: Allen and Unwin, 1969); E. O. Wilson, *Sociobiology: The New Synthesis* (Cambridge: Harvard University Press, 1975); J. Z. Young, *An Introduction to the Study of Man* (Oxford: Oxford University Press, 1971).
36. Cf. H. T. Engelhardt, "Introduction," in *Morals, Science and Sociality,* ed. by H. T. Engelhardt, Jr., and D. Callahan (Hastings-on-Hudson: The Hastings Center, 1978), p. 3.
37. The distinction of three worlds of perception stems from the work of Merleau-Ponty. The scientific world is a world of objectified symbols (the world of "it" and "they") such as laws, theories, concepts, institutions, and so forth. The everyday world is the lifeworld (*Lebenswelt*) of Husserl. It is the realm of figure-ground, of images which are objective-subjective, the realm of practice and experience which is the condition for the truth of the scientific world. The condition of the lifeworld is a world of originary prearticulated experience. In early works, Merleau-Ponty referred to the lifeworld and the originary world as one and the same, or distinguished them in a confused way. However, later writings show that the originary world is the logically prior realm of the body, organizing its experiences prior to any subjective-objective distinction. In his last work, *L'Visible et L'Invisible,* Merleau-Ponty identified the origin of truth in the originary world as "l'etre brut ou sauvage," an act of illumination not unlike Aquinas' agent intellect or Heidegger's *Sein.* Truth in all relationships, for Merleau-Ponty, ultimately depends on a "logos prophoricho" or a "logos endiathetos." Whatever this may mean, it definitely places the condition of truth not in

concepts but in a prearticulated realm of bodily organization of perception.

38. The distinction between lived self and lived body is not unlike that between person and individual. This distinction was originally drawn by the Christian theologians in attempting to understand the union in Christ of God and man. Thus Aquinas distinguished human nature, held in common, from individuals (matter "signed" by quantity in a unique way), and from persons (individual substances of a rational nature).
39. E. Cassell, "Disease as an 'It'," *Social Science and Medicine,* Vol. 10 (1976), 143–46.
40. Disease categories and classifications are all measured against the "normal range" or normal limits of common characteristics of bodies.
41. Medicine may also just know a therapy which allows the body to heal itself without a knowledge of the cause, as in the case of a common cold.
42. E. D. Pellegrino, "From the Rational to the Radical: The Sociocultural Impact of Modern Therapeutics," presented at the University of Pennsylvania, 2–4 December 1976.
43. A simple comparison of Garrison's *Principles of Internal Medicine* and a standard text in biology will reveal this difference. It could be a mistake to conclude that medicine is just an applied biology, because the requirement of specificity also leads to the realm of *praxis*. Thus the very theory of medicine is infused with practice on behalf of individual bodies. As Aquinas noted, the theory of medicine is theory about how to act.
44. E. Jokl, "Three Olympic Champions," in W. Von Baeyer and R. Griffith, eds., *Conditio Humana* (Berlin: Springer-Verlag, 1966), pp. 115–35, notes that rehabilitation introduces an anthropological concept into clinical pathology, because the wisdom of the body is a preordained pattern of autonomic responses to physiological changes. The wisdom of the body varies with each individual to the extent of the individual's response and capacity to break through barriers set by corporeal existence.
45. J. B. Burgers, "Causality and Anticipation," *Science,* Vol. 189 (1975), 194–98), argues that even cellular structures exhibit this anticipatory capacity. For this reason, purely mechanical causality is insufficient even for a philosophy of biology.
46. Gorovitz and MacIntyre, "Towards a Theory."
47. *Praxis* is another one of the many classical philosophical terms given specific meaning by an early philosopher, such as Aristotle, and then appropriated by many others throughout the history of ideas, each time with new connotations. Originally the Greek term *praxis* applied to ways in which one speaks of actions and doing,

and is usually translated in English into "practice." But the English word is vaguer than the Greek meaning. Aristotle, for example, used *praxis* to apply in a general way to accomplished actions and many biological activities. But he also used it as a philosophical term to apply to the freedom of man in activities covered by disciplines such as ethics and politics. (Cf. R. J. Bernstein, *Praxis and Action: Contemporary Philosophies of Human Action* [Philadelphia: University of Pennsylvania Press, 1971], p. ix). Earlier we distinguished two forms of *tekné,* one which had the goal of the action within itself (*praxis*) and the other which brings into effect an action outside itself (*poesis*). Hence the use of *praxis* intended by us does very little violence to its historical meaning. We intend by *praxis* to mean the organized activity of human beings taken as a whole, as distinct from that class of random actions Aristotle might have meant by acts of man. *Praxis* is an aspect of the everyday world, previously described, in which the organized activity of human beings reveals upon philosophical examination an internal structure capable of being formulated in the realm of theory.

48. If so, physicians would be held responsible for all environmental causes of disease and would become the high priests of culture. While this view is a healthy corrective to entitative concepts of disease, it is characterized by a lack of appreciation for the role of the living body in clinical relationships.
49. P. Lain-Entralgo, *Mind and Body,* p. xv, declares: "Whether it be skillful or unskillful, the curative activity of the physician is always determined by the reality of the human being towards which it is directed, that is, by the 'personal' conditions of the disease and of the patient."
50. *An Essay on Man* (New York: Bantam Books, 1970), p. 25.
51. Buchanan, *The Doctrine of Signatures,* p. 147.
52. Cf. Herbert Spiegelberg, "On the Motility of the Ego," in *Conditio Humana,* pp. 136–50.
53. This activity of bodies led John Dewey to say that " the body is the bodying forth of the soul" ("Soul and Body," in S. Spicker, ed., *The Philosophy of the Body* [Chicago: Quadrangle Books, 1970], p. 119).
54. The term is borrowed from K. E. Rothschuh, "Zu einer Einheitstheorie der Verursachung und Ausbildung von somatischen, psychosomatischen, and psychischen Krankheiten," *Hippokrates,* Vol. 44 (1973), 3–17.
55. Cf. Von Weizsäcker, *Grundfragen Medizinischer Anthropologie* (Tübingen: Max Niemeyer Verlag, 1948); P. Lain-Entralgo, "The Health and Perfection of Man," *Diogenes,* No. 31 (1960), 1–18.
56. Portmann, p. 3.
57. M. Scheler warns, "In no other period of human knowledge has man ever become more problematical to himself than in our own

day. We have a scientific, a philosophical, and a theological anthropology that know nothing of each other. Therefore we no longer possess any clear and consistent idea of man. The evergrowing multiplicity of the particular sciences that are engaged in the study of men has confused rather than elucidated our concept of man." *Die Stellung des Menschen in Kosmos* (Darmstadt: Reiche, 1928), pp. 13ff. The translation is modified from Cassirer, *An Essay*, p. 24.

CHAPTER SIX

1. Aristotle, *Metaphysics*, IV, 1006a.
2. R. Cabot, *Differential Diagnosis* (Philadelphia: Saunders, 1916), Vol. I, p. 19.
3. E. A. Murphy, *The Logic of Medicine* (Baltimore: Johns Hopkins University Press, 1976); A. Feinstein, *Clinical Judgment* (Baltimore: Williams and Wilkins, 1967): J. A. Jacquez, ed., *The Diagnostic Process* (Ann Arbor, Mich.: University of Michigan Press, 1964); H. R. Wulff, *Rational Diagnosis and Treatment* (Oxford: Blackwell Scientific Publications, 1976); R. S. Ledley and L. B. Lusted, "Reasoning Foundation of Medical Diagnosis," *Science*, Vol. 130 (1959), 9–21; D. A. K. Black, *The Logic of Medicine* (Edinburgh: Oliver & Boyd, 1968).
4. W. Jaeger, *Paideia: The Ideals of Greek Culture,* Gilbert Mighet, tr. (New York: Oxford University Press, 1944), Vol. III, pp. 17–19.
5. A. S. Elstein, "Clinical Judgment: Psychological Research and Medical Practice," *Science,* Vol. 194 (1976), 696–700.
6. Examination of human actions according to the ends was proposed by Aristotle. Teleological analysis fell into disrepute with the rise of modern science but was reintroduced by American pragmatists who, unlike Aristotle, insisted that human actions could be analyzed only in terms of finite ends, or to use Dewey's phrase, the "end in view." Since we maintain the conviction that medicine is distinguished by its end in view from other disciplines, the analysis that follows highlights the role of the end of medicine, its purpose, in determining its form.
7. E. D. Pellegrino, "Philosophy of Medicine: Problematic and Potential," *Journal of Medicine and Philosophy,* Vol. 1, No. 1 (1976), 5–31.
8. K. E. Rothschuh, "Zu einer Einheitstheorie," op. cit., discusses this concept of patient in great detail.
9. A. MacIntyre, "Patients as Agents," in H. T. Engelhardt, Jr. and S. Spicker, eds., *Philosophical Medical Ethics: Its Nature and Significance* (Dordrecht/Boston: D. Reidel, 1977) pp. 197–212.
10. L. M. Koran, "The Reliability of Clinical Methods, Data, and Judgments," first of two parts, *New England Journal of Medicine,* Vol.

293, No. 13 (1975), 642–46, and second of two parts, Ibid., No. 14 (1975), 695–701.

11. B. J. McNeil, E. Keeler, and S. J. Adelstein, "Primer on Certain Elements of Medical Decision-Making," *New England Journal of Medicine,* Vol. 293, No. 5 (1975), 211–15.
12. Feinstein, *Clinical Judgment,* p. 214.
13. W. B. Schwartz, G. A. Gorry, J. P. Cassiere, and A. Essig, "Decision Analysis and Clinical Judgment," *American Journal of Medicine,* Vol. 55 (1973), 459–72; H. Raiffa, *Decision Analysis: Introductory Lectures on Choices under Uncertainty* (Reading, Mass.: Addison-Wesley, 1968); A. R. Feinstein, "The Haze of Bayes, the Aerial Palaces of Decision Analysis, and the Computerized Ouija Board" (*Clinical Biostatistics,* XXXIX, forthcoming). A discussion of the role of values in determining models of disease explanation, and the role of clinical diagnostic procedures leading to these different models can be found in D. D. Copeland, "Concepts of Disease and Diagnosis," *Perspectives in Biology and Medicine,* Vol. 20, No. 4 (Summer 1977), 528–38.
14. Wulff, op. cit., pp. 101–17; Buchanan, *The Doctrine of Signatures* (London: Kegan Paul, Trench, Trubner & Co., 1938), pp. 61–63; R. I. Engle, "Medical Diagnosis: Past, Present and Future," *Archives of Internal Medicine,* Vol. 112 (1963), Part I, with B. J. Davis, 512–19, Part II, 520–29. This problem calls for what Toulmin has called a "need for an epistemology of a multivalued enterprise" ("On the Nature of the Physician's Understanding," *Journal of Medicine and Philosophy,* Vol. 1, No. 1, [1976], 49).
15. M. J. Adler, *Dialectic* (New York: Harcourt, Brace, 1927), p. 31, footnote 1, pp. 24–47.
16. E. Sober, "Learning Theory and Clinical Practice," presented at the Fifth Trans-Disciplinary Symposium on Philosophy and Medicine: Clinical Judgment, University of California School of Medicine, 14–16 April 1977.
17. Cf. The entire issue of *Journal of Medicine and Philosophy,* Vol. 1, No. 4 (1976), which is devoted to a discussion of causality in medicine.
18. A. R. Feinstein and C. K. Wells, "Randomized Trials vs. Historical Controls: The Scientific Plagues of Both Houses" (Washington, D.C.: Association of American Physicians, forthcoming).
19. C. C. Chambers, J. A. Inciardi, and H. A. Siegal, *Chemical Coping: A Report on Legal Drug Use in the U.S.* (New York: Spectrum Publishers, 1975), p. 141.
20. R. Weaver, *The Ethics of Rhetoric* (Chicago: Henry Regnery, 1968), esp. Chap. 2, pp. 27–28.
21. M. L. J. Abercrombie, *The Anatomy of Judgment* (London: Penguin Books, 1974); Engle, "Medical Diagnosis," pp. 520–29. T. S.

Kuhn seemed to exclude medicine from the sciences in his terms precisely because he recognized that its *raison d'etre* is an external social need, unlike other sciences (*The Structure of Scientific Revolutions* [Chicago: University of Chicago Press, 1962], p. 19). Charles Davison, a student in philosophy under one of us, is currently examining the relevance of Kuhn for the debate about whether clinical medicine is a science or not. We are indebted to him for this reference.

22. C. Bernard, *An Introduction to the Study of Experimental Medicine* (New York: Macmillan, 1927), p. 203.
23. A. Tversky, "Elimination by Aspects: A Theory of Choice," *Psychological Review,* Vol. 79, No. 4 (1972), 281–99; Elstein, loc. cit.
24. J. Kroger, "Polanyi and Lonergan on Scientific Method," *Philosophy Today* (Spring 1977), pp. 2–20.
25. R. R. Sokal, "Numerical Taxonomy and Disease Classification," in J. A. Jacquez, ed., *The Diagnostic Process* (Ann Arbor, Mich.: University of Michigan Press, 1964).
26. E. McMullin, "Two Faces of Science," *Review of Metaphysics,* Vol. 27, No. 4 (1974), 655–76.
27. Sober, loc. cit.
28. T. S. Kuhn, *The Structure of Scientific Revolutions* 2d. ed. (Chicago: University of Chicago Press, 1970).
29. S. Toulmin, "From Form to Function: Discoveries and Interpretations," Studies in Contemporary Scholarship, *Daedalus* Vol. 1 (1977), 154.
30. P. Feyerabend, *Against Method: Outline of an Anarchistic Theory of Knowledge* (Atlantic Highlands, N.J.: Humanities Press, 1975).
31. E. McMullin, commentary on J. L. Gedye, "Simulating Clinical Judgment," presented at the Fifth Trans-Disciplinary Symposium on Philosophy and Medicine: Clinical Judgment, University of California School of Medicine, 14–16 April 1977.
32. A. Einstein, *Out of My Later Years* (Secaucus, N.J.: Citadel Press, 1974), p. 24.
33. S. Buchanan, *Embers of the World,* loc. cit., argued that the liberal arts were the power of handling symbols. Minimally, then, the liberal arts and medicine are necessarily linked in the handling of symbols about history–the former, the history of the human condition, the latter, the history of individual patients.
34. Aristotle, *Metaphysics,* VI, 3, Ch. 3, p. 1140, a10.
35. J. Maritain, *Art and Scholasticism with Other Essays* (New York: Scribners, 1949), p. 7, notes 4 and 5; Saint Thomas Aquinas, *Summa Theologiae,* Ia2ae, Question 57, art. 3–4.
36. Aristotle, *Metaphysics* VI, Ch. 4, 1140b, 5–6.
37. Saint Thomas Aquinas, *Summa Theologiae,* ibid.
38. E. D. Pellegrino, "Educating the Humanist Physician: An Ancient

Ideal Reconsidered," *Journal of the American Medical Association,* Vol. 227, No. 11 (1974), 1288–94.

39. D. Thomasma, "Training in Medical Ethics: An Ethical Work-Up," *Forum on Medicine,* Vol. I (Dec. 1978), 33–36.
40. E. D. Pellegrino, "Preface," in T. K. McElhinney, ed., *Human Values Teaching Programs for Health Professionals,* 3rd ed. (Philadelphia: Society for Health and Human Values, 1976).
41. S. Buchanan, *The Doctrine,* p. 174. The role of the healing end of medicine is, as Fritz Hartmann observes, the measure of the quality of the classification system and whether the system fulfills its purpose. Cf. "What Could and Should Doctors Learn from Their Experiences with Computers in Medicine?" in *Medinfo* (Amsterdam: North-Holland Publishing Co., 1974), p. 1158.

Chapter Seven

1. W. Jaeger, *Paideia: The Ideals of Greek Culture,* Gilbert Mighet, tr. (New York: Oxford University Press, 1944), Vol. III, p. 17.
2. E. D. Pellegrino, "Toward an Expanded Medical Ethics: The Hippocratic Ethic Revisited," in Roger J. Bulger, M.D., ed., *Hippocrates Revisited* (New York: MEDCOM Press, 1973), pp. 133–47.
3. E. Ackerknecht, "Medicine and Ethnology: Selected Essays," in H. H. Wlaser and H. M. Koelbing, eds., *Primitive Medicine's Social Function* (Bern: Verlag Han Huber, 1971), p. 170.
4. I. Illich, *Medical Nemesis* (New York: Pantheon, 1975).
5. A. MacIntyre, "Patients as Agents," in S. F. Spicker and H. T. Engelhardt, Jr., eds., *Philosophical Medical Ethics: Its Nature and Significance* (Dordrecht: Reidel, 1977), pp. 179–212.
6. K. Arrow, "Government Decision Making and the Preciousness of Life," in L. Tancredi, ed., *Ethics of Health Care* (Washington, D.C.: National Academy of Sciences, 1974), pp. 33–47.
7. E. D. Pellegrino, "Interdisciplinary Education in the Health Professions: Assumptions, Definitions and Some Notes on Teams," *Report of a Conference: Educating for the Health Team* (Washington, D.C.: National Academy of Sciences, Institute of Medicine, 1972), pp. 4–18; Pellegrino, "The Ethical Implications of Changing Patterns of Medical Care," *North Carolina Medical Journal,* Vol. 26 (1965), 73–76.
8. Public Law 93-641, Section 1502.
9. M. Lalonde, *A New Perspective on the Health of Canadians* (Ottawa: Government of Canada, 1974); Illich, op. cit., R. Carlson, *The End of Medicine* (New York: Wiley, 1975).
10. J. Hitchcock, "The Dynamics of Popular Intellectual Change," *American Scholar,* Vol. 45 (Autumn 1976), 522–35.
11. H. Sigerist, *A History of Medicine,* Vol. 1: *Primitive and Archaic Medicine* (New York: Oxford University Press, 1961), p. 161.

CHAPTER EIGHT

1. For example, see F. Kudlein, "Medical Ethics and Popular Ethics in Greece and Rome," *Clio Medica,* Vol. 5 (1976), 91–121. Also C. Burns, ed., *Legacies in Ethics and Medicine* (New York: Science History Publications, 1977), which traces important ethical theories and codes throughout the history of medicine.
2. We share this concern with D. Callahan, "The Emergence of Bioethics," in *Science, Ethics, and Medicine,* D. Callahan and H. T. Engelhardt, Jr., eds. (Hastings-on-Hudson: Hastings Center, 1976), pp. x–xxvi.
3. Thus H. T. Engelhardt's study of abortion, for it rests on a claim that a fetus is not a person because it does not manifest rational or self-conscious activity. Be it noted that Engelhardt makes an attempt to ground the ethics of abortion in an ontology, and the ontology reflects the way society and medicine actually act toward fetuses. Additional work is needed on such an ontology, however, if it is to truly convey a contemporary anthropology ("The Ontology of Abortion," *Ethics,* Vol. 84 [1974], 217–34).
4. Cf., for example, R. M. Hare, "Survival of the Weakest," in S. Gorovitz, et al., eds., *Moral Problems in Medicine* (Englewood Cliffs, N.J.: Prentice-Hall, 1976), pp. 364–69.
5. H. Jonas, "Philosophical Reflections on Experimenting With Human Subjects," in Paul Freud, ed., *Experimentation With Human Subjects* (New York: George Braziller, 1969), pp. 1–31. See also L. Mumford, *The Myth of the Machine* (New York: Harcourt Brace Jovanovich, 1970).
6. This situation is described by D. Callahan, "The Ethics Backlash," *Hastings Center Report,* Vol. 5 (1975), 18.
7. We do not regard as untenable the position that medical ethics is a branch of ethics, if by that is understood that medical ethics is a philosophy of value questions, clarification, and prioritization, as Clouser argues is the proper task of medical ethics ("Medical Ethics: Some Uses, Abuses and Limitations," *Arizona Medicine,* Vol. 33 [1976], 44–49). However, applications of previously formulated ethical theory to medicine we prefer to call "ethics of medicine" rather than "medical ethics," a term we reserve for an ethics arising from the medical situation. For example, the ethical problems posed by research on recombinant DNA is presently an issue in the ethics of biology or medicine (if impact on persons is connoted). It is not a medical ethics issue because it does not presently arise from the medical event.
8. We make a distinction between these terms later in the chapter.
9. "Introduction," The Humanities and Medicine: *Texas Reports on Biology and Medicine Special Issue,* Vol. 32 (Spring 1974), ix.
10. J. Dewey, *Experience and Nature* (New York: Dover, 1958),

p. 399. It is because of this that Dewey identifies philosophy as a moral task (pp. 396–99) and as a method of discriminating among goods and consequences.

11. MacIntyre and Gorovitz, "Toward a Theory of Medical Fallibility," *Journal of Medicine and Philosophy,* Vol. 1 (1976), 51–71.
12. See their positions as collected in R. Lepley, ed., *The Language of Value* (New York: Columbia University Press, 1957).
13. The development of the three kinds of values can be found in H. N. Lee, "The Meaning of 'Intrinsic Value'," in Lepley, ed., *The Language,* pp. 178–96.
14. Lee, "Intrinsic Value," p. 189.
15. These distinctions are borrowed from R. S. Hartman, *The Structure of Value* (Carbondale, Ill.: Southern Illinois University Press, 1967).
16. Cf. E. D. Pellegrino, "Humanism in Human Experimentation: Some Notes on the Investigator's Fiduciary Role," in C. Burns and H. T. Engelhardt, eds., *The Humanities and Medicine, Texas Reports on Biology and Medicine,* Vol. 32 (1974), 311–25.
17. Hippocrates, *Epidemiae* I, 11.
18. We are indebted to E. L. Erde for sharing his "The Place of 'Good' in the Science and Art of Medicine," a paper as yet unpublished. Dr. Erde explores the manifold judgments about the good which enter the medical enterprise. See also K. D. Clouser, "Some Things Medical Ethics Is Not," *Journal of the American Medical Association,* Vol. 223, No. 7 (1973), 787–89. Clouser argues that medical ethics cannot be prescriptive.
19. This is the belief of Aristotle, for example. In his view, ethics respects the good of all of human life, while medicine respects bodily health (*Nichomachean Ethics,* I, 2, 1094b6–11; I, 7, 1097a15–24). Hence, health would be viewed as a means and a necessary condition of the good life.
20. J. Owens, "Aristotelian Ethics, Medicine, and the Changing Nature of Man," in S. Spicker and H. T. Engelhardt, Jr., eds., *Philosophical Medical Ethics: Its Nature and Significance* (Dordrecht/Boston: Reidel, 1977), pp. 129–30, points out that for Aristotle, moral knowledge changes with the changing conditions of a human being because it is worked into the cultural, habitual, physical and psychic conditions of human life. Persons make judgments according to the kind of life they lead (Aristotle, *Nichomachean Ethics,* I, 5, 1095b14–1096a7). The relative ranking of various goods will be further examined in our final chapter when we deal with the clash between economic and other values in health care.
21. It is our view that moral norms are flexible enough to allow for absolute norms in certain situations and relative ones in others. The degree to which persons adhere to the professed value of medicine is therefore the degree to which the axioms developed from the phy-

sician-patient relationship acquire absolute force. The degree to which persons do not adhere to the axioms is the degree to which they acquire only relative force. This flexibility of moral norms is apparently the position of Aristotle (see Owens, "Aristotelian Ethics," p. 133). The position about flexibility of moral norms is conditioned by the recognition that health is often only a means to other ends. Hence axioms developed from health as a value must sometimes be secondary, sometimes primary, depending upon the situation. Indeed, many medical ethics issues, such as prolonging life, abortion, distribution of resources, experimentation on children, and so on involve the clash between the absolute ranking of health by the profession of medicine and its relative ranking by persons who participate as patients or experimental subjects.

22. Cf. Owens, pp. 136–37. The physical disposition of the patient has a great deal to do with the ranking of goods. Of course, other factors also contribute to the relativity of norms in ethics. R. M. Hare notes these as follows: "Premises [for claims] can be denied; the argumentation towards [the norms] is simply invalid; or it is expressed in an ambiguous way, so that if you take the words one way, the premises can be denied, but if you take them in a way in which the premises cannot be denied, the conclusion does not follow from them," ("Can the Moral Philosopher Help?" in Spicker and Engelhardt, *Philosophical Medical Ethics,* pp. 50–51). Of course, Hare uses this observation to argue that ethics is merely a study of words, at least, in helping medicine. We have argued differently.
23. The use of the deontological and counsel of prudence interpretations of the axiom of nonharm stems from A. Jonsen's description of four senses in which the principle of non-harm can be taken in medicine: medicine as moral enterprise; due care; risk-benefit ratio; benefit-detriment equation. Jonsen describes these senses as deontological, counsel of prudence, a calculation of susceptibility, and a rule of double effect. Jonsen correctly observes that each of these senses of nonharm leads to different kinds of moral arguments "Do No Harm: Axiom of Medical Ethics," in *Philosophical Medical Ethics,* pp. 29–38.) Note that our interpretation of the axiom of "do no harm," or the other axioms developed in the previous section of this chapter, follows none of the four senses developed above by Jonsen.
24. Cf. R. M. Hare, op. cit., p. 57; S. Morgenbesser, "Experimentation and Consent: A Note," in *Philosophical Medical Ethics,* p. 97.
25 Hare, op. cit.; P. Ramsey, *The Patient as Person* (New Haven: Yale University Press, 1970), pp. 1–50; "The Enforcement of Morals: Non-Therapeutic Research on Children," *Hastings Center Report,* Vol. 6 (1976), 21–30; R. McCormick, "Proxy Consent in the Experimental Situation," *Perspectives in Biology and Medicine,* Vol.

18 (1974), 2–20; and "Experimentation in Children: Sharing in Sociality," *Hastings Center Report,* Vol. 6 (1976), 41–46.

26. *On Human Care* (Nashville: Abingdon Press, 1977), pp. 19–21.
27. T. Ackerman, "The Specialty of Medical Ethics and Its Role in Medical Care," *Forum on Medicine,* in press.
28. "Legalism and Medical Ethics," *Journal of Medicine and Philosophy,* Vol. 4 (1979), 70–71.
29. The National Commission for the Protection of Human Subjects, *The Belmont Report* (Washington, D.C.: U.S. Government Printing Office, 1978: OS 78-0012), distinguishes three "prescriptive principles" governing medical research: respect for persons, beneficence, and justice (pp. 5–10), and then discusses the application of these principles to practice through secondary principles such as informed consent, risk-benefit assessments, and the selection of subjects. The process of applying general principles through middle principles can be duplicated for medical practice as well as for research.
30. "How Virtues Become Vices," 111–12.
31. J. S. Mill, "Dr. Whewell on Moral Philosophy," in J. B. Schneewind, ed., *Mill's Ethical Writings* (New York: Macmillan, 1965), p. 178.

Chapter Nine

1. This is the very real question posed by MacIntyre, "How Virtues Become Vices: Values, Medicine and Social Context," in H. T. Engelhardt, Jr. and S. Spicker, eds., *Evaluation and Explanation in the Biomedical Sciences* (Dordrecht/Boston: D. Reidel, 1975), pp. 97–112, in calling attention to the cultural basis of medical ethics. He argues that no foundation currently exists for medical ethics.
2. C. Burns shows how the code of professional standards in American medicine in the eighteenth and nineteenth centuries depended explicitly on a Christian code of gentlemanly behavior ("American Medical Ethics: Some Historical Roots," in S. Spicker and H. T. Engelhardt, eds., *Philosophical Medical Ethics, Its Nature and Significance* (Dordrecht/Boston: Reidel, 1977), pp. 21–25). In the later part of the nineteenth and the early twentieth centuries, as cultural pluralism rose in importance, the religious base was replaced by a psychological or behavioristic one. Burns further points out that during the eighteenth and nineteenth centuries a philosophical basis for professional ethics was specifically ruled out as "godless" or the result of heathen speculation.
3. L. Edelstein, "The Hippocratic Oath: Text, Translation and Interpretation," Supplement to the *Bulletin of the History of Medicine,* No. 1 (Baltimore, Johns Hopkins Press, 1943). This superb piece of textual criticism established the provenance of the oath as a

Pythagorean document and seems more cogent in every way than W. H. S. Jones, *Philosophy and Medicine in Ancient Greece* (Baltimore: Johns Hopkins Press, 1946).

4. We have drawn heavily for all of the foregoing on the excellent William Osler Oration in the History of Medicine, "The Professional Ethics of the Greek Physician," in L. Edelstein, *Ancient Medicine,* O. Temkin and C. L. Temkin, eds. (Baltimore: Johns Hopkins Press, 1967), pp. 319–48.
5. Burns, ibid.
6. W. Hooker, *Physician and Patient, A Practical View of Medical Ethics,* 1849), Chap. VIII.
7. S. Largus, *Compositions,* G. Helmreich, ed. (Lipsiae, 1887); also, *Professio medici Zum Vorwort des Scribonius Largus,* Karl Deichgraber, both cited by L. Edelstein, op. cit. 18 supra. It is Edelstein's interpretation of Scribonius which stimulated our own thoughts about the possibility of an ethics specific to medicine. We have translated the relevant portions for ourselves and concur with Edelstein's reading.
8. *Cicero on Moral Obligation; A New Translation of Cicero's De Officiis,* with introduction and notes by John Higginbotham (Berkeley: University of California Press, 1967), Books I and II.
9. T. Percival, *Medical Ethics* (Baltimore: Williams and Wilkins); reprinted Huntington, N.Y.: Robert A. Krieger, 1975).
10. We have already noted the philosophical problems associated with this approach as underlined by MacIntyre and Gorovitz.
11. P. Ramsey, *The Patient as Person* (New Haven: Yale University Press, 1970), pp. 1–18.
12. P. Lain-Entralgo, "La Relacion medica en el cuadro de las relaciones interhumana," in *La Relacion medico-enferma* (Madrid: Ediciones de Revista de Occidente, 1964), pp. 235–58. Lain-Entralgo speaks of a special love, *iatrikê philia,* which the physician evidences for his patient in the special inter-human relationship of healing.
13. Cf. Aristotle on this point of dedication to craftsmanship, *Metaphysics,* I, I, 11–12.
14. *Hippocrates,* trans. W. H. S. Jones, *The Loeb Classical Library* (Cambridge: Harvard University Press, 1923), "Epidemica."
15. Hippocrates, ibid., "On Diseases."
16. Hippocrates, ibid., "On Decorum," XIV.
17. L. Edelstein, "The Professional Ethics of the Greek Physician," op. cit.
18. Hippocrates, op. cit., "Decorum," XVI.
19. Hippocrates, op. cit., "The Physician."
20. Hippocrates, op. cit., "On Joints."
21. L. Edelstein, "The Professional Ethics of the Greek Physician," op. cit.

22. The Stoics were the first philosophers to suggest that taking an oath or professing a human service was a hallmark of personal integrity and necessarily led one to an acceptance of a code of ethics. In this regard, see M. Aurelius, *Meditations* (Garden City, N.Y.: Doubleday Paperbacks, 1960), p. 37.
23. L. Edelstein, "The Professional Ethics of the Greek Physician," op. cit.
24. M. Levey, "Medical Ontology in Ninth Century Islam," in *Legacies in Ethics and Medicine,* C. Burns, ed. (New York: Science History Publications, 1977), p. 144; A. Ba-Sela and H. E. Hoff, "Isaac Israeli's Fifty Admonitions to the Physician," in ibid., pp. 145–57.
25. Hippocrates, op. cit., "Decorum," XIII, and "Laws," V.
26. B. Nortell, "AMA Judicial Activities," *Journal of the American Medical Association,* Vol. 239, No. 14 (1978), 1396–97. A synopsis of the proposed changes follows:

    The first three principles stress competence and scientific medicine. Omitted from the immediately preceding version are references to "service to humanity," "meriting the confidence of the patient," and "rendering a full measure of service and devotion."

    The fourth principle, which calls for protection of the public by exposing the incompetent and immoral physician, is essentially unchanged.

    The fifth principle accords the physician the right to treat whom he chooses except in emergencies and forbids abandonment of the patient once treatment is initiated.

    The sixth principle calls for resistance to restraints deleterious to the quality of care.

    The seventh principle deals with "fair" compensation and forbids acceptance of a fee for referral. The new version omits "limiting income," "adjusting fee to patients' ability to pay," and the reference to dispensing drugs.

    The eighth principle, which deals with consultation, omits reference to "doubtful or difficult" cases and previous mention of quality of care.

    The ninth principle deals with preservation of confidences, except when required by law, or in the interest of public good or safety.

    The tenth principle imposes the social responsibility to "participate" in activities to improve the health of the community.
27. It is this aspect of illness we find underdeveloped in Ramsey's account of the covenant between patient and physician, for the illness of the body, by that very fact, determines the need for the relationship and the patient's obligations to future generations. One is not as "free" in the relationship as Ramsey supposes.
28. We have established that ethics in medicine is not a relative piety adopted by its practitioners but a necessary and productive basis

for action. In this respect, see E. Cassell, "Autonomy and Ethics in Action," *New England Journal of Medicine,* Vol. 6 (1977), 333–34, Editorial.

29. "It is essential that the patient be made to believe that he is an independent, worthy person entitled to the most clearly stated information possible." (M. Benarde and E. W. Mayerson, "Patient-Physician Negotiation," *Journal of the American Medical Association,* Vol. 239, No. 4 (1978), 1413. In our view, the position taken is not only a claim derived from the principle of respect for persons but a necessary moral principle of the physician-patient relationship.
30. Cf. further discussion in R. Cabot, "The Use of Truth and Falsehood in Medicine, An Experimental Study," reprinted in S. Reiser et al., eds., *Ethics in Medicine* (Cambridge: MIT Press, 1977), pp. 213–20; H. W. Hooker, "Truth in Our Intercourse with the Sick," ibid., pp. 206–12; I. Kant, "Ethical Duties Towards Others: Truthfulness," in his *Lectures on Ethics* (New York: Harper Torchbooks, 1963), pp. 224–34; and D. Oken, "What to Tell Cancer Patients," in S. Gorovitz et al., eds., *Moral Problems in Medicine* (Englewood Cliffs, N.J.: Prentice-Hall, 1976), pp. 109–15.
31. Although we have developed this golden rule from the philosophical reflections on the physician-patient relationship, it does have similarities to general ethical points of view, particularly that principle of liberty developed by John Stuart Mill (*On Liberty*) which argues that one cannot interfere with the freedom of another unless they are a danger to others, and the ethical reflections of Gert, *The Moral Rules* (New York: Harper Torchbooks, 1973).
32. The importance of truth-telling obligations for patients can be seen in the recent case of leukemia in a small child handled by the Massachusetts courts, Massachusetts Appeals Court, Plymouth, Mass., May 23, 1978: "In Re Custody of a Minor," *Family Law Reporter,* Vol. 4 (1978) 2432. In this case, the parents explicitly lied to the physician about how the child had relapsed while taking his cancer medications, thus leading the physician to consent to discontinue treatment (as the chance of recovery from relapse while taking anticancer drugs is very low). In fact, the parents, as the physician later found out, had discontinued the drugs themselves. The child had a much better chance to recover than originally assessed, leading the physician to bring the case to court. The court decided with the physician and against the parents to continue the treatment of the child.

Chapter Ten

1. D. E. Konold, "History of the Codes of Medical Ethics," *Encyclopedia of Bioethics* (New York: The Free Press, 1978).

2. M. B. Etzioni, "The Physician's Creed," *An Anthology of Medical Prayers, Oaths and Codes of Ethics Written and Recited by Medical Practitioners Through the Ages* (Springfield, Ill.: Charles C. Thomas, 1973). This book illustrates the many and varied historical expressions of medical morality in a variety of documents of different provenance.
3. The debate surrounding the current revision of the AMA Code of Ethics is revealing. One charge is that the proposed revision replaces individual responsibility with a "new collectivism." This problem will be more centrally addressed in the next chapter ("AMA to Restudy Ethics Changes," *American Medical News,* June 30–July 7, 1978, p. 3.)
4. Particular to this point, see D. B. Marquis, "Medical Ethics: Danger or Help to Clinicians?" *Dialogue* (A Kansas Journal of Health Concerns), Vol. 3, No. 4 (1976), 35–38.
5. E. D. Pellegrino, "Toward an Expanded Medical Ethics, The Hippocratic Ethic Revisited," in R. J. Bulger, ed., *Hippocrates Revisited* (New York: MEDCOM Press, 1973), pp. 133–47.
6. A. MacIntyre, "Patients as Moral Agents," in S. Spicker and H. T. Engelhardt, Jr., eds., *Philosophical Medical Ethics: Its Nature and Significance* (Dordrecht: Reidel, 1977), pp. 197–212.
7. C. Burns, "Richard Clarke Cabot (1868–1939) and the Reformation of American Medical Ethics," *Bulletin of the History of Medicine,* Vol. 51, No. 3 (1977), 357–58.
8. L. Edelstein, "The Hippocratic Oath: Translation and Interpretation," *Bulletin of the History of Medicine,* Supplement No. 1, 1943.
9. C. Burns, ed., *Legacies in Ethics and Medicine* (New York: Science History Publications, 1977), pp. 129–284. These pages contain a series of articles by various authors tracing the influence of Hippocratic ethics in medieval and more recent times.
10. R. Veatch, "Models for Ethical Medicine in a Revolutionary Age," *Hastings Center Report,* Vol. 2, No. 3 (1972), 7.
11. P. Ramsey, *The Patient as Person* (New Haven: Yale University Press, 1970), pp. xii–xiii.
12. *Primary Care in Medicine: A Definition,* Interim Report of a Study. (Washington, D.C., Institute of Medicine, National Academy of Sciences, 1977).
13. C. F. Fried, "Equality and Rights in Medical Care," in J. G. Perpich, ed., *Implications of Guaranteeing Medical Care* (Washington, D.C.: National Academy of Sciences, Institute of Medicine, 1975).
14. Perpich, *Implications;* D. Mechanic, ed., *A Right to Health: The Problem of Access to Primary Medical Care* (New York: Wiley, 1976); R. M. Veatch and R. Branson, eds., *Ethics and Health Policy* (Cambridge, Mass.: Ballinger, 1976); M. Zubkoff, *Health: A Victim or Cause of Inflation?* (New York: Milbank Memorial

Fund, 1976); Gene Outka, "Social Justice and Equal Access to Health Care," *Journal of Religious Ethics,* Vol. 2, No. 1 (1974), 11.

15. It was in light of concerns like these that we noted the limits of the principles of medical ethics in Chapter Eight.
16. U.S. Congress. Senate. *National Health Planning and Resources Development Act of 1974* (Washington, D.C.: U.S. Printing Office, 1975); Public Law 93–641, 93rd Congress, 1st session, 1975, S. 2994.

CHAPTER ELEVEN

1. We are indebted to Prof. L. H. Newton of Fairfield University for noting the development of collective ethics in relation to the Vietnam War in a private communication. We have incorporated some of her citations about this problem in the pages to follow, but of course, have applied these to the problems of hospitals and health care teams.
2. This is explicitly noted by A. Jonsen and A. Hellegers, "Conceptual Foundations for an Ethics of Medical Care," in *Ethics in Medicine,* S. Reiser, et al., eds. (Cambridge: MIT Press, 1977), pp. 129–36.
3. Philosophical literature is unanimous in supporting the individual's moral obligation to express and act upon values held. Difficult moral problems in medicine, as in other endeavors, occur when individuals will not or cannot conform to the morality of the group. Among the "values" offered protection by philosophical thought (though not always in the law) are: scruples (prohibitions against morally wrong action); imperatives (prescripts of one's own moral persuasion); confessional beliefs (prescripts held publicly with others); and one's autonomy. In view of this protection, the individual must always be able to dissent from the group's moral decision without prejudice to autonomy and legal rights. Currently, however, in team health care decisions, interprofessional conflicts about moral principles often lead to suppression of the opinions of those held to be "lower" in the medical hierarchy.
4. This claim needs further amplification. Many contemporary philosophers argue that nothing new is created when a collective is formed. We call this the atomistic view of collectives. In this view, any predicate made of a collective must be able to be made of all individuals within it. Statements made about collectives, according to methodological individualism, are really statements made about each and every individual within the collective. Other philosophers are willing to admit that collectives stand as logical substances, that is, as that which can stand as a subject of a sentence. Caution about reifying collectives is important, but it may not apply when considering actually existing institutions and health care teams.

5. It should be noted that establishing moral obligations of groups is a difficult task, however. Some sociologists have paid attention to collective purpose, usually concluding that purpose must respect some consensus or agreement formed by the group. In the case of health care, the goals of institutions and teams are rather explicit, compared, for example, to an informal group with implied or unexpressed aims. What is important for this discussion is the fact that the aims of teams and hospitals are the values surrounding healing. See: A. Etzioni, *Modern Organizations* (Englewood Cliffs, N.J.: Prentice-Hall, 1964); E. Gross, "The Definition of Organizational Goals," *British Journal of Sociology,* Vol. 20 (1969), 282; J. Ladd, "Morality and the Ideal of Rationality in Formal Organizations," *The Monist,* Vol. 54 (1970), 488–517.
6. The values one brings to any new collective stem from other previous collectives, even if they remain unanalyzed. Family, home, church, society, and political structure have all contributed to our values. When an individual enters a team or an institution, therefore, the values should be reexamined to discern to what extent they might have to be modified or adjusted, and to what extent they will be protected and enhanced.
7. This relationship immediately creates obligations on the part of the group and the patient. Looking at the group, one must distinguish the many forms of obligations, tasks, responsibilities, culpabilities, liabilities, and accountabilities (cf. K. Baier, "Guilt and Responsibility," in P. French, ed., *Individual and Collective Responsibility* (Cambridge, Mass.: Schenkman, 1974). It is the position of John Ladd, op. cit., that collectives or organizations are governed by their own rules of decision making such that actions of individuals within them are attributed to the group and not to an individual moral agency. Consequently, good decisions are those judged as following the rational rules of the organization and its purpose and not the determinants of moral action (pp. 488ff.). However, we have argued that the purposes of hospitals and teams are the same as those of the discipline of medicine: healing; further, we have held that this aim is beneficial or good. As a result, a well-designed health care institution or team aimed at the good of healing would be following the rules of medical morality. Group decisions would be based not upon bureaucratic norms but moral guidelines. Clearly, the difference between Ladd's and our point of view is the difference between description of what is often the case and a description of what *ought* to be.
8. There is a confusion in the law. Civil law does impute moral responsibility to groups, while criminal law always considers individual responsibility.
9. This concept of profession by institutions and teams is useful because it allows us to remove the objection of philosophers, such as

John Ladd, that institutions are by their nature amoral. Even if one did not agree that institutions and teams for health care are designed for a moral purpose, the profession of these groups to healing requires a moral commitment. Because health care providers each bring to the institution and team the sum of their individual personal and professional moral integrities, the institution is, in this sense, a public profession of these integrities. Failure to foster and support these integrities is failure to reach the healing aims of the group itself.

10. C. Fried, "Rights and Health Care–Beyond Equity and Efficiency," *New England Journal of Medicine,* Vol. 293, No. 5 (1975), 241–45; and *Medical Experimentation, Personal Integrity and Social Policy* (New York: American Elsevier, 1974).
11. D. Crane, *The Sanctity of Social Life: Physicians' Treatment of Critically Ill Patients* (New York: Russell Sage Foundation, 1975).
12. J. Katz and A. M. Capron, *Catastrophic Diseases: Who Decides What?* (New York: Russell Sage Foundation, 1975).
13. A. Kantrowitz, "Controlling Technology Democratically," *American Scientist,* Vol. 63, No. 5 (1975), 505–9.
14. R. C. Fox, "Ethical and Existential Developments in Contemporaneous American Medicine: Their Implications for Culture and Society," *Milbank Memorial Fund Quarterly* (Fall 1974), 445–83.

CHAPTER TWELVE

1. Cf. "Health as a Human Value," Winning Essays of the Medical Student and House Staff Essay Contest (Philadelphia: Society for Health and Human Values, 1977).
2. Despite improvements in health worldwide as well, the basic need of the human race is still primary health care. See G. T. Harrell, "Change in the Role and Education of Doctors," *The Changing Roles of Education of Health Care Personnel Worldwide* (Philadelphia: Society for Health and Human Values, 1977), pp. 241–45.
3. See H. L. Abrams and B. J. McNeil, "Medical Implications of Computerized Tomography–'CAT Scanning'," *New England Journal of Medicine,* Vol. 293 (1978), 255–61; J. Ambrose and D. Ottley, "EMI Scan in the Management of Head Injuries," *Lancet,* Vol. 1 (1976), 847–48.
4. The principle of the common good developed in Chapter Eight requires consent on the part of the patient, for as we noted, it is an expression of both altruism and recognition of membership in the "common structures of living bodies." Unless a moral policy is discussed and evolved from public policy on this point, the neglect of a presently ill person in favor of a future social benefit would violate the other two principles of medical ethics also previously developed. In our view, it would be morally reprehensible.

5. This point is especially pertinent when the economic and moral issues are focused on the future of medical education. See E. D. Pellegrino, "Medical Education," in *Encyclopedia of Bioethics* (New York: The Free Press, 1978), Vol. II, 863–69.
6. For example, of the $10 billion going to scientific research in 1977–78, $9 billion was earmarked for medical research. The largest portion of this amount was further earmarked for cancer research. It is clear that the American people do value research on life-threatening diseases. One could very well imagine a growth in allocation to preventive medicine as the causes of cancer and heart disease become more fully known.
7. In early chapters we cited Aristotle, and later, the Alexandrian commentaries on Galen which highlight the importance of health for man's freedom and well-being.
8. An idea of the form this moral policy might take can be gleaned from the intergenerational axioms formulated in another context by R. M. Green, "Intergenerational Distributive Justice and Environmental Responsibility," *BioScience,* Vol. 27, No. 4 (1977), 260–65.

Index

Index

Index